BRAIN MAPPING RESEARCH DEVELOPMENTS

BRAIN MAPPING RESEARCH DEVELOPMENTS

LARS N. BAKKER
EDITOR

Nova Biomedical Books
New York

LIBRARY OF CONGRESS CATALOGING-IN-PUBLICATION DATA

Brain mapping research developments / Lars N. Bakker, editor.
p. ; cm.
Includes bibliographical references and index.
ISBN 978-1-60456-007-7 (hardcover)
1. Brain mapping. I. Bakker, Lars N.
[DNLM: 1. Brain Mapping. 2. Brain--physiology. 3. Diagnostic Imaging--methods. WL 335 B81428 2008]
RC386.6.B7B63 2008
612.8'2--dc22

2007035858

Published by Nova Science Publishers, Inc. ✢ New York

Contents

Preface vii

Expert Commentary Neural Activation Due to Olfactory Stimulation Measured by Near Infrared Spectroscopy 1
Hiroaki Shoji, Noriko Sato and Hisaki Ozaki

Research and Review Studies 11

Chapter I Mapping the Auditory Brain Using Magnetoencephalography (MEG) 13
Christopher J. Brignell, Deborah A. Hall and Caroline Witton

Chapter II Cortical Organization of Cat Licking Fine Tongue Movements during Cat Licking Executed by Bilateral Cortical Control 43
Hisao Hiraba, Takako Sato and Koichiro Ueda

Chapter III Role of the Corpus Callosum in the Interhemispheric Transfer of Somatosensory Information: An fMRI Study 73
Mara Fabri and Gabriele Polonara

Chapter IV Laboratory Memory Tasks and Autobiographical Recollection: Cognitive and Neurofunctional Evidence for Differential Forms of Episodic Memory 101
Martina Piefke

Chapter V Real-Time Functional Magnetic Resonance Imaging and Its Applications 129
Shaolin Yang, Thomas J. Ross and Yihong Yang

Chapter VI Brain Functional Asymmetry Based on Brain BOLD Signal Dynamic Model 155
Huafu Chen and Dezhong Yao

Chapter VII Multi-Parametric Mapping of Gliomas: Demonstration of Segmentation Strategies **177**
Kathryn M. McMillan and Ronald R. Price

Chapter VIII The Emotional S1-S2 Paradigm for Exploring Brain Mechanisms Underlying Affective Modulation of Expectancy **197**
Francisco Mercado, Jose Antonio Hinojosa, Cecilia Peñacoba and Luis Carretié

Chapter IX Brain Electric Source Imaging by an Iterative Correlation Matrix Based Multiple Signal Classification Approach **211**
Dezhong Yao

Index **231**

PREFACE

Brain mapping is a set of neuroscience techniques predicated on the mapping of (biological) quantities or properties onto spatial representations of the (human or non-human) brain resulting in maps. All neuroimaging can be considered part of brain mapping. Brain mapping can be conceived as a higher form of neuroimaging, producing brain images supplemented by the result of additional (imaging or non-imaging) data processing or analysis, such as maps projecting (measures of) behaviour onto brain regions (see fMRI). Brain Mapping techniques are constantly evolving, and rely on the development and refinement of image acquisition, representation, analysis, visualization and interpretation techniques. Functional and structural neuroimaging are at the core of the mapping aspect of Brain Mapping. This book presents the latest research in the field.

Chapter I - The use of magnetoencephalography (MEG) as an imaging technique for auditory brain mapping research has rapidly grown over the past decade to take advantage of its excellent temporal resolution (sub millisecond) and reasonable spatial resolution (sub centimetre). MEG can be used to study evoked transient deflections such as the energy onset or pitch onset responses, sustained responses and stimulus-induced oscillations through a wide range of techniques including amplitude and latency analysis, dipole source modelling and beamformer analysis. The wide range of approaches to data analysis ensures MEG is a highly flexible tool for brain mapping.

In this chapter, the authors review the contribution of MEG to advances in auditory brain mapping, seeking to explore its advantages and limitations and clarifying some misconceptions regarding its use. In the first section the authors describe the method and discuss some of the technical issues related to the optimal design of auditory experiments. In the second section, the authors introduce different strategies for the analysis of MEG data. In the third section the authors present a review of published studies that have mapped central auditory function using MEG.

Chapter II - Mastication is accomplished by the cooperative movement produced by various striated muscles in the face, jaw and tongue. Their movements are generally credited with activations organized by the central pattern generator (CPG) existing in the brain stem depending on commands from the cerebral cortex.

However, studies concerning outputs from cerebral cortex generating the CPG have been rarely reported. Firstly, the authors explored the properties of neurons related to mastication (MRNs) using single unit recording and intracortical microstimulation (ICMS) in various areas of the cat frontal cortex. The authors identified the mastication-related cortical areas (MRCAs) of one orofacial SI (the facial and intraoral primary somatosensory cortex) and four motor cortical areas (area C in the anterior part of coronal sulcus, MA in the masticatory area, area M in the ventral bank of cruciate sulcus and area P in the lateral wall of presylcian sulcus). Next, the authors examined changes in orofacial behaviors induced by localized lesions in respective area. These results showed that the cortical control for appropriate feeding behaviors was organized by two distinct cortical regions for facial and masticatory (jaw and tongue) movements.

Facial movements are unilaterally controlled by the facial SI (area 3b), area C (area 3a) and area M (area 4∂), whereas masticatory movements are bilaterally controlled by the intraoral SI (areas 3b and 3a), masticatory cortex (area 43) and area P (area 6aß). Although the unilateral cortical processing for facial movements is the same as the one for the limb movement, bilateral networks for movements of jaw and tongue remain unclear. However, since the jaw movement of cats consists of jaw- opening and -closing only, the authors focused on the tongue movement.

The authors showed the characteristic change in the abnormal tongue-protrusion with the increased genioglossus muscle activities during licking after the unilateral motor cortical area (area P) lesion, and the abnormal protrusion without deviation, as well as the protrusion evoked by the ICMS.

On the other hand, the unilateral hypoglossal nerve cutting showed deviation toward the affected side (Hiraba and Sato 2004), and pyramidal neurons (PT) in the unilateral area P projected to the bilateral hypoglossal nuclei at the brain stem, as shown in anatomical data. These findings suggested that tongue muscles in the left and right sides were supplied by the hypoglossal nuclei in the left and right sides, and also that the unilateral area P contained two kinds of PTs projecting to left or right nuclei. Furthermore, the authors assumed the relay circuit of inhibitory interneuron between connections of both hemispheres based on the abnormal tongue protrusion after the unilateral lesion.

Chapter III - This chapter reviews the functional magnetic resonance imaging (fMRI) studies carried out by the authors' group in the past 10 years to elucidate the role of the human corpus callosum (CC) in the interhemispheric transfer of somatosensory information.

Functional studies using various techniques (somatosensory evoked potentials, magneto-encephalography, positron emission tomography) have shown that unilateral tactile stimulation evokes bilateral activation in two cortical regions involved in the processing of tactile stimuli: the posterior parietal (PP) cortex in the postcentral gyrus, containing the first somatic sensory area, and the parietal operculum in the upper bank of the Sylvian sulcus, containing the second somatic sensory area (SII).

The pathways by which sensory afferents reach the ipsilateral cortices are still unknown. It is a widely held view that the CC transfers sensory information by relaying it to the somatic sensory areas of the contralateral hemisphere. The "callosal recrossing" hypothesis is supported by experiments on the callosal connectivity of homologous cortical regions of non-human primates and other mammals.

The fMRI researches described here were organized as follows:

[1] a "normal" activation pattern was established by investigating cortical somatic sensory areas in normal volunteers, who received unilateral moving tactile stimulation of the hand and fingers or of the ventral trunk surface;

[2] the "callosal recrossing" hypothesis was tested by performing the same studies in patients subjected to surgical resection of the CC to control medically intractable epilepsy;

[3] the possible role of the CC in mediating pain-related ipsilateral cortical activation was investigated by analyzing the pattern of cortical activation evoked by painful mechanical stimulation in normal volunteers and in three patients with complete CC resection.

Results point to the following conclusions: the CC is mainly responsible for somatic sensory cortex bilateral activation evoked by unilateral tactile stimulation of the hand and fingers. Callosal fibres carrying activation to the ipsilateral PP cortex and SII cross in the posterior third of the body of the commissure, anterior to the splenium. By contrast, ipsilateral activation evoked by tactile trunk and painful hand stimulation is at least partially independent of callosal transmission, being probably mediated by extracallosal pathways: uncrossed subcortical pathways, subcortical commissures, or both.

Chapter IV - The classic model of episodic memory refers to both laboratory tasks requiring the conscious recall or recognition of experimental materials and autobiographical recollection of one's personal past experiences. Recent research in cognitive neuroscience, however, showed evidence that laboratory and autobiographical memory may share aspects of conscious retrieval and reference to the temporal and spatial context at the time of encoding of information, but are different from each other in some important respects. The autobiographical memory domain is characterized by self-referential information processing, subjective emotional evaluation of memories, and the accompanying autonoetic conscious awareness. In contrast, laboratory episodic memory requires the effortful search for impersonal target information and the intentional use of retrieval strategies. Subregions of the prefrontal, medial temporal, and retrosplenial cortices appear to be differentially involved in the neural processing of each type of episodic memory, thus suggesting that they are supported by anatomically and functionally overlapping, but also segregated neural circuits. The empirical data reviewed here support the view that laboratory and autobiographical episodic memory can at least in part be distinguished on the cognitive-behavioral and the neurofunctional levels. Accordingly, the review proposes an integrated view of laboratory and autobiographical forms of episodic memory which accounts for an overlap, but also emphasizes the unique features distinguishing the two memory types.

Chapter V - Functional magnetic resonance imaging (fMRI) is a noninvasive imaging technique that is able to detect hemodynamic changes associated with neuronal activity in vivo. In the past decade, it has been used extensively for mapping functional neuroanatomy in basic neuroscience and clinical applications. A typical fMRI study includes acquisition of a time series of images (during which the subject is instructed to perform certain tasks) and offline processing and analysis of the image series. In real-time fMRI (rtfMRI), however, image processing and analysis start shortly after the beginning of the scan and then follow the image acquisition procedure as closely as possible. Real-time fMRI provides not only a useful tool for effective quality assurance of fMRI studies, but also opportunities for designing functional examinations with interactive controls and feedback.

In this chapter, the authors describe the basic concept and technical solution of rtfMRI, with a focus on a technique that the authors have recently developed and implemented on a Siemens 3T MRI scanner. The authors then demonstrate potential applications of rtfMRI techniques for neurofeedback and motion artifact reduction. In particular, the authors present a novel method of voluntary head-motion suppression using the feedback of the subject's own motion information in real time. This method was tested and the possible influence on the performance of tasks in fMRI study was assessed utilizing a commonly used working memory task. The authors experiments showed that significant suppression of head motion was achieved consistently while the influence on the performance of task and the interference to brain activation could be minimized by careful design of the feedback system.

Chapter VI - Blood oxygenation level-dependent (BOLD) contrast-based functional magnetic resonance imaging (fMRI) has been widely utilized to detect brain neural activities and great efforts are now stressed on the hemodynamic processes of different brain regions activated by a stimulus. The focus of this paper is the comparison of Gamma and Gaussian dynamic convolution models of the fMRI BOLD response. The convolutions are between the perfusion function of the neural response to a stimulus and a Gaussian or Gamma function. The parameters of the two models are estimated by a nonlinear least-squares optimal algorithm for the fMRI data of eight subjects collected in a visual stimulus experiment. The results show that the Gaussian model is better than the Gamma model in fitting the data. The model parameters are different in the left and right occipital regions, which indicate that the dynamic processes seem different in various cerebral functional regions. Further, the asymmetry of the left-right and upper-lower visual field is investigated by the differences of the Gaussian model parameters. The results from eight subjects show that reaction time is significant shorter and the response is significant stronger when the lower field is stimulated than that when the upper field is stimulated. For the left and right fields, the response is different. These results provide the fMRI BOLD response evidence of the asymmetry of spatial visual fields.

Chapter VII - While MRI is well suited for examining post-treatment gliomas, there are often ambiguous results when attempting to interpret T1- and T2-weighted images, even with the use of an extravascular contrast agent. To provide additional clarity when distinguishing recurrent disease from radiation necrosis, edema, and normal tissue, a host of MRI parameters that probe physiology have been developed and continue to be optimized. These include specialized MR sequences that yield descriptive maps of tissue perfusion and diffusion [1-4]; chemical shift imaging that provides biochemical measures (choline, creatine, N-acetyl aspartate, lactate) [5]; and a blood oxygenation level dependent (BOLD)-based scan that provides hypoxia maps [6, 7].

The multi-parametric techniques now being used for recurrent Glioblastoma Multiforme (GBM) patients could be applied to many cancer management situations (e.g. diagnosis, surgical and radiation planning, monitoring therapy). When prescribing radiation therapy, for example, greater knowledge of the tumor environment would allow advances in radiation delivery systems (e.g. Intensity Modulated Radiotherapy) to deliver more focused, patient-specific treatment [8]. However, the imaging techniques yield a variety of maps that all require interpretation. The quantity of parameter maps and complexity of the dataset obtained from multi-parametric approaches emphasizes the need for further work to make these techniques more user-friendly in clinical settings.

Chapter VIII - From the past decade to date, research on the interactive brain mechanisms between attention and emotion studied through event-related potentials (ERPs) has increasingly grown. This brain signal reflects fast and swift cognitive processing due to its excellent temporal resolution and it has become a suitable tool in order to study several issues concerning cognitive processing. In this chapter the authors present a detailed description of an 'emotional variant' of the S1 (cue)-S2 (target) task that has been typically used to explore vigilance-related attention. The application of the emotional S1-S2 paradigm elicits an affective modulation effect on a brainwave that has been related to expectancy, the early Contingent Negative Variation (eCNV). In this chapter the authors will present several issues concerning different methodological aspects to take into account when applying this paradigm and some details related to the procedures of quantification and analysis of the ERP data. Finally, some findings obtained through the use of the emotional S1-S2 protocol are summarized and some of its different application possibilities (e.g., clinical samples) are proposed.

Chapter IX - How to localize the neural electric activities effectively and precisely from the scalp EEG recordings is a critical issue for clinical neurology and cognitive neuroscience. In the past 80s and 90s, suggested approaches included the dipole localization, cortical imaging, scalp Laplacian and 3D tomography. The 3D tomography may be realized by a direct linear inversion, or an indirect algorithm such as the subspace projection scanning method named MUltiple SIgnal Classification (MUSIC). However, the classical MUSIC algorithm is limited for its assumption of random noise. In this work, the authors propose to use a delay-correlation matrix instead of the previous zero-delay-correlation matrix in the signal-subspace estimate of the MUSIC algorithm to get a better performance over a spatial coherent but temporal random noisy disturbance. Then an Iterative application of the Delay-correlation MUSIC (IDM) is emphasized to derive a reasonable reconstruction of the multi-sources. The present simulation and empirical data experiment show that final promising results are obtained.

In: Brain Mapping Research Developments
Editor: Lars N. Bakker, pp. 1-9

ISBN 978-1-60456-007-7

Expert Commentary

NEURAL ACTIVATION DUE TO OLFACTORY STIMULATION MEASURED BY NEAR INFRARED SPECTROSCOPY

Hiroaki Shoji, Noriko Sato and Hisaki Ozaki
Laboratory of Physiology, Faculty of Education,
Ibaraki University, Mito 310-8512, Japan

ABSTRACT

The present study examined hemodynamic brain activities due to olfactory stimulation, using near infrared spectroscopy (NIRS). Participants in the experiment, 9 healthy adults, sat on a chair with their eyes closed during the measurement of cerebral blood flow. The concentration changes of oxy- and deoxy-hemoglobin were measured from 22 channels over the forehead. Odorized air was puffed into the right nostril for 30 seconds through an injector in which a cotton pad with lemongrass essential oil had been placed. The olfactory stimulation was interrupted by non-odorized air spurted from another injector for 30 seconds. Odorant presentation was repeated 3 times. In order to examine olfactory processing with minimal interference from respiration, participants were requested to breath through their mouth during the measurements. Following odorant presentation, the concentration of oxy-hemoglobin increased significantly in the orbito-frontal regions, while deoxy-hemoglobin slightly decreased. The present results suggest that orbito-frontal activation might be due to an odorant stimulus. Topographic implications for odorant detection are discussed.

1. INTRODUCTION

After air inhaled into the nostrils goes through the nasal cavity, the olfactory receptors in the upper part of the nasal cavity transduce odorant stimuli into electrical signals. Odorant signals reach the olfactory bulbs, from which odorant information is sent to the primary olfactory cortex. Recently, cerebral activity in human olfactory processing has been examined using modern brain imaging techniques, for instance, positron emission tomography (PET: Zatorre et al., 1992) and functional magnetic resonance imaging (fMRI: Sabri et al., 2005; Sobel et al., 1998). Published studies have reported that many brain structures are concerned with olfactory processing. At present, the human primary olfactory cortex is thought to be the piriform cortices of the temporal lobes. Furthermore, it has been demonstrated that more conscious smell perception might be treated at the associative olfactory cortex in the orbito-frontal region (Sobel et al., 1998; Zatorre et al., 1992).

Near-infrared spectroscopy (NIRS) is a noninvasive method for detecting relative concentration changes in oxygenated hemoglobin (oxy-Hb) and deoxygenated hemoglobin (deoxy-Hb). NIRS allows monitoring of cerebral blood flow in an unshielded room, e.g., bedside or classroom. In addition, participants are not required to constrain their body movements. Therefore, NIRS is widely applicable for exploring cerebral functions in various populations, including infants, children, people with developmental disabilities, and hospitalized patients.

In recent years, several NIRS studies have demonstrated cerebral activation due to odor stimulation in the olfactory cortex, e.g., the orbito-frontal area (Ishimaru et al., 2004; Kobayashi et al., 2007) and the temporal area (Fladby et al., 2004). Our long-range research goal is to evaluate olfactory perception objectively in people with profound and/or multiple disabilities. People with profound and/or multiple disabilities, especially people who need special health care, often have poor spontaneous respiration. For example, artificial respiration after a tracheotomy operation might restrict respiratory airflow in the nasal cavity. We cannot perceive odors without airflow, even if odorants fill the nasal cavity (Mainland and Sobel, 2006). For that reason, in people with poor spontaneous respiration, unless the odorized air is forced by airflow from outside into the olfactory receptor in the nasal cavity, odors can hardly be perceived. However, to our knowledge, no previous NIRS study has examined neural activation due to forced injection of olfactory stimuli into the nostrils.

The aim of the present study is to clarify olfactory activation in the orbito-frontal regions in normal adults under the condition of forced odor presentation.

2. Methods

2.1. Participants

9 healthy volunteers (2 males and 7 females; 8 right-handed; mean age 22.1 years, ranging from 21.2 to 23.0 years) participated in the present experiment. Prior to the start of the experiment, the purpose and procedure of the experiment was explained, and their informed consent for participation was obtained.

2.2. Stimuli

Lemongrass essential oil (Prevail essential oil; Biken Co. LTD, Japan) was used as the olfactory stimulus in the present study. A cotton pad (2.5 × 3.0 cm) soaked with 0.15 ml of oil was placed in an injector, and odorized air was puffed into the right nostril through the injector. For the comparison stimulus, air that had not been odorized was presented via another injector that had only a dry cotton pad in it.

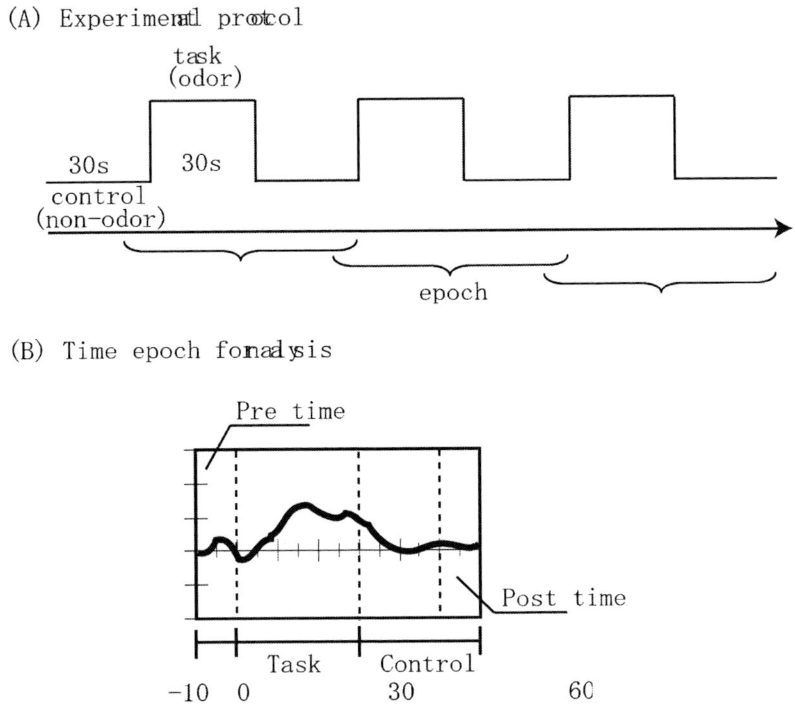

Figure 1. Experimental protocol and time epoch for analysis. (A) After the non-odorized air was injected for 30 seconds as a baseline in the first epoch, odorized air and non-odorized air were presented alternately for 30 seconds. One session was composed of 3 epochs. (B) The time epoch for analysis was 70 seconds, including the 10-second epoch prior to the odorant stimulus onset, the 30-second epoch during the task period, and the 30-second epoch beginning from the odorant stimulus offset. Baseline correction was done by linear fitting according to the mean value of the 10-second epoch prior to the task (pre-time) and that of the 10-second epoch between 20 seconds and 30 seconds after the task (post-time).

2.3. Procedure

During the measurement of brain blood flow, the participants sat on a chair with their eyes closed. Prior to the odorant injection, non-odorized air was spurted into the right nostril for 30 seconds. Then, a task period followed, in which odorized air was puffed into the right nostril for 30 seconds through the injector. The olfactory stimulation was terminated by non-odorized air spurted from the other injector for 30 seconds (control period; Figure 1). This sequence was repeated 3 times. At each stroke, 10 ml of odorized or non-odorized air was manually pushed out. Each stroke took 2 seconds; a 2-second silent period was inserted between each stroke. The air stream was injected 7 times during each 30-second trial. In order to examine olfactory processing with minimal interference from respiration, participants were requested to breath through their mouth during the measurements.

2.4. Near-Infrared Spectroscopy (NIRS) Measurement

We used a 24-channel NIRS instrument (ETG-100 Optical Topography System; Hitachi Medical Co., Japan) to measure relative concentration changes in oxy-Hb and deoxy-Hb from 2-3 cm beneath the scalp, i.e., the cerebral cortices. The ETG-100 generated 2 wavelengths of near-infrared light: 780 and 830 nm. Changes in the concentration of oxy-Hb and deoxy-Hb were calculated from the difference between the absorption of oxy-Hb and deoxy-Hb for the 2 near-infrared wavelengths due to the Beer–Lambert law. The sum of oxy-Hb and deoxy-Hb was the total-Hb.

Probes with 8 emitters and 7 detectors in a 3×5 array were placed over the forehead (see Figure 2). The distance between the probes was 3.0 cm. This array allowed measurement of hemoglobin concentration changes at 22 sites. The center probe of the bottom row was placed at the Fpz of the international 10/20 system for electroencephalography.

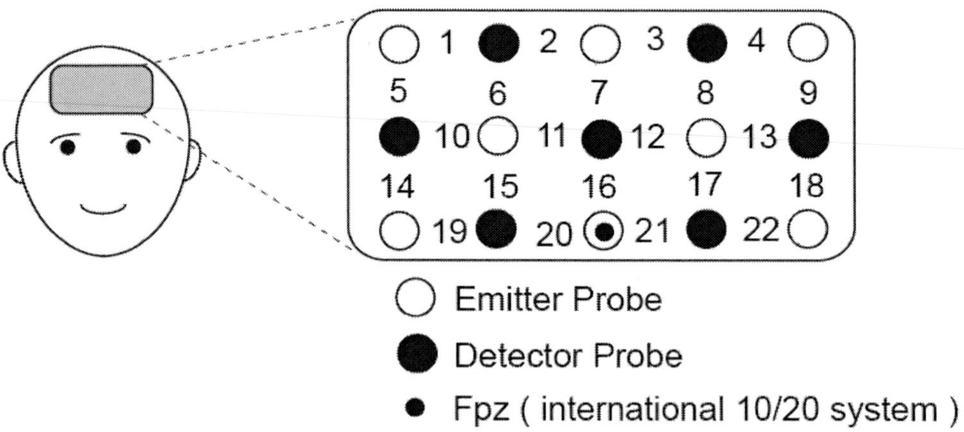

Figure 2. Probe locations in the frontal area. Open and closed circles indicate emitters and detectors through the optical fiber, respectively. The location of the probe indicated by a small circle (Fpz) was decided according to the international 10/20 system for EEG recording. The numbers between the probes indicate the recording channels for NIRS.

2.5. Analysis

The NIRS data were low-pass-filtered at 0.1 Hz. The time epoch for analysis was 70 seconds, including the 10-second epoch prior to odorant stimulus onset, the 30-second epoch during the task period, and the 30-second epoch beginning at odorant stimulus offset (Figure 1). In order to exclude the steady trend of hemodynamic increase/decrease, baseline correction was done by linear fitting according to the mean value of the 10-second epoch prior to the task (pre-time) and that of the 10-second epoch between 20 seconds and 30 seconds after the task (post-time). Then, waveforms of blood flow were averaged over all trials, excluding any epochs with artifacts.

The mean value of each 5-second epoch after the odorant stimulation was calculated for each participant. These 5-second epoch data in the cortical regions of interest, i.e., channels 14-22 corresponding to the orbito-frontal region, were compared with the mean 10-second epoch data before the task, using Fisher's exact test.

Furthermore, in order to clarify the hemispheric difference of the orbito-frontal area, data from the lower frontal channels were averaged for each hemisphere, i.e., channels 14, 15, 19, and 20 for the right hemisphere, and channels 17, 18, 21, and 22 for the left. Fisher's exact test was applied for the comparison of the hemispheric difference. Because the concentration changes of oxy-Hb and total-Hb are more sensitive and responsive to cerebral activation than those of deoxy-Hb, these statistical analyses were performed on the data of oxy-Hb and total-Hb.

3. Results

Figure 3 shows the grand averaged waveforms of oxy-Hb, deoxy-Hb and total-Hb after the odorant stimulation. In the inferior frontal region, which covers the orbito-frontal area, oxy-Hb and total-Hb increased immediately after the onset of olfactory stimulation, and reached maximal value at around 15 seconds after the olfactory stimulation. On the other hand, in the orbito-frontal area, the concentration of deoxy-Hb decreased slightly after the olfactory stimulation.

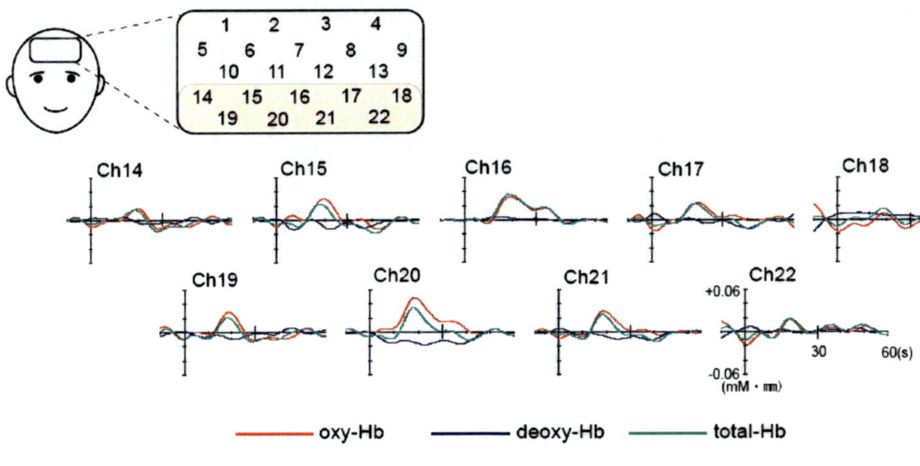

Figure 3. Grand average waveforms of hemoglobin concentration changes in the inferior frontal region. The concentration changes in the channels marked in red in the upper part of the Figure are displayed in the lower part of the Figure. The grand mean data from all 9 participants are shown. Red, blue and green lines indicate the concentration of oxy-Hb, deoxy-Hb and total-Hb respectively.

In order to examine neural activation due to the odorant stimulus excluding effects of the injected air, the concentration changes in the odorant stimulation during the task period were compared with those in the control period (non-odorant stimulation). The concentration changes in oxy-Hb during the task period significantly increased during 15-20 seconds after olfactory stimulation in channels 16 (Z= -2.073, p=0.039) and 20 (Z= -2.191, p=0.027), compared to those in the control period prior to the odorant stimulation. The concentration of total-Hb at channel 16 (Z= -2.191, p=0.027) significantly increased during the epoch 15-20 seconds after the olfactory stimulation.

Figure 4 shows a map series of the hemoglobin concentration changes at each second from 15 seconds to 20 seconds after the olfactory stimulation. An increase in the concentration of oxy-Hb and total-Hb was observed in the right inferior frontal area. At the same time, the concentration of deoxy-Hb decreased slightly in the similar cerebral region. The mean values of oxy-Hb and total-Hb in the right hemisphere (channels 14, 15, 19, 20) were compared with those in the left hemisphere (channels 17, 18, 21, 22). For both oxy-Hb and total-Hb, 8 of the 9 participants showed a larger oxy-Hb and total-Hb concentration in the right hemisphere than in the left. Quantitative statistical analysis revealed a right-hemispheric-dominant tendency (oxy-Hb: Z= -1.836, p=.074; total-Hb: Z= -1.838, p=.070).

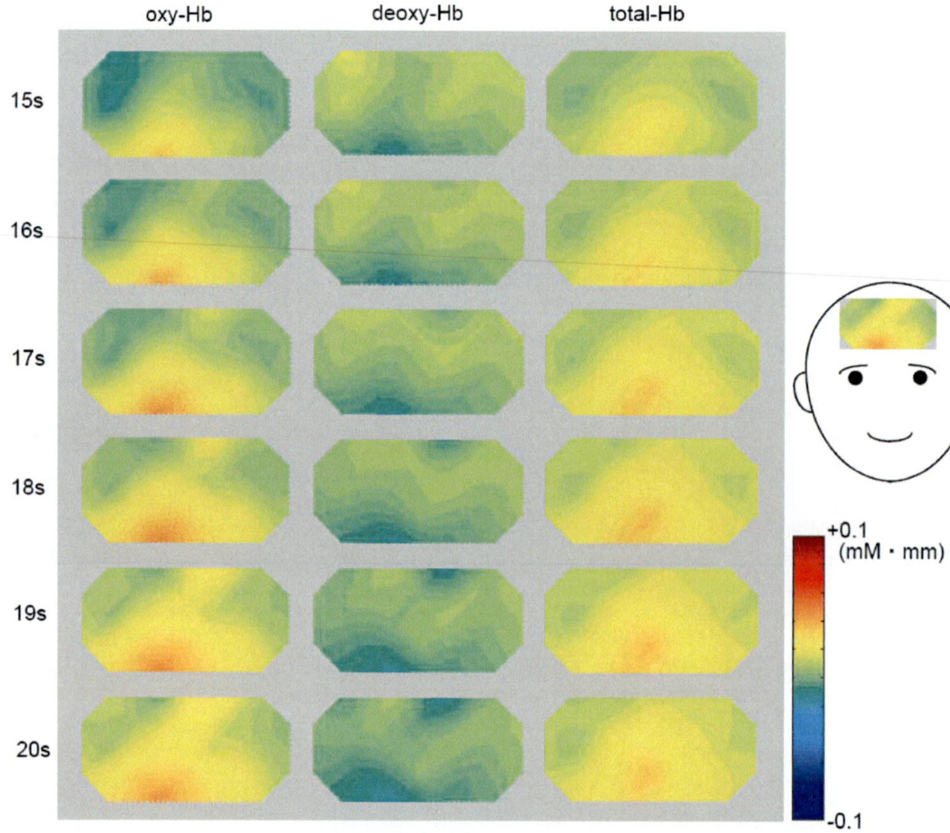

Figure 4. Map series of hemoglobin concentration. The grand mean data for oxy-Hb, deoxy-Hb, and total-Hb from the epoch 15 to 20 seconds after the onset of odorant stimulation are displayed in 1-second intervals.

4. Discussion

We normally sense smells as a consequence of odorant airflow in the nostrils. However, people who need artificial respiration, e.g., after a tracheotomy operation, and individuals with profound and/or multiple disabilities might find it difficult to perceive odors spontaneously because of restriction of the respiratory airflow in their nasal cavity. In such cases, forced injection of odorants might be an efficient way to enable them to sense the smell of an odorant. If individuals with profound and/or multiple disabilities have some residual ability to sense smell when an odorant is presented in this way, activation of the olfactory system might be a channel for promoting their functional development.

However, it was not clear that olfactory activation due to the forced injection could be evaluated by NIRS. Therefore, we examined the hemodynamic activation due to the forced injection of odorants in adults without disabilities.

Previous functional neuroimaging studies have shown that the orbito-frontal gyri of the frontal lobe and the piriform cortex of the temporal lobe are responsible for olfactory processing in the human brain (Sobel et al., 1998; Zatorre et al., 1992), and that the anterior orbito-frontal cortex is primarily activated by the presentation of odors.

In the present study, the concentration of oxy-Hb and total-Hb significantly increased in the lower part of the frontal cortex, which might correspond to the orbito-frontal region. On the other hand, the concentration of deoxy-Hb slightly decreased along a similar time course. Such hemodynamic changes are the typical neuronal activation traced by NIRS (Matsuo et al., 2003). The increases in oxy-Hb and total-Hb concentration reached a plateau within about 18 seconds after the odorant stimulation. This is also in line with previous NIRS studies on olfactory response in the orbito-frontal region, in which the concentration changes of oxy-Hb and total-Hb were shown to reach a peak with a similar time course (Harada et al., 2006; Kobayashi et al., 2007).

In the present study, hemodynamic brain activities due to odorant stimulation during the task period were compared with those due to non-odorant stimulation in the control period. Therefore, the effect of the air injected into the nasal cavity is thought to be subtracted from hemodynamic activity in the orbito-frontal region during the task. The present results indicate that activation of the olfactory cortex in humans was detectable by NIRS under the condition of the forced injection of odorants.

Right hemisphere dominance of olfactory discrimination in each nostril has been reported in a behavioral study by Zatorre and Jones-Gotman (1990). Prominent activation of the right orbito-frontal cortex has been demonstrated in brain imaging studies, e.g., in fMRI (Sobel et al., 1998) and PET (Zatorre et al., 1992). In the present study, topographical concentration changes seemed to be more prominent in the right orbito-frontal area than in the left, even though the inter-hemispheric difference in hemoglobin concentration did not reach statistical significance. This bilateral activation in the orbito-frontal area corresponds to previous NIRS findings on olfactory stimulation (Ishimaru et al., 2004; Kobayashi et al., 2007).

The discrepancy between the findings in the fMRI/PET studies and the present NIRS study might be caused by the different principle of hemodynamic brain imaging. In addition, since cerebral projection of the olfactory nerve is ipsilateral, the slightly right-sided lateralization may be due to the olfactory stimulation through the right nostril. With respect to monorhinal stimulation, although a magnetoencephalogram study showed ipsilateral activation (Tonoike et al., 1996), a PET study revealed activation in the right orbito-frontal cortex, regardless of nostril side (Savic and Gulyas, 2000). Thus, this question is still open. Future research should examine hemodynamic changes due to olfactory stimulation to each nostril, i.e., on both sides.

Conclusion

In the present study, the concentration of oxy-Hb and total-Hb significantly increased in the lower part of the frontal cortex during odorant stimulation. This finding suggests that the olfactory response in human brain can be evaluated by NIRS even when forced injection of odorants is used. Therefore, NIRS may be useful for an objective evaluation of the olfactory cortex.

Acknowledgements

This work was supported by a grant-in-aid from the Mitsubishi Foundation to H. Shoji and a grant-in-aid from the Japan Society for the Promotion of Science (18653116) to H. Ozaki.

References

Fladby, T., Bryhn, G., Halvorsen, O., Rosé, I., Wahlund, M., Wiig, P., and Wetterberg, L. (2004). Olfactory response in the temporal cortex of the elderly measured with near-infrared spectroscopy: a preliminary feasibility study. *Journal of Cerebral Blood Flow and Metabolism*, 24, 677-680.

Harada, H., Tanaka, M., and Kato, T. (2006). Brain olfactory activation measured by near-infrared spectroscopy in humans. *The Journal of Laryngology and Otology*, 120, 638-643.

Ishimaru, T., Yata, T., Horikawa, K., and Hatanaka, S. (2004). Near-infrared spectroscopy of the adult human olfactory cortex. *Acta Oto-Laryngologica. Supplementum*, 553, 95-98.

Kobayashi, E., Kusaka, T., Karaki, M., Kobayashi, R., Itoh, S., and Mori, N. (2007). Functional optical hemodynamic imaging of the olfactory cortex. *Laryngoscope*, 117, 541-546.

Mainland, J., and Sobel, N. (2006). The sniff is part of the olfactory percept. *Chemical Senses*, 31, 181-196.

Matsuo, K., Kato, T., Taneichi, K., Matsumoto, A., Ohtani, T., Hamamoto, T., Yamasue, H., Sakano, Y., Sasaki, T., Sadamatsu, M., Iwanami, A., Asukai, N., and Kato, N. (2003). Activation of the prefrontal cortex to trauma-related stimuli measured by near-infrared spectroscopy in posttraumatic stress disorder due to terrorism. *Psychophysiology*, 40, 492-500.

Sabri, M., Radnovich, A. J., Li, T. Q., and Kareken, D. A. (2005). Neural correlates of olfactory change detection. *Neuroimage*, 25, 969-974.

Savic, I., and Gulyas, B. (2000). PET shows that odors are processed both ipsilaterally and contralaterally to the stimulated nostril. *Neuroreport*, 11, 2861-2866.

Sobel, N., Prabhakaran, V., Desmond, J. E., Glover, G. H., Goode, R. L., Sullivan, E. V., and Gabrieli, J. D. (1998). Sniffing and smelling: separate subsystems in the human olfactory cortex. *Nature*, 392, 282-286.

Tonoike, M., Maeda, A., Kawai, H., and Kaetsu, I. (1996). Measurement of olfactory event-related magnetic fields evoked by odorant pulses synchronized with respiration. *Electroencephalography and Clinical Neurophysiology. Supplement*, 47, 143-150.

Zatorre, R. J., and Jones-Gotman, M. (1990). Right-nostril advantage for discrimination of odors. *Perception and Psychophysics*, 47, 526-531.

Zatorre, R. J., Jones-Gotman, M., Evans, A. C., and Meyer, E. (1992). Functional localization and lateralization of human olfactory cortex. *Nature*, 360, 339-340.

RESEARCH AND REVIEW STUDIES

In: Brain Mapping Research Developments
Editor: Lars N. Bakker, pp. 13-42

ISBN 978-1-60456-007-7

Chapter I

Mapping the Auditory Brain Using Magnetoencephalography (MEG)

***Christopher J. Brignell*[1]*, Deborah A. Hall*[1,*] *and Caroline Witton*[2]**
[1]MRC Institute of Hearing Research, Nottingham, UK
[2]School of Life and Health Sciences, Aston University, Birmingham, UK

Abstract

The use of magnetoencephalography (MEG) as an imaging technique for auditory brain mapping research has rapidly grown over the past decade to take advantage of its excellent temporal resolution (sub millisecond) and reasonable spatial resolution (sub centimetre). MEG can be used to study evoked transient deflections such as the energy onset or pitch onset responses, sustained responses and stimulus-induced oscillations through a wide range of techniques including amplitude and latency analysis, dipole source modelling and beamformer analysis. The wide range of approaches to data analysis ensures MEG is a highly flexible tool for brain mapping.

In this chapter, we review the contribution of MEG to advances in auditory brain mapping, seeking to explore its advantages and limitations and clarifying some misconceptions regarding its use. In the first section we describe the method and discuss some of the technical issues related to the optimal design of auditory experiments. In the second section, we introduce different strategies for the analysis of MEG data. In the third section we present a review of published studies that have mapped central auditory function using MEG.

* Corresponding author: MRC Institute of Hearing Research, University Park, Nottingham, NG7 2RD, UK. Tel.: +44 115 9223431; fax: +44 115 951 8503. E-mail address: d.hall@ihr.mrc.ac.uk.

1. Introduction

1.1. Methodological Issues in Magnetoencephalography (MEG)

Synchronous neuronal firing in the human brain produces a net electrical current flow which induces a change in the magnetic field. The ability to record such small disturbances in the natural magnetic field was first demonstrated by Cohen (1968). The measurements of the electrical current and the magnetic field are known as electroencephalography (EEG) and magnetoencephalography (MEG) respectively. The use of MEG as a neuroimaging technique was somewhat restricted until technological advances in the 1990s produced the first half-head and whole-head systems, with an array of sensors arranged over the scalp. Subsequently, there has been an exponential growth over the past decade in the use MEG for a wide range of clinical and research applications.

Neural magnetic fields are tiny in amplitude and measurements are typically quoted in femtoTeslas (fT). This makes them a billion times smaller than the earth's natural magnetic field and several orders of magnitude smaller that the magnetic field induced by urban noise, such as a moving car. Measurements are therefore collected inside a magnetically shielded room. The sensors are known as superconducting quantum interference detectors (SQUIDs), which operate at a temperature of -260°C and are cooled using liquid helium. The total number of sensors in the helmet varies according to the manufacturer, but currently up to about 300 can be positioned equidistant from one another in a head-shaped array, with more sensors allowing greater spatial resolution. Figure 1 shows a 275 channel whole-head MEG system (CTF Systems Inc., Vancouver, Canada) in operation. MEG is reliant upon the neural activity generating a magnetic field which is measurable outside the head; deeper sources are therefore more difficult to record than superficial ones, as are those in a radial orientation.

The maximum sampling rate for SQUIDs is approximately 12 kHz, but MEG is usually recorded at about 500-1000 Hz, still providing excellent time resolution to study responses in the millisecond range. MEG signals are also recorded across a spectral power range which spans the typical frequency bands of brain activity (<100 Hz). Perhaps the greatest advantage of MEG compared to EEG is its improved spatial resolution of around 5 mm on most systems. The magnetic field is undisturbed when passing through grey-matter, cerebro-spinal fluid, skull or skin; all of which influence the strength and location of EEG signals recorded using scalp electrodes. The excellent temporal resolution and reasonably precise spatial resolution makes MEG suitable for recording stimulus evoked fields and spontaneous brain activity with great accuracy. MEG has additional advantages over functional magnetic resonance imaging (fMRI), which measures the relative blood oxygenation level rather than neuronal firing. This indirect measurement results in poor temporal resolution, in the order of seconds, and limits the spatial precision due to the contribution of venous and capillary influences on the signal. Importantly for carefully controlled auditory studies, MEG is acoustically silent and subjects are not affected by MR scanner noise. Subjects also do not experience the discomfort of EEG scalp electrodes.

To obtain accurate spatial resolution, the location of the subject's head must be monitored in relation to the position of the MEG sensors. In most systems, at least three small electrical coils are taped to the subject's head to define a spatial coordinate system.

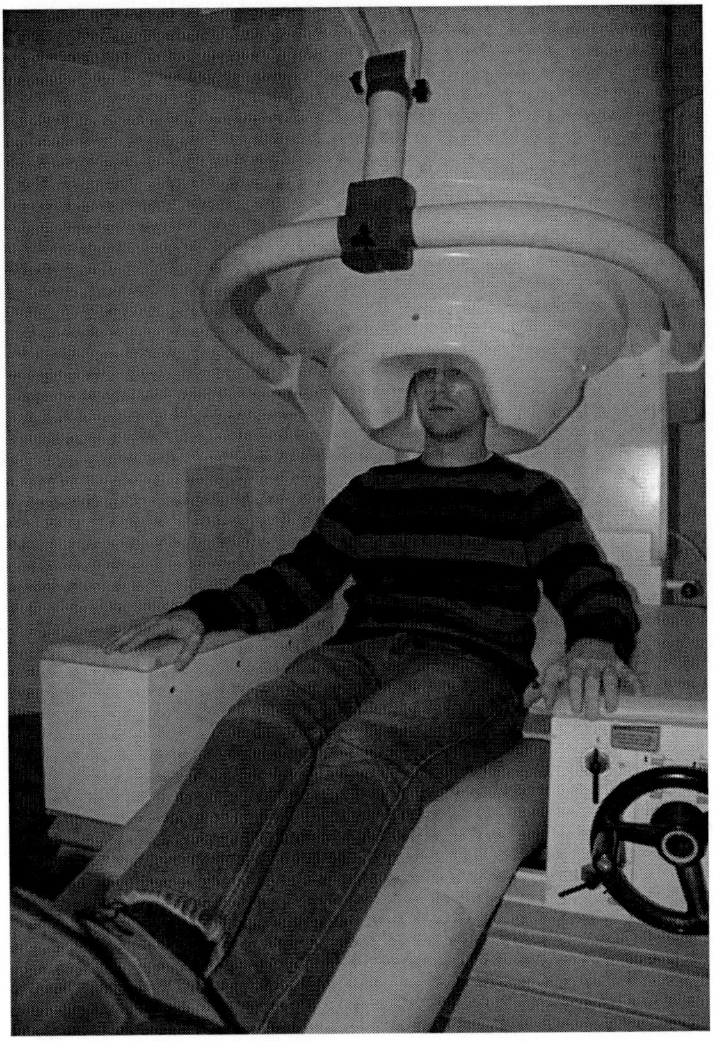

Figure 1. A subject participating in an MEG experiment at the Wellcome Trust Laboratory for MEG Studies at Aston University. The scanner is located inside a magnetically shielded room, with the SQUID sensors arranged over the scalp surface.

A known magnetic field is induced by sending a small electrical pulse to these coils throughout the experiment and this procedure establishes the distance of each sensor from each electrical coil at all times. A dataset may be discarded if subject movement exceeds the desired spatial resolution during the experiment. Precise anatomical localisation of neural brain activity also requires the acquisition of a magnetic resonance image (MRI) to provide a detailed anatomical image of the subject's brain and scalp surface. The coordinate system determined by the coils can be imposed on the MRI, either by making the coil locations visible during the MR scanning (e.g. by using oil capsules taped in the coil position) or by taking a digitised representation of the actual scalp surface and coregistering this to the scalp observed in the MRI. If a subject's MRI is unavailable, Holliday et al. (2003) showed that the use of a substitute MRI with similar scalp surface, can provide a coregistration with a modal error of only 6 mm.

The structure of MEG data is a time-series of magnetic field values for each sensor. Data analysis usually involves a number of pre-processing steps. Perhaps the most important is to screen for artefacts, which may either be extraneous to the recording, or physiological in origin. The high sensitivity of the MEG sensors to electrical interference means that power-line comb filtering is usually necessary to remove the effect of alternating current in electrical power cables (at 50 Hz in Europe or 60 Hz in North America). Physiological artefacts include the magnetic fields caused by eye-blinks, muscle activity and resting rhythms. Screening can be manual or automated. Automated algorithms detect trials in which the signal exceeds a given amplitude or rate of change threshold. Eye-movement artefacts can also be identified using electrodes placed around the eye muscles (Palomäki et al., 2005). Identified data segments or channels can either be removed from the dataset, or can be corrected to some extent using principal components analysis (PCA, Sieroka et al., 2003) or independent components analysis (ICA), without the loss of any trials or channels. ICA identifies, after training, components that represent the artefacts which can be subtracted from the original data (Delorme et al., 2007). MEG data also need to be corrected for the effects of slow drifts in the recording baseline, by removal of linear trends or, for data recorded in epochs, by subtracting the mean of a pre-stimulus period from the post-stimulus time of interest.

1.2. Issues for the Design of Auditory MEG Experiments

The human auditory system encodes a wide variety of sounds, including those with complex spectro-temporal patterns such as speech and music. These natural sounds have many changing variables that make them ill-suited for use as stimuli in neuroimaging experiments and so they are commonly replaced with synthesised sounds such as clicks, tones and white noise. Such stimuli enable greater experimental control for identifying how one particular sound feature (such as intensity, duration, pitch or spatial location) influences the neuronal response in the auditory cortex. The simplest experimental paradigm contrasts two stimuli that differ only in a single acoustic feature. For example, Hertrich et al. (2005) compared the neural response to 333 Hz and 400 Hz pitches. Another paradigm systematically varies the value of that feature across conditions. Tiitinen et al. (2006), for example, presented sounds from eight equidistantly spaced azimuth direction angles (-135°, -90°, -45°, 0°, 45°, 90°, 135°, 180°), separated by 45 degree steps.

One challenge for auditory MEG research concerns the method of stimulus delivery. Sound stimuli must be presented to the subject's ears without perturbing the natural, shielded, magnetic field. Conventional headphones, with their electrical and moving components, naturally induce changes in the magnetic field that correspond to the acoustic signal rather than to the evoked neural activity. The most common solution is to deliver sounds using tubephones. The sound is delivered as an electrical signal to two small transducers fixed at least half a metre from the MEG sensors. These convert the signal into sound that is sent down a tube, 0.5-1 m in length, and into the subject's ears. The end of the tube is sheathed with a foam ear plug to attenuate ambient acoustic noise. The length, diameter and material of the tube are designed to maximise the accuracy of the delivered sound across the frequency spectrum but some calibration may be required. For example, the E-A-R TONE system (Aearo Company, Indianapolis, USA), shown in Figure 2, can produce 110 dB HL at standard audiometric frequencies between 500 and 4000 Hz. Synchronising the data acquisition with the stimuli is achieved by recording a trigger coincident with the onset of each stimulus event in an additional channel, using (where possible) a different label for each type of stimulus event. There is a delay, however, in the subject hearing the sound of around 3 ms depending on the length of the tube (Gutschalk et al., 2005), although this is rarely acknowledged.

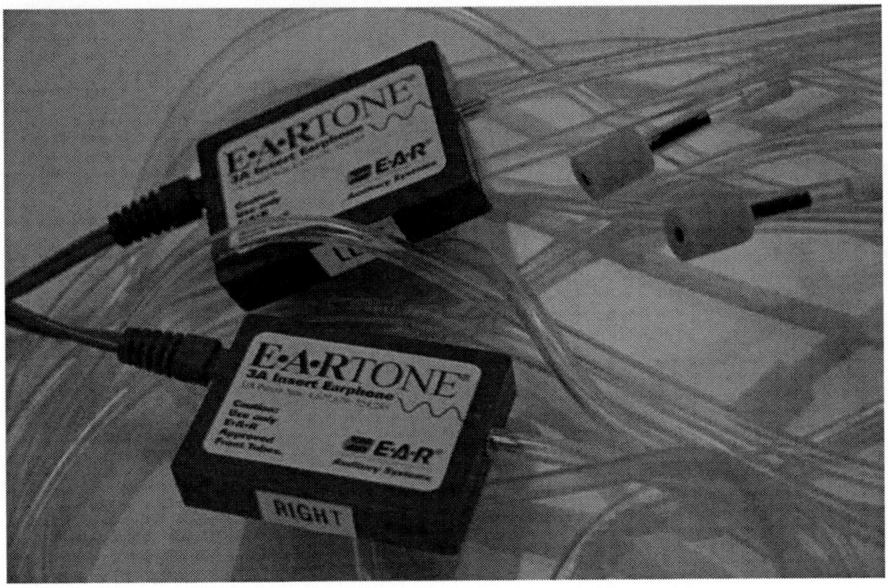

Figure 2. An example of the tube-phone system used to deliver sound stimuli in MEG scanners.

The process of identifying the sources of activity can be made more challenging when there are multiple sources distributed across the brain, especially when the sound stimulus is presented binaurally. One solution to this problem is to present stimuli monaurally. Monaural presentation typically elicits a much stronger response in the contralateral hemisphere compared to the ipsilateral hemisphere, reducing the number of sources that have a large response amplitude. Monaural presentation is sometimes beneficial for dipole source modelling and beamformer analysis, see later for details. However, if hemispheric asymmetries are of interest then a distinct disadvantage is a doubling in the number of conditions required and hence in the total duration of the experiment. Monaural presentation is also obviously unsuitable for any dichotic listening study (in which two sets of sound stimuli are presented separately to left and right ears) and for auditory percepts that require binaural integration, such as a lateralised sound or a dichotic pitch which can only be perceived by computing interaural differences between the signals at the two ears.

An MEG recording session is typically limited in overall duration to approximately 15-20 minutes because the spatial resolution of MEG is partly dependent on minimising subject movement throughout the experiment. Any longer than 20 minutes and subject fatigue tends to increase the amount of head movement. The length of each individual stimulus condition is influenced by the desire to maximise the signal-to-noise ratio (SNR); achieved by averaging over many repetitions of each condition. An average transient evoked response is typically generated from at least 50 trials per condition (Soeta et al., 2006), although the improved SNR of modern recording systems may mean this figure can be reduced. The need to include periods of silence or another control condition for use as a baseline comparison is a further limiting factor to the number of repetitions possible in any single experimental session. Choice of inter-stimulus interval should be taken with care to avoid the phase-locking of stimulus responses with intrinsic rhythms such as the alpha rhythm.

The task that the subjects are asked to perform during the MEG experiment can exert an important influence on the quality of the data that are acquired. Some studies do not employ any explicit task and subjects can be asked to 'close their eyes' (Soeta et al., 2004) or to 'fixate on a visual dot' (Rosburg et al., 2002a) while listening to the sounds. In the absence of an explicit task, subjects find it difficult to remain vigilant for long periods of time and the MEG data can be dominated by bursts of oscillatory power in the alpha band (8-12 Hz) (personal observation). Alpha oscillations are modulated by having the eyes closed or open and by drowsiness. These problems can partially be overcome by presenting a subtitled silent movie to subjects while the auditory experiment is being conducted (Rupp et al., 2002). Certainly, this strategy can help to reduce the boredom of the MEG experiment but is less suitable when behavioural responses to the sound stimuli are required; a factor that may be important in studies where the MEG signal is contingent upon performance (Palomäki et al, 2005). Behavioural responses can also be used as a way simply to engage and maintain auditory selective attention; for example by asking subjects to press a button in response to a target sound (Palomäki et al., 2000).

2. Auditory MEG Data Analysis

In a typical auditory experiment, MEG data (like EEG data) will contain both stimulus-evoked and stimulus-induced brain activity. Evoked activity is phase-locked to the time structure of the stimulus and is most commonly seen as a transient deflection in response to a sensory, cognitive or task-related event. By contrast, induced activity is not time-locked to the stimulus and therefore does not "average in" like an evoked potential. This is more frequently characterised by a change in spectral power of the response within a specific frequency band. Evoked and induced activity can be characterised both by their time-course and their spatial location. We provide a brief description of the range of analysis techniques below, together with examples of their application in the published auditory MEG literature.

2.1. Transient Deflection Analysis

An evoked response is usually elicited by the sudden onset or offset of a stimulus, or a sudden change in one of its characteristics such as its amplitude, location or pitch, and caused by the synchronous activity of a large number of neurons. It is usually identified by averaging over a number of trials with an identical stimulus, to maximise the SNR. Figure 3A shows a typical average evoked energy onset and offset response to a pure tone in a sensor channel positioned over the temporal cortex.

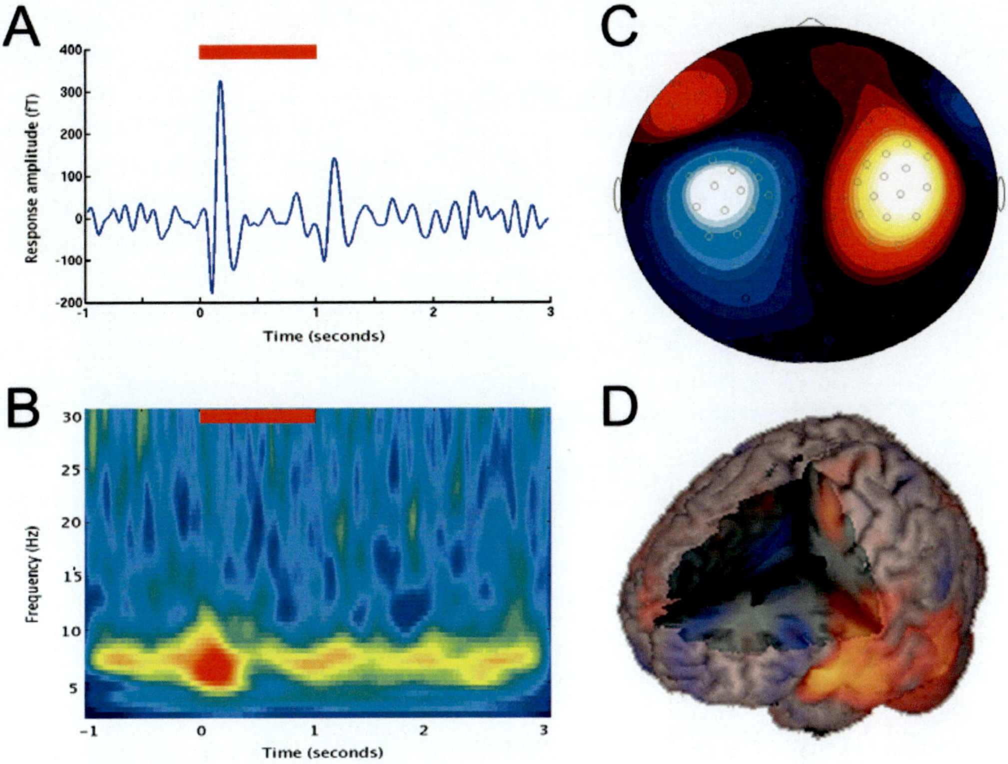

Figure 3. The response to a 500 Hz pure tone of 1 second duration (with 1 ms cosine rise and fall times) starting at time 0. (A) The response to the stimulus of one left temporal channel averaged over 70 trials. The duration of the stimulus is indicated by the red bar. The energy onset (N100m/P200m) response and a similar energy offset response can be clearly observed. (B) An average spectrogram in the 1-30 Hz range from a virtual electrode in the left temporal lobe. A burst of theta and alpha activity is observed coincident with stimulus onset. (C) A field map showing the average response of all 151 channels at 100 ms after stimulus onset. The red/blue (source/sink) pattern in each hemisphere indicates bilateral sources of the N100m. (D) A SAM image of the comparison between an active pure tone condition (300 ms post-stimulus onset) and a passive silence condition (300 ms pre-stimulus onset). The red region in the left temporal lobe indicates an increase in oscillatory power.

Although most of the published literature focuses on averaged evoked responses, there has been increasing interest in assessing response latencies for these types of stimulus from single-trial data using filters (Salajegheh et al., 2004; Burghoff et al., 2005). Evoked activity can also be examined by computing the difference in the averaged waveforms elicited by two classes of stimuli. Analysis of difference waveforms is particularly important in mismatch negativity (MMNm) studies where the response to a deviant compared to a control is of interest (Mathiak et al., 2005).

The amplitude and latency of a transient deflection can be analysed independently of any source localisation technique, based on data from single MEG channels, or through global field power, which is the root-mean-square (RMS) of all channels or a subset of channels.

Either of these approaches provides a gross measure of activity through time, which can be informative of neural processing even if source localisation is not to be attempted. If it is, then the latency of the transient deflection can be used to establish a time-window for a source localisation technique, such as dipole source modelling (e.g. Lütkenhöner et al., 2003b). The amplitude and latency of the dipole source moment can then also be analysed.

Automating the search for transient peaks requires a good SNR. In addition to averaging, Rosburg et al. (2004) increased the SNR of their MEG waveform data by examining the first four components of a singular value decomposition, cutting off the components that were most likely to represent noise. In order to ensure the detection of global signal peaks from local random fluctuations due to noise, constraints are often imposed on the location, width and height of estimated peaks. For example, after manually establishing the peak latency after tone onset across all sessions, Lütkenhöner et al. (2001) conducted an automatic search of peak latency in each session, constraining the solution to be within 20 ms of the manually derived value. Instead of just searching for the largest RMS value, Seither-Preisler et al. (2003) used a measure of amplitude that was the average of five values sampled over a 15 ms window centred on the maximum value. This should average out the noise, thus making the measure of signal amplitude more robust. Multiple time windows are commonly used for testing the latency of transient deflections to different stimulus conditions. For example, Hertrich et al. (2005) use four time windows centred on 130, 180, 225 and 275 ms after pitch onset to examine the response to two different types of pitch-evoking stimulus. One can deduce aspects of the underlying signal processing, such as hemispheric asymmetries and neural adaptation, from statistical analysis of the amplitude and latency of transient deflections.

The effect of the stimulus condition on the peak amplitude and latency values is often assessed through standard statistical tests, such as the ANOVA (e.g. Seither-Preisler et al., 2006b) or regression analysis (e.g. Borgmann et al., 2001). *Post-hoc* comparisons can also be performed to assess which conditions contribute to the significant main effect of condition (Seither-Preisler et al., 2004). As an alternative to parametric testing, non-parametric methods, such as a permutation test, have also been applied. These tests are valid without making any assumptions about the underlying distribution and correlation (Rupp et al., 2004). Bootstrap resampling procedures (Ritter et al., 2005) or Greenhouse-Geisser correction of degrees of freedom (Gutschalk et al., 2007) can also be used to set significance levels. Chait et al. (2006) noted that parametric and bootstrap methods produced similar results for their analysis of peak latency data, despite the tendency for positive skew and outliers in this type of data.

It is also informative to study normalised amplitude values, often a ratio such as (test sound amplitude)/(control sound amplitude). This controls for natural variation in amplitude among subjects, so that group analyses observe the changes within individuals rather inter-subject variability. For example, Pantev et al. (2004) used this ratio to demonstrate neural adaptation was present in the response to two repetitions of a stimulus when the masking sound between the repetitions contained different frequencies to the stimulus. Ross et al. (2005b) introduced a normalised laterality index (LI) to assess hemispheric dominance, LI = (R-L)/(R+L) where R and L are the amplitudes of responses in the right and left hemispheres, respectively. Although most subjects showed either a right or left hemispheric dominance in their transient and steady state responses to an amplitude modulated tone, only the steady state response (see Section 3.5) was significantly right lateralised across the group of subjects.

A peak stimulus-related deflection is typically determined by averaging the MEG data over multiple presentations of the same stimulus; presented in succession or as part of a randomised sequence. However, one cannot assume that the response is the same across each presentation because the neural response can change over time. Typically, the response reduces in amplitude over successive presentations and the amount of adaptation is determined by the characteristics of the stimulus and the inter-stimulus timing. Gutschalk et al. (2004b) tested for adaptation by comparing subsets of trials, taken in chronological order through the recording session. They noted the amplitude of the negative transient deflection 90-180 ms after the onset of a click train significantly decreased with time during a 32 minute experiment. They also reported a weaker adaptation of the sustained field. The reproducibility of peak amplitude and latency data can be analysed by repeating the experiment and analysis on the same subjects on different days. Fujioka et al. (2002) found no significant difference in the response to tone onset, using paired t-tests and six subjects.

As well as absolute or relative amplitude measures, some studies have examined the RMS of the first derivative with respect to time (e.g. Lütkenhöner and Steinsträter, 1998). This measure reveals the temporal window of the averaged data segment that contains the greatest change in signal over time (either a rise or a fall), and in turn this is informative of the timing and speed of the initial response. The neural sources that contribute to the slope may differ from those contributing to the peak. Computing the first derivative reduces the SNR and, consequently, the stability of a source location estimate. Lütkenhöner et al. (2003a) propose improving the stability using regularisation, a compromise between fitting the data and minimising the model energy. Another alternative is the residual RMS, computed using the difference between measured and modelled values from a dipole fit (Lütkenhöner et al., 2003b). This provides an estimate of a particular dipole's contribution to the overall RMS over time.

2.2. Sustained Response Analysis

The sustained field is the prolonged absence from baseline of the magnetic field for the duration of the sound, representing the on-going processing of the stimulus. A crude measure is the RMS value averaged over the duration of the stimulus. Source localisation of a sustained field is problematic due to the extended time period and comparatively small amplitudes (Seither-Preisler et al., 2006b). Lammertmann and Lütkenhöner (2001) propose fitting the models, $M(t) = a + b \exp(-(t-1)/\tau)$, for $t > 1$ seconds after stimulus onset, and $M(t) = c \exp(-(t-0.75)/\tau)$, for $t > 0.75$ seconds after stimulus offset, where $M(t)$ is a fixed-dipole moment amplitude and a, b, c and τ are model parameters.

Obtaining accurate measurements of sustained responses, with their slowly varying amplitudes, is problematic because magnetically shielded rooms are not efficient in preventing low-frequency fluctuations in the background magnetic field. Such fluctuations are typical of the earth's natural magnetic field. Mackert et al. (1999) introduced an interesting solution by moving the subject horizontally relative to the speakers at 0.4 Hz, hence the sustained field is superimposed on top of a fluctuating baseline that lies within a frequency range which has better protection from external sources.

A related phenomenon is the steady state response (SSR), often recorded in response to sinusoidal frequency modulation (FM) and amplitude modulation (AM); see Section 3.5.

2.3. Spectral Power Analysis

Behavioural state-dependent changes in the oscillatory power spectrum of brain activity were first reported more than 100 yeas ago from intracranial recordings (Caton, 1875), and such changes can be measured with MEG. The functional role of cortical oscillations is still not clear but their presence is thought to indicate the synchronisation of neuronal firing within and across areas of cortex (Gross et al., 2001). The oscillations are modulated by task and external stimuli and the spectral power in each frequency band can be suppressed or activated during sound processing (Hari and Salmelin, 1997). The main frequency bands typically described in the EEG literature are θ (2-8 Hz), α (8-15 Hz), β (15-30 Hz) and γ (30-70 Hz) (Schadow et al., 2007). Activity in the 10 Hz range in auditory cortex, measured with MEG, has also been termed the τ rhythm. Their presence in the spectral domain can be detected using wavelet analysis or a fast Fourier transform. Figure 3B shows changes in oscillatory power in the 1-30 Hz range in response to a pure tone stimulus. Changes in spectral power can be evoked by an auditory stimulus, where the onset and phase of oscillations is locked to the time-structure of the stimulus. Alternatively they can be induced, where the power change is not strongly stimulus-locked. Changes in synchronisation can occur without altering the mean neuronal firing rate or the haemodynamic flow, although patterns of spectral power change recorded with MEG have been shown to be spatially coincident to the BOLD signal (Singh et al., 2002). While evoked and induced changes in spectral power have been explored in great detail for cognitive tasks, and in other sensory systems, using both MEG and EEG, the role of such activity in auditory cortex remains poorly understood.

2.4. Dipole Source Modelling

As has already been mentioned, the likely source of a particular transient deflection can be identified using some sort of source localisation method. To date, the most common analysis method for mapping the source of the evoked responses is dipole source modelling. Dipoles can also be fitted to a field created by the difference of two fields, indicating the source of processing for the sound feature that changes between the two conditions (Gutschalk et al., 2004a). A sensible model for an active patch of cortex is a dipole current sheet. The mathematical model can be simplified if this is reduced to a dipole point source. The dipole source is defined in terms of its location, orientation and strength. Using a suitable head model, such as a sphere, the forward problem determines the anticipated field strength, F_{model}, at a sensor, s, for any given dipole moment, M, via a weighting matrix, W, defined by the relative location of the dipole from the sensor, d. This model can be either fixed in time, $F_{model}(s) = W(s,d)\ M$, or allowed to change in amplitude over time $F_{model}(s,t) = W(s,d)\ M(t)$. The choice of head model is not as critical for MEG data as it is for EEG data, because MEG signals are unaffected by the different electrical conductance properties found in the head. Most studies position the sphere to minimise the distance between the surface and the true scalp but some centre the sphere in relation to a specific anatomical feature, such as the posterior commissure (Gutschalk et al., 2002).

The stumbling block for all source reconstruction techniques is that the measured field could be created by an infinite number of different configurations of cortical activity. This issue is known as the "inverse" problem. Solving the inverse problem requires recreating the measured magnetic field during a given time window. At each time point, the difference between observed and modelled magnetic fields must be minimised over six parameters per dipole: three location coordinates, two orientation angles and the dipole strength. The generic method takes a starting estimate of the six parameters and computes $F_{model}(s,t)$. The model is assessed by calculating the sum-of-squares error (SSE), $\sum(F_{model} - F_{data})^2$, summing over sensors and time. If the difference is less than a user-specified error tolerance, then the parameters are accepted, otherwise the parameters are adjusted and the procedure iterates until an acceptable solution is reached. Anatomical constraints, such as the location being greater than 3 cm from the midsagittal plane, can also be used (Draganova et al., 2002). Several algorithms exist for implementing this iterative procedure. The main difference between the algorithms is how they non-linearly update the parameter estimates between iterations. Traditional model-fitting techniques include the Levenberg-Marquardt method, the simplex method and simulated annealing (see Press et al., 1992, for details of their implementation). An alternative maximum-likelihood method has also been advocated, with reduced error measurements compared to least squares fit techniques (Lütkenhöner, 1998a, b). All methods are dependent on the starting values and multiple starting points should be tried to ensure the global minimum is achieved. Various software packages exist for implementing dipole source modelling, including Brain Electrical Source Analysis (BESA, MEGIS Software GmbH, Gräfelfing, Germany)

The error of source locations can be estimated by testing the same subjects in separate sessions. Lütkenhöner and Steinsträter (1998) use the median location across sessions as a point estimate because it is more robust than the mean. Lütkenhöner et al. (2003b) provides a comparison between the fixed dipole approach (fixed location and orientation but changing moment) and the moving dipole approach (estimating all parameters for each time point). They advocate the fixed-dipole approach because the moving-dipole location can move several centimetres during a 100 ms period. The locations estimated with a moving dipole approach can be made more robust by estimating over a moving-time window rather than individual time points.

One of the main limitations for dipole source modelling is that initial assumptions about the number of sources and their initial locations must be made by the user. A priori knowledge can come from mathematical models, the literature or neuroimaging data. The number of dipoles is usually specified as one or two per hemisphere. A dipole can explain the majority of the topographical distribution of activity when it clearly forms a canonical dipole pattern (i.e. a clear source-sink pair that is contained within the hemisphere), as seen in

Figure 3C. If bilateral sources are fitted simultaneously, it is possible to constrain them to have hemispheric symmetry in terms of their location, orientation or strength. In the case of fitting bilateral dipoles, it is important to reduce the bias caused by the order of fitting. For example, such bias can be overcome by alternately fitting one dipole while holding the other fixed, and repeating the process until no further change is found (Ross et al., 2005a). Alternatively, a dipole can be fit to the MEG data for each hemisphere separately (Soeta et al., 2005b), using the channels in each hemisphere independently. However, this means the left dipole fit does not take into account the data in the right hemisphere and vice-versa. In reality, a number of sources are usually active and several neighbouring cortex structures may contribute to a source, making interpretation difficult. Minimum current estimation (MCE) is an alternative to the equivalent current dipole method, which can describe multiple local sources (Tiitinen et al., 2006).

Conventionally, the estimated source location is plotted on an MR structural scan, either an individual scan or a representative scan. However, meaningful comparisons between the locations of different sources are still possible without an MR scan (Ross and Pantev, 2004). They showed the steady-state response to an amplitude-modulated tone was anterior, medial and inferior of the transient deflection to a pure tone onset. A further problem for dipole modelling is that generalisations across individuals are confounded by variations in cortical folding, meaning the activity in the same cortical region can be perceived at different orientations and depths in each subject. Individual differences in auditory activation may also be due to individual differences in sensory perception. These issues make group analyses for MEG and EEG data more problematic than for other neuroimaging techniques such as fMRI and positron emission tomography (PET). There has been a growing trend in fMRI and MEG studies to report individual analyses, with qualitative visual comparisons between subjects, instead (e.g. Lütkenhöner et al., 2003a; Hall et al., 2002). Hertrich et al. (2004) take the unusual approach of fitting dipoles *after* averaging across subjects in sensor space. This strategy ignores differences in head position and shape but is noise insensitive, therefore optimising the SNR. The loss of spatial resolution is tolerable if the temporal dynamics are of primary interest.

2.5. Beamformer Analysis

A recent addition to the analysis of induced oscillations in MEG data is the beamformer (van Veen and Buckley, 1988). Beamformer analysis can reveal increases and decreases in induced oscillations, known as event-related synchronisation (ERS) and event-related desynchronisation (ERD), even when no evoked response is recorded. A beamformer is essentially a spatial filter, which weights the contribution of each sensor to the overall output for each potential source location within a head volume usually derived from an MR structural scan (Hillebrand and Barnes, 2005). Let N be the number of sensors and V the number of user-specified voxels within the head volume. The data, D, a $N \times 1$ vector of sensor recordings at a given time point, is related to the neuronal activity, A, an unknown $V \times 1$ vector, by the lead field matrix, L, such that $D = LA$. Each column of the lead field matrix is the magnetic field that would be recorded at the sensors if a source of unit strength was generated at that source. The lead field requires assumptions regarding the volume conductor, either a single-sphere or multi-sphere, and the source model, usually an equivalent current dipole. The generalised linear inverse solution to determining the neuronal activity is $A = C_S L^T C_D^{-1} D$, where C_S is the estimated source current covariance matrix and C_D is the estimated data covariance matrix. The assumption of no linearly correlated sources constrains C_S to be diagonal. The calculations are based on either the orientation of the dipole being estimated to maximise the output (a non-linear beamformer) or the sum of the dipole in tangential orientations (a linear beamformer). See the appendix of Hillebrand and Barnes (2003) for a full derivation.

The normalised beamformer for location θ, expressed as a squared pseudo-Z statistic, is the ratio of $P_\theta = W_\theta^T C_D W_\theta$ and $N_\theta = W_\theta^T \Sigma W_\theta$, where W_θ are the estimated weights and Σ is the estimated sensor noise covariance matrix. When comparing active and control conditions, the output is a pseudo-T statistic $T_\theta = (P_\theta^{active} - P_\theta^{control})/(N_\theta^{active} + N_\theta^{control})$, see Vrba and Robinson (2001). A further variant is regularisation, replacing C_D with $C_D + \mu\Sigma$ where μ is a scalar parameter, to spatially smooth the covariance matrix, which gains a reduction of sensitivity to correlated sources at the expense of a loss of spatial resolution. As this brief introduction shows, there are several possible variants of beamformer algorithm. The method described here is synthetic aperture magnetometry (SAM), see Robinson and Vrba (1999) for details and Huang et al. (2004) for a comparison of different algorithms. SAM has been successfully applied to transient and steady-state responses to auditory stimuli, localising the source of activity to superior temporal plane in a similar position to dipole source modelling (Herdman et al., 2003).

The null hypothesis of the beamformer analysis is that, averaged across epochs, there is no difference in the power at each location between active and control conditions. This hypothesis is tested at each time/frequency/location combination and a correction for multiple comparisons is necessary. For each time/frequency comparison, it is possible to plot a statistical parametric map (SPM) for each subject, known as a SAM image. Figure 3D shows an example of a SAM image. The normalisation of each subject's structural MR scan to a template can be applied to their SAM image and an average across subjects taken as the basis of a group analysis. Again, multiple comparisons causes a problem and either a parametric (Singh et al., 2002) or non-parametric (Singh et al., 2003) approach can be adopted. For each location comparison, a spectrogram can be plotted showing the power of cortical oscillations at each time/frequency bin (Leiberg et al., 2006). Statistical analysis of data from beamformer techniques is non-trivial due to the inhomogeneous smoothness of SAM images and the desire to make meaningful comparisons between subjects at the voxel or cluster level. Various software packages for implementing beamformer techniques have been developed, with no one package being widely accepted as the gold standard at the moment.

From the analyst's viewpoint, beamformer techniques are advantageous because they require little user intervention after specifying the time window and frequency band that are of interest. Unlike dipole source modelling, the user needs to make no initial assumptions about the number of sources or their initial locations. However, the beamformer technique is only valid when its main assumptions are met by the data. The critical assumption is that no two distant cortical areas generate a coherent pattern of local magnetic field changes over a long time period. It has been shown that this assumption is plausible based on anatomical and electrophysiological data, especially when active and control conditions are both of long duration (Hillebrand et al., 2005).

A further variant of beamformer analysis is signal-space projection (SSP, sometimes known as source-space projection). This method uses a linear combination of the sensors to create a time-series of a magnetic dipole moment at a particular source location and orientation. Such signal-space projections are independent of sensor position and can, therefore, be averaged across subjects and sessions, enhancing the SNR (Ross et al., 2003). A derivative of SSP is response source weighting (RSW) for the average, with the weights based on the transient deflection amplitude of each sensor when averaged across trials (Mäkinen et al., 2005b). Dynamic imaging of coherent sources (DICS) is another beamformer technique that examines cortico-cortical interactions through the complex cross spectral density matrix (Gross et al., 2001). Although this method can measure coherence with a second brain region, localising an initial reference brain area is partly subjective.

3. Review of Auditory MEG Literature

In this section we review the contribution over the past decade of MEG research to the functional mapping of the auditory brain. After an initial introduction to the measurement of auditory evoked and sustained responses, we focus on contributions of MEG to understanding the mechanisms of pitch coding, spatial processing, sound detection, gap detection and stream segregation. A more limited number of publications consider the effect of more cognitively demanding listening tasks by assessing auditory attention and auditory working memory, and these remain potential areas for future research. We have not sought to include studies with clinical or language applications and refer the reader to Salmelin (2007) for a review.

3.1. Transient Responses to Energy Onset

In response to sound energy onset, the early auditory evoked activity occurring in the brain stem cannot be measured using MEG due to the depth of these anatomical structures from the cortical surface. The first evoked MEG response that is consistently recorded is the set of "middle-latency" responses that occur 10-60 ms after stimulus onset. These typically represent the initial processing of the sound in the primary auditory cortex. The most common deflections are known as the P30m, N40m and P50m. The initial letter reflects their oscillating polarity and the number indicates the approximate latency. The small "m" indicates a magnetic response. These deflections have their analogues in EEG, where they have been widely reported (e.g. Picton et al., 1974). Consistent with EEG, Borgmann et al. (2001) placed the middle latency MEG responses in primary auditory cortex, along Heschl's gyrus. They also demonstrated greater amplitudes and decreased latencies of the middle latency responses following an increase in intensity, up to a saturation level of 60 dB SPL, again consistent with EEG.

Believing that the P30m received input from more than one cortical area, Lütkenhöner et al. (2003a) probed earlier responses by analysing the waves' first temporal derivative, showing waves denoted dN13m and dP20m. The dP20m is the point of greatest slope on the P30m. By using dipole source modelling, Lütkenhöner and colleagues located the source of this response to the retroinsular part of Heschl's gyrus (primary auditory cortex). It was suggested that the dN13m arose from a sub-cortical auditory structure. Although using the point of greatest slope may have advantages in reducing the number of cortical areas contributing to the signal, some caution must exist due to the reduced SNR.

The "late-latency" responses occur 60-300 ms after stimulus onset and are influenced by interactions between brain regions and the cognitive operations performed by the subject. The largest and most consistently reported deflection in response to sound onset is the N100m. The most comprehensive study that has modelled the source of the N100m to date suggests that this deflection is sourced in planum temporale, posterior of the middle latency responses and the subsequent P200m (Lütkenhöner and Steinsträter, 1998). During the 30 ms window around the peak of the N100m, Rosburg et al. (2002a) reported an anterior and inferior movement of the corresponding dipole. The amount of movement was proportional to the duration (up to 200 ms) of the stimuli. There remains debate regarding the neurophysiological mechanism for generating the N100m response. Hamada (2006) proposes a model which implies that the natural ongoing oscillations above 6 Hz in the areas near the auditory cortex become phase-locked at the onset of the auditory stimulus for the duration of the transient deflections. Conversely, Mäkinen et al. (2005b) found no reorganisation of ongoing activity, with evidence suggesting the N100m is a linear summation of an increased spectral power event related response and the ongoing oscillations with randomly distributed phase. The controversy will probably remain until better methods are developed for studying single-trial data or until a better understanding is gained of how the MEG response reflects neuronal network activity. To examine the functional role of the N100m, a number of researchers have explored the type of sound features that modulate this deflection. The amplitude of the N100m is affected by bandwidth, with amplitude increasing with bandwidth for harmonic complex tones (Seither-Preisler et al., 2003) but decreasing with bandwidth for noise (Soeta et al., 2005c). The N100m amplitude in response to noise is inversely proportional to the inter-aural cross-correlation (Soeta et al., 2006).

A later component of the energy onset response is the P200m. To date, this transient deflection has been relatively neglected, although it is thought to play an important role in spatial sound localisation, see Section 3.6.

3.2. Sustained Responses to Energy Onset

In addition to the transient energy onset response, which lasts up to 300 ms post-stimulus onset, pure tones tend to elicit a sustained response. This sustained activity continues throughout the duration of the stimulus. Dipole source modelling shows that the sustained field arises from activity in a similar area to the N100m, posterior to the P200m (Lammertmann and Lütkenhöner, 2001). They also report that the magnitude of the sustained field returns to baseline after approximately 3.6 seconds, perhaps caused by long-term neural adaptation in the auditory pathway.

3.3. Pitch Coding

Initial attempts to analyse pitch processing using MEG focussed on the prominent N100m deflection. However, more recent studies have implemented a new paradigm of continuous stimulation to separate the transient energy onset deflection from that for the pitch onset. Studies have also used this paradigm in combination with a long train of regular click stimuli which elicit a clear pitch to generate a sustained field.

Until recently it was accepted that the N100m latency was an index of pitch. Using a regular click train, Forss et al. (1993) showed that the latency of the N100m was inversely proportional to the pitch. This was also demonstrated by Lütkenhöner et al. (2001), who also noted the latency of the N100m was unchanged in response to complex tones compared to pure tones, regardless of the stimulus duration. Roberts et al. (2000) reported a latency difference of 30 ms between the N100m response to 100 Hz and 1 kHz pure tones. They also showed that the latency is affected by hemisphere (the right hemisphere has a shorter latency), the inclusion of harmonic frequencies in a complex tone (increasing latency) and is inversely proportional to sound level intensity. Seither-Priesler et al. (2006a) recently showed the latency was due to the period, rather than the phase. These findings suggest that the N100m response to pitch is confounded by other sound attributes.

Despite the N100m being affected by other spectral characteristics, many other studies have probed the N100m response to a variety of pitch stimuli. Soeta et al. (2005b) showed that the amplitude of the N100m increases with the pitch salience of iterated ripple noise (IRN). IRN takes random white noise and introduces the perception of pitch by delaying and adding the same noise segment to increase the regularity of time intervals between peaks (Yost, 1996). An advantage of using IRN is that the perceived pitch value and its salience can easily be manipulated. Another use of IRN in pitch studies is to create a dichotic stimulus by playing IRN to one ear and noise to the other. Hertrich et al. (2004) noted a tendency for pitch processing in the right hemisphere and noise processing in the left hemisphere through examining the N100m. The IRN generates a right lateralised N100m, with a stronger amplitude at higher pitch values.

Soeta et al. (2006) noted the highest amplitudes and shortest latencies were observed near 1-2 kHz, compared with extremely low pitches (250 Hz) or high pitches (8 kHz), using narrowband noise. To the authors' knowledge, Fujioka et al. (2002) is the only study to have focussed on the N100m response to high audible frequencies (4-14 kHz) and inaudible ultrasound (20-40 kHz) in the auditory cortex. An N100m deflection was only recorded in response to the audible frequencies, confirming the N100m response to be a physiological part of a hearing mechanism rather than pure frequency detection. In the audible range, significantly larger amplitude responses were seen in the right hemisphere, compared to the left, and in response to lower frequencies, compared to higher frequencies.

Pitch coding has also been studied using the magnetic mismatch negativity (MMNm) effect. The MMNm refers to the difference waveform computed from the difference between the response to a standard stimulus and a deviant stimulus. The MMNm is a negative deflection between 120-250 ms post sound onset and can be elicited using an oddball design, where a deviant pitch has a low probability of occurrence relative to the standard pitch. The MMNm has been shown to be larger with a shorter latency in response to left ear pitch deviants, compared to right ear pitch deviants (Mathiak et al., 2002). These insights are still of limited scientific benefit if the N100m response to pitch is confounded by other sound attributes.

Krumbholz et al. (2003) introduced a new experiment paradigm to separate the energy onset response from the pitch onset response (POR) by preceding the pitch with a period of noise. In this study, the pitch was created using IRN. The energy and spectral profile of the noise and pitch are well-matched, so that the critical difference at the transition from noise to pitch is in the temporal structure of the sound. The continuous stimulation paradigm demonstrated that the POR has a different shape to the N100m, with the POR having a latency of over 130 ms, compared with around 100 ms for the N100m. The latency decreased from over 350 ms to just 130 ms as pitch increased from 15 Hz to 250 Hz. (Ritter et al., 2005, demonstrate the same correlation using perceived psycho-acoustic measures of pitch.) The POR amplitude was found to increase with both pitch value and pitch salience. Using dipole source modelling, the POR source location was found in Heschl's gyrus, anterior and inferior of the N100m, demonstrating some functional independence between the neurons responsible for these two responses. Additional studies have shown a positive correlation between the amplitude of the POR and the length of noise preceding the transition, up to a period of 4000 ms (Seither-Preisler et al., 2004) and an increase in amplitude/decrease in latency with frequency band width (Seither-Priesler et al., 2006b).

The POR can also be elicited by replacing IRN with a different type of pitch-eliciting stimulus. Two types of pitch stimuli that have been used are a Huggins pitch (HP), created by shifting the interaural phase of noise by 180° in a narrow frequency band about the desired frequency, and a single-frequency tone presented in a simultaneous noise-masker (TN). Figure 4 shows the RMS of channels in response to HP using the continuous stimulation paradigm. Hertrich et al. (2005) found that the POR for both IRN and HP to be left lateralised with a peak at 180 ms, with a greater amplitude for higher pitches. Chait et al. (2006) also used HP to find a POR peak at 160 ms, 30 ms earlier than using a pure tone in noise (TN). The POR was, again, left lateralised and close to primary auditory cortex for both types of pitch-eliciting stimulus. Replacing the initial correlated noise with uncorrelated noise, increased the latency of the POR to HP by 30 ms. This is probably due to the additional processing of the change in noise correlation, which provides an explanation for an earlier smaller peak seen at 130 ms. Chait et al. (2005) had previously shown that the amplitude of this peak, caused by a change in noise correlation, is proportional to the amount of correlation change, and is generally smaller when switching from uncorrelated to correlated noise than vice-versa.

Another type of pitch-evoking stimulus is the regular click train, which generates a pitch equal to the reciprocal of the inter-click interval (ICI). Gutschalk et al. (2004a) alternated between periods of regular and irregular click trains, in a version of the continuous stimulation paradigm. In addition to generating a transient response 130-190 ms after the regularity onset, this paradigm also generated a negative sustained field, with both originating in lateral Heschl's gyrus. The sustained field, known as the sustained pitch response (SPR), was shown to emerge 70 ms after regularity onset. It increases in amplitude until it asymptotes at 450 ms, before starting to decay 70 ms after the regularity ceases.

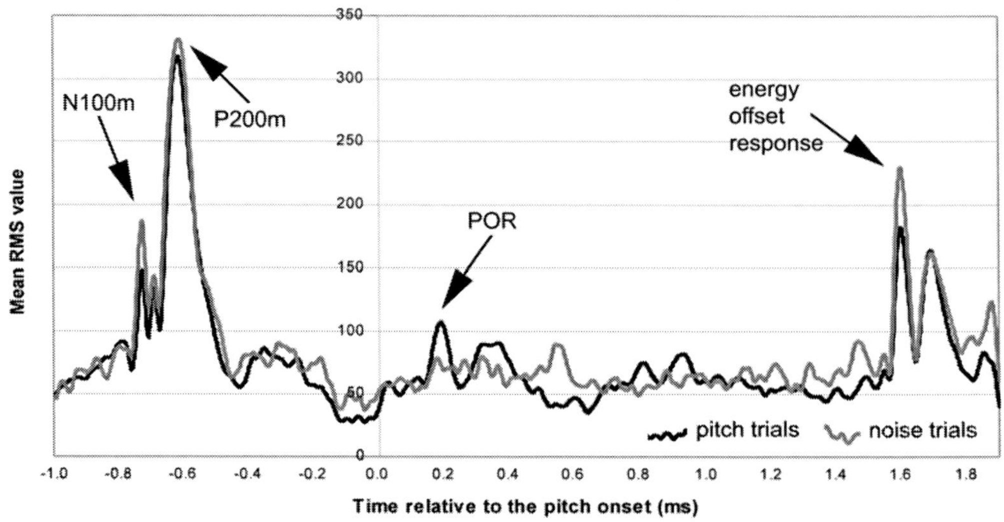

Figure 4. The root mean square response of 275 channels to a broadband noise (0-4 kHz) from -0.8 to 1.5 secs (grey line). Transient energy onset and offset responses can be observed. An additional pitch onset response (POR) is observed if the broadband noise is transformed to create a Huggins pitch from 0 to 0.5 secs (black line).

The sustained field has a time-scale that is too long to represent the primary stage of pitch coding. However, it is interesting to note that Gutschalk and colleagues found that varying the pitch by manipulating the ICI of the regular click train produced an SPR that appeared to originate from a similar location (lateral Heschl's gyrus) to that for the POR generated previously using IRN. This pitch-related response dissociated from the response to varying the sound intensity, which was located in planum temporale (Gutschalk et al., 2002). The amplitude of the SPR depends on the distinctiveness of the regular click train from the irregular click train. Gutschalk et al. (2007) showed that the amplitude can be decreased by increasing the regularity in the control condition or lengthening the proportion of regular click trains, indicating an element of neural adaptation.

3.4. Frequency Coding

The auditory system is tonotopically organised, such that sound frequencies that are close to each other are processed in neighbouring cells or nerves, with each neuron responding to a specific frequency. This spatial organisation has been plotted within different sites of the auditory pathway from the cochlea to the cortex. A principal aim of auditory neuroimaging studies has been to establish a similar tonotopic map of neurons in the auditory cortex. Early attempts focussing on the N100m conjectured a variety of theories: deeper sources for higher frequencies (e.g. Romani et al., 1982), posterior sources for higher frequencies (e.g. Elberling et al., 1982), anterior sources for higher frequencies (e.g. Hari and Makela, 1986) or no consistent pattern at all (e.g. Stufflebeam et al., 1998). An association between deeper sources and higher frequencies is still, perhaps, the most widely held belief (e.g. Tecchio et al., 2000; Rojas et al., 2002). However, the majority of studies have either failed to show a significant relationship between pitch and location or an anterior-posterior organisation (Rosburg et al., 1998). Fujioka et al. (2003) noted higher frequencies were more medially located for both pure and complex tones, but produced conflicting results in the superior-inferior direction for the two groups. This, combined with a longer latency for complex tones, might indicate a different tonotopic processing path for pure and complex tones.

Lütkenhöner et al. (2003b) dipole source modelled the N100m responses to four specific frequencies in ten listeners and could establish no orderly alignment in most listeners. They also noted a substantial inter-subject variability, despite high within-subject reproducibility, indicating that no generic tonotopic map may ever be established. Indeed, the various proposed theories for the tonotopic organisation of the auditory cortex may simply reflect the variability in subjects, experiment paradigms and analysis techniques used.

3.5. Coding of Amplitude and Frequency Modulated Tones

Responses elicited by repeating stimuli, such as click trains, or periodic modulations, such as sinusoidal amplitude modulation (AM) or frequency modulation (FM), are referred to as steady-state responses (SSR). Like the sustained field, see Section 3.2, the SSR exists for the duration of the sound, increasing in amplitude between 40-240 ms post stimulus onset and ceases within 50 ms of sound offset. The sustained field and the steady-state response, however, should not be confused. An AM pure tone will create both a sustained field and a SSR, whereas a non-modulated pure tone will only create the former. For example, Ross et al. (2002) use a 1-24 Hz filter to extract transient deflections and sustained fields and a 24-60 Hz filter to examine the SSR. The SSR is phase-locked to the envelope of the stimulus.

The SSR originates in primary auditory cortex, anterior of the transient N100m, with Pantev et al. (1996) suggesting that both the N100m and SSR have a more medial location at higher carrier frequencies. The N100m, sustained field and SSR all generate a contra-lateral dominance when monaural stimulation is used, but only the non-transient responses have a right hemisphere dominance (Ross et al., 2005b), perhaps indicating they are sensitive to stimulus periodicity.

Ross et al. (2000) demonstrated that while the SSR exists for 10-98 Hz rates of AM, the maximum amplitude is achieved in the region of 40 Hz. The amplitude is proportional to intensity and modulation depth. The amplitude decreases as the carrier frequency increases, in the range 250-4000 Hz, and also in the presence of a second AM tone, especially if the interfering sound has a higher carrier frequency (Ross et al., 2003). A suppression also exists if two different modulation rates are applied to the same carrier frequency (Draganova et al., 2002). A gap detection threshold of around 3 ms can be seen in the SSR (Ross et al., 2004) and the amplitude can be reduced for 250 ms following the introduction of a concurrent noise stimulus (Ross et al., 2005a).

The SSR can also encode the rate of frequency modulation (FM). For FM rates less than 5 Hz, the phase of the SSR tracks the envelope of frequency modulations (Luo et al., 2006).

3.6. Spatial Sound Localisation

Sounds presented in free field contain several acoustic cues for determining their spatial origin, in terms of azimuth angles. These cues can be recreated in the laboratory over headphones by using interaural time differences (ITD), interaural level differences (ILD), head-related transfer functions (HRTF) and individualised binaural recordings (BAR). Palomäki et al. (2000), Palomäki et al. (2005) and Tiitinen et al. (2006) have all investigated the auditory processing of sounds from eight locations (-135°, -90°, -45°, 0°, 45°, 90°, 135°, 180°), evenly separated by 45° in the azimuth plane, using a variety of these spatial cues.

These studies showed that both hemispheres demonstrate directional tuning, with the P50m and N100m deflections being most prominent (earlier peak and higher amplitude) at the contralateral direction and least prominent at the ipsilateral direction. The data also showed the N100m amplitude variation and the average N100m amplitude across angles to be larger in the right hemisphere, suggesting that the right hemisphere is implicated more in spatial processing than the left. The N100m amplitude, in particular, is correlated to behavioural measures of correctly identifying sound origin, implying that the richness of spatial cues in the sound is reflected in the level of brain activity. Parietal lobe activation, corresponding to a motor response in the contralateral hand, was also observed when subjects made a physical response to sound location, compared to passive listening.

The effect of different spatial sound cues can also be seen in the N100m and P200m. Both are sensitive to the richness of spatial cues present, with increased amplitude for individualised BAR compared to ITD alone. The N100m amplitude systematically responded to sound location for BAR, HRTF and ITD+ILD but not for ITD or ILD alone. Additionally, the N100m was sourced further anterior for the former group. The P200m, though, shows a stronger response to the speed of simulated auditory motion, through continuously changing the ITD (Soeta et al., 2005a).

3.7. Gap Detection

Psychoacoustic measurements show that subjects can detect a silent period in a long duration broadband noise burst, providing the gap is greater than approximately 2 ms in length (Forrest and Green, 1987). Rupp et al. (2002) demonstrated that gaps as short as 3 ms evoke a transient response in primary auditory cortex approximately 37 ms after the resumption of sound. Rupp et al. (2004) showed that the gap duration necessary to elicit the P37m increases if the gap shortly follows the onset of the initial sound. An increase to 5.3 ms gap duration following an initial 5 ms noise burst replicates psychoacoustic measurements. The P37m is only observed by examining the difference waveform of subtracting the noise onset response (without gaps) from the response following a gap.

Gutschalk et al. (2004b) considered inserting a gap in a regular click train. They noted neural adaptation on a shorter time scale, with a reduced P50m response to the second click train after a short gap. The sustained field, conversely, produced by the second click train was enhanced 150-350 ms after the gap, indicating that the sustained response to a regular click train may be a means of monitoring continuity.

3.8. Stream Segregation

A key function, known as stream segregation, of the auditory system is to separate sounds from distinct sources, such as different talkers in a noisy environment. A common paradigm for examining this in the laboratory is to play a sequence of tones, ABA, where tone A and tone B have different frequencies (Bregman and Steiger, 1980). If the frequency difference is small and the inter-stimulus interval long, then the listener generally perceives one stream. If the frequency difference is large and the inter-stimulus interval short, then two streams are perceived. Gutschalk et al. (2005) showed that the amplitude of the P50m and N100m evoked by tone B is proportional to the frequency difference. A larger amplitude was also recorded for subjects who perceived two streams, as opposed to one, for a fixed frequency difference. This stream segregation is likely to occur in non-primary auditory cortex and the strength of the late-latency responses contains a physiological correlate of reported behavioural measures.

3.9. Sound Detection

The N100m, although elicited in response to sound onset, is a poor reflection of sound detection because its amplitude and latency does not correlate with behavioural response times or stimulus intensity. An alternative transient response can be seen when smoothly increasing the intensity of a pure tone from -10 to 60 dB SPL over varying lengths of time. The transient response consistently precedes the behavioural response by 180 ms, with a comparable variation in deflection latency and reaction times (Mäkinen et al., 2004).

3.10. Neural Adaptation

Rosburg et al. (2002b) provides evidence for neural adaptation, with the amplitude decreasing and the latency increasing, during the course of the experiment, independent of stimulus duration. Neural adaptation is less if the frequency of the stimuli is changed, although a significant amplitude decrease is also seen between first and second repetitions of each frequency (Rosburg et al., 2004). Using an oddball paradigm, Rosburg et al. (2003) showed the magnetic mismatch negativity (MMNm) dipole to be anterior, inferior and medial of the N100m dipole in response to changes in frequency, duration and intensity, with three distinct MMNm dipole locations for each class of deviant.

The competing theories of neural adaptation and inhibition have also been probed using 40 Hz modulated pure tones. If successive stimuli are played, a decreased response to the second stimulus may be caused by familiarity if the two stimuli are identical (adaptation) or a tuning to the first stimulus if the second is different (inhibition). Pantev et al. (2004) preceded the AM pure tone with a filtered noise band. A larger N100m amplitude was seen if the AM tone and noise contained the same frequencies compared to different frequencies, providing evidence that inhibition is stronger than adaptation in non-primary auditory cortex. The difference was maximised if the silence between noise and AM tone was minimised (Okamoto et al., 2004). No difference was observed, however, in the SSR.

4. Conclusion

To date, the majority of auditory MEG studies have used dipole source modelling to localise auditory processing, with the analysis of transient deflections frequently based on the dipole moment. While these studies have produced significant advances in understanding auditory processing, they are limited by dipole source modelling's assumptions that cortical activity can be represented as a finite number of single point sources.

As acknowledged in the introduction, MEG is less sensitive to sources that are deep or have a radial direction. Although the former limits the spatial resolution of detecting activity in the brainstem, the latter has raised concerns that MEG cannot accurately model sources on the crests of gyri. Hillebrand and Barnes (2002) demonstrated that these regions are limited to strips approximately 2 mm in width, with only 5% of cortical areas being within 15° of the radial direction, and are adjacent to regions of tangential cortex. They also showed that large deflections, such as the N100m, are caused by large areas of cortical activity, implying that single dipole models provide an inaccurate representation of the true underlying activity. The fitted dipole's location and orientation, therefore, will be an average and may not truly reflect any of the contributing sources. See also Lütkenhöner et al. (2003b).

The greatest theoretical challenge to using beamformers for auditory MEG is the underlying assumption that there are no linear long-term interdependencies between sources. In certain cases, this assumption may not be valid for modelling the bilateral auditory cortices. Although long-term correlations are inefficient, transient correlations may provide a means of neural coding. Hadjipapas et al. (2005) examined the effect of transient correlations using coherence, phase synchronisation and mutual information. They showed that beamformer source reconstruction was accurate as long as the transient correlations composed less than 30-40% of the time duration. Further, beamformer methods preserved the phase synchronisation of interacting non-linear sources.

Despite this reassurance, there remains the possibility that correlated bilateral auditory sources may be suppressed by standard beamformer techniques. A number of solutions have been proposed to this problem. One crude method is to construct the beamformer weights in each hemisphere independently by only applying the data from sensors in the corresponding hemisphere (Herdman et al., 2003). A second method is to increase the regularisation parameter, spatially smoothing the covariance matrix (Hillebrand and Barnes, 2005). Both methods give broadly similar patterns of activation as the basic SAM algorithm with, usually, a small increase in the significance (personal observation). More recently, Brookes et al. (2007) have developed the dual-source beamformer to accurately reconstruct two spatially separate but temporally correlated sources. An application to the auditory steady-state response increased the statistical significance compared to a single-source beamformer and localised the sources to within 5 mm of the single-source beamformer and 4.5 mm of a 2-dipole model. The dual-source beamformer requires, however, recursive searches of the source-space to find the two most correlated sources which is computationally demanding. Separating the estimated time-course into the two separate sources is also difficult if they are only partially correlated.

Theoretical misconceptions, like those outlined above, are not the only reason for few auditory MEG studies using beamformers. There has also been a delay in the development of robust statistical techniques but the majority of these challenges have now been met. Barnes and Hillebrand (2003) showed that beamformer images have highly inhomogeneous smoothness, compared to fMRI images, due to the correlation in weights between adjacent voxels. The images are least smooth near to sources of high source strength, but accurate measurement can yield correct false-positive error rates for beamformer images. In a visual experiment, the majority of 1 mm cubic voxels have a full-width half-maximum smoothness of less that 10 mm (Barnes et al., 2004).

The use of SAM as a beamformer technique was validated by Singh et al. (2002), who conducted the same experiment using fMRI and MEG and noted the remarkable consistency in localisation between the haemodynamic response and the event-related synchronisations and desynchronisations (ERS/ERD), using both letter fluency and visual motion discrimination tasks. There was simultaneous activity in frontal, parietal and occipital areas, which would be difficult to model using dipoles due to the a priori assumption on the number of sources.

Singh et al. (2002) also provided a method for conducting group MEG analyses resulting in a statistical parametric map (SPM) analogous to the SPM from group fMRI (Friston et al., 1995). The method involves normalising each individual beamformer SAM image to a reference template and averaging across subjects. Unfortunately, this simple average contains no statistical test at the voxel or cluster level. A subsequent paper reported a non-parametric permutation test that identifies significant voxels, in cases where an application of Gaussian field theory to a parametric test failed (Singh et al., 2003).

Another move towards an fMRI-style of analysis, has been the development of a general linear model (GLM) for beamformer images (Brookes et al., 2004). The beamformer weights and spectral filter are applied to compute a single virtual electrode for each voxel. The envelope of cortical activity is given by a Hilbert transform and is the data for the GLM, analogous to the haemodynamic response used in fMRI studies. The GLM has found favour in fMRI studies because its flexibility can be applied to complex experimental designs, and a move away from standard active versus control paradigms is now possible for beamformer analysis.

The most important reason for auditory MEG studies to embrace beamformer analysis is, perhaps, that ERS and ERD have been shown to play an important role in a variety of sensory-motor and cognitive tasks (Hillebrand et al., 2005) and some have suggested cortical oscillations underlie consciousness (Engel et al., 2001). Beamformer algorithms, such as

SAM, have been successfully applied to auditory transient and steady-state responses (Herdman et al., 2003) despite the bilateral correlation in auditory cortex. It is clear, therefore, that beamformer techniques can contribute to our understanding of auditory processing, if applied correctly alongside dipole source modelling of auditory evoked stimulus-locked averaged responses. The analysis of induced changes in auditory cortical oscillatory power remains a largely untapped field of study.

REFERENCES

Barnes, G. R., and Hillebrand, A. (2003). Statistical flattening of MEG beamformer images. *Hum. Brain Mapp., 18*(1), 1-12.

Barnes, G. R., Hillebrand, A., Fawcett, I. P., and Singh, K. D. (2004). Realistic spatial sampling for MEG beamformer images. *Hum. Brain Mapp., 23*(2), 120-127.

Borgmann, C., Ross, B., Draganova, R., and Pantev, C. (2001). Human auditory middle latency responses: influence of stimulus type and intensity. *Hear Res., 158*(1-2), 57-64.

Brookes, M. J., Gibson, A. M., Hall, S. D., Furlong, P. L., Barnes, G. R., Hillebrand, A., et al. (2004). A general linear model for MEG beamformer imaging. *Neuroimage, 23*(3), 936-946.

Bregman, A. S., and Steiger, H. (1980). Auditory streaming and vertical localization: interdependence of “what” and “where” decisions in audition. *Percept Psychophys, 28*(6), 539-546.

Brookes, M. J., Stevenson, C. M., Barnes, G. R., Hillebrand, A., Simpson, M. I., Francis, S. T., et al. (2007). Beamformer reconstruction of correlated sources using a modified source model. *Neuroimage, 34*(4), 1454-1465.

Burghoff, M., Link, A., Salajegheh, A., Elster, C., Poeppel, D., and Trahms, L. (2005). A template-free approach for determining the latency of single events of auditory evoked M100. *Phys. Med. Biol., 50*(3), N43-N48.

Caton, R. (1875). The electric currents of the brain. *Br. Med. J., 2,* 278.

Chait, M., Poeppel, D., de Cheveigné, A., and Simon, J. Z. (2005). Human auditory cortical processing of changes in interaural correlation. *J. Neurosci., 25*(37), 8518-8527.

Chait, M., Poeppel, D., and Simon, J. Z. (2006). Neural response correlates of detection of monaurally and binaurally created pitches in humans. *Cereb. Cortex, 16*(6), 835-848.

Cohen, D. (1968). Magnetoencephalography: evidence of magnetic fields produced by alpha-rhythm currents. *Science, 161*(843), 784-786.

Delorme, A., Sejnowski, T., and Makeig, S. (2007). Enhanced detection of artifacts in EEG data using higher-order statistics and independent component analysis. *Neuroimage, 34*(4), 1443-1449.

Draganova, R., Ross, B., Borgmann, C., and Pantev, C. (2002). Auditory cortical response patterns to multiple rhythms of AM sound. *Ear Hear, 23*(3), 254-265.

Elberling, C., Bak, C., Kofoed, B., Lebech, J., and Saermark, K. (1982). Auditory magnetic fields: source location and 'tonotopical organization' in the right hemisphere of the human brain. *Scand. Audiol, 11*(1), 61-65.

Engel, A. K., Fries, P., and Singer, W. (2001). Dynamic predictions: oscillations and synchrony in top-down processing. *Nat. Rev. Neurosci., 2*(10), 704-716.

Forrest, T. G., and Green, D. M. (1987). Detection of partially filled gaps in noise and the temporal modulation transfer function. *J. Acoust. Soc. Am., 82*(6), 1933-1943.

Forss, N., Makela, J. P., McEvoy, L., and Hari, R. (1993). Temporal integration and oscillatory responses of the human auditory cortex revealed by evoked magnetic fields to click trains. *Hear Res., 68*(1), 89-96.

Friston, K. J., Holmes, A. P., Worsley, K. J., Poline, J. P., Frith, C. D., and Frackowiak, R. S. J. (1995). Statistical parametric maps in functional imaging: A general linear approach. *Hum. Brain Mapp., 2,* 189-210.

Fujioka, T., Kakigi, R., Gunji, A., and Takeshima, Y. (2002). The auditory evoked magnetic fields to very high frequency tones. *Neuroscience, 112*(2), 367-381.

Fujioka, T., Ross, B., Okamoto, H., Takeshima, Y., Kakigi, R., and Pantev, C. (2003). Tonotopic representation of missing fundamental complex sounds in the human auditory cortex. *Eur. J. Neurosci., 18*(2), 432-440.

Gross, J., Kujala, J., Hämäläinen, M., Timmermann, L., Schnitzler, A., and Salmelin, R. (2001). Dynamic imaging of coherent sources: Studying neural interactions in the human brain. *Proc. Natl. Acad. Sci. USA, 98*(2), 694-699.

Gutschalk, A., Micheyl, C., Melcher, J. R., Rupp, A., Scherg, M., and Oxenham, A. J. (2005). Neuromagnetic correlates of streaming in human auditory cortex. *J. Neurosci., 25*(22), 5382-5388.

Gutschalk, A., Patterson, R. D., Rupp, A., Uppenkamp, S., and Scherg, M. (2002). Sustained magnetic fields reveal separate sites for sound level and temporal regularity in human auditory cortex. *Neuroimage, 15*(1), 207-216.

Gutschalk, A., Patterson, R. D., Scherg, M., Uppenkamp, S., and Rupp, A. (2004a). Temporal dynamics of pitch in human auditory cortex. *Neuroimage, 22*(2), 755-766.

Gutschalk, A., Patterson, R. D., Scherg, M., Uppenkamp, S., and Rupp, A. (2007). The effect of temporal context on the sustained pitch response in human auditory cortex. *Cereb. Cortex, 17*(3), 552-561.

Gutschalk, A., Patterson, R. D., Uppenkamp, S., Scherg, M., and Rupp, A. (2004b). Recovery and refractoriness of auditory evoked fields after gaps in click trains. *Eur. J. Neurosci., 20*(11), 3141-3147.

Hadjipapas, A., Hillebrand, A., Holliday, I. E., Singh, K. D., and Barnes, G. R. (2005). Assessing interactions of linear and nonlinear neuronal sources using MEG beamformers: a proof of concept. *Clin. Neurophysiol., 116*(6), 1300-1313.

Hall, D. A., Johnsrude, I. S., Haggard, M. P., Palmer, A. R., Akeroyd, M. A., and Summerfield, A. Q. (2002). Spectral and temporal processing in human auditory cortex. *Cereb. Cortex, 12*(2), 140-149.

Hamada, T. (2006). A model for the mechanism of generating the auditory evoked field. *Biol. Cybern., 94*(2), 143-148.

Hari, R., and Makela, J. P. (1986). Neuromagnetic responses to frequency modulation of a continuous tone. *Acta Otolaryngol. Suppl., 432*, 26-32.

Hari, R., and Salmelin, R. (1997). Human cortical oscillations: a neuromagnetic view through the skull. *Trends Neurosci.*, 20(1), 44-49.

Herdman, A. T., Wollbrink, A., Chau, W., Ishii, R., Ross, B., and Pantev, C. (2003). Determination of activation areas in the human auditory cortex by means of synthetic aperture magnetometry. *Neuroimage, 20*(2), 995-1005.

Hertrich, I., Mathiak, K., Lutzenberger, W., and Ackermann, H. (2004). Time course and hemispheric lateralization effects of complex pitch processing: evoked magnetic fields in response to rippled noise stimuli. *Neuropsychologia, 42*(13), 1814-1826.

Hertrich, I., Mathiak, K., Menning, H., Lutzenberger, W., and Ackermann, H. (2005). MEG responses to rippled noise and Huggins pitch reveal similar cortical representations. *Neuroreport, 16*(2), 193-196.

Hillebrand, A., and Barnes, G. R. (2002). A quantitative assessment of the sensitivity of whole-head MEG to activity in the adult human cortex. *Neuroimage, 16*(3 Pt 1), 638-650.

Hillebrand, A., and Barnes, G. R. (2003). The use of anatomical constraints with MEG beamformers. *Neuroimage, 20*(4), 2302-2313.

Hillebrand, A., and Barnes, G. R. (2005). Beamformer analysis of MEG data. *Int. Rev. Neurobiol., 68*, 149-171.

Hillebrand, A., Singh, K. D., Holliday, I. E., Furlong, P. L., and Barnes, G. R. (2005). A new approach to neuroimaging with magnetoencephalography. *Hum. Brain Mapp., 25*(2), 199-211.

Holliday, I. E., Barnes, G. R., Hillebrand, A., and Singh, K. D. (2003). Accuracy and applications of group MEG studies using cortical source locations estimated from participants' scalp surfaces. *Hum. Brain Mapp., 20*(3), 142-147.

Huang, M. X., Shih, J. J., Lee, R. R., Harrington, D. L., Thoma, R. J., Weisend, M. P., et al. (2004). Commonalities and differences among vectorized beamformers in electromagnetic source imaging. *Brain Topogr., 16*(3), 139-158.

Krumbholz, K., Patterson, R. D., Seither-Preisler, A., Lammertmann, C., and Lütkenhöner, B. (2003). Neuromagnetic evidence for a pitch processing center in Heschl's gyrus. *Cereb. Cortex, 13*(7), 765-772.

Lammertmann, C., and Lütkenhöner, B. (2001). Near-DC magnetic fields following a periodic presentation of long-duration tonebursts. *Clin. Neurophysiol., 112*(3), 499-513.

Leiberg, S., Kaiser, J., and Lutzenberger, W. (2006). Gamma-band activity dissociates between matching and nonmatching stimulus pairs in an auditory delayed matching-to-sample task. *Neuroimage, 30*(4), 1357-1364.

Luo, H., Wang, Y., Poeppel, D., and Simon, J. Z. (2006). Concurrent encoding of frequency and amplitude modulation in human auditory cortex: MEG evidence. *J. Neurophysiol., 96*(5), 2712-2723.

Lütkenhöner, B. (1998a). Dipole source localization by means of maximum likelihood estimation I. Theory and simulations. *Electroencephalogr. Clin. Neurophysiol., 106*(4), 314-321.

Lütkenhöner, B. (1998b). Dipole source localization by means of maximum likelihood estimation. II. Experimental evaluation. *Electroencephalogr. Clin. Neurophysiol., 106*(4), 322-329.

Lütkenhöner, B., Krumbholz, K., Lammertmann, C., Seither-Preisler, A., Steinsträter, O., and Patterson, R. D. (2003a). Localization of primary auditory cortex in humans by magnetoencephalography. *Neuroimage, 18*(1), 58-66.

Lütkenhöner, B., Krumbholz, K., and Seither-Preisler, A. (2003b). Studies of tonotopy based on wave N100 of the auditory evoked field are problematic. *Neuroimage, 19*(3), 935-949.

Lütkenhöner, B., Lammertmann, C., and Knecht, S. (2001). Latency of auditory evoked field deflection N100m ruled by pitch or spectrum? *Audiol Neurootol., 6*(5), 263-278.

Lütkenhöner, B., and Steinsträter, O. (1998). High-precision neuromagnetic study of the functional organization of the human auditory cortex. *Audiol Neurootol, 3*(2-3), 191-213.

Mackert, B. M., Wubbeler, G., Burghoff, M., Marx, P., Trahms, L., and Curio, G. (1999). Non-invasive long-term recordings of cortical 'direct current' (DC-) activity in humans using magnetoencephalography. *Neurosci Lett., 273*(3), 159-162.

Mäkinen, V., May, P., and Tiitinen, H. (2004). Transient brain responses predict the temporal dynamics of sound detection in humans. *Neuroimage, 21*(2), 701-706.

Mäkinen, V., Tiitinen, H., and May, P. (2005). Auditory event-related responses are generated independently of ongoing brain activity. *Neuroimage, 24*(4), 961-968.

Mathiak, K., Hertrich, I., Lutzenberger, W., and Ackermann, H. (2002). Functional cerebral asymmetries of pitch processing during dichotic stimulus application: a whole-head magnetoencephalography study. *Neuropsychologia, 40*(6), 585-593.

Mathiak, K., Hertrich, I., Zvyagintsev, M., Lutzenberger, W., and Ackermann, H. (2005). Selective influences of cross-modal spatial-cues on preattentive auditory processing: a whole-head magnetoencephalography study. *Neuroimage, 28*(3), 627-634.

Okamoto, H., Ross, B., Kakigi, R., Kubo, T., and Pantev, C. (2004). N1m recovery from decline after exposure to noise with strong spectral contrasts. *Hear Res, 196*(1-2), 77-86.

Palomäki, K., Alku, P., Mäkinen, V., May, P., and Tiitinen, H. (2000). Sound localization in the human brain: neuromagnetic observations. *Neuroreport, 11*(7), 1535-1538.

Palomäki, K. J., Tiitinen, H., Mäkinen, V., May, P. J., and Alku, P. (2005). Spatial processing in human auditory cortex: the effects of 3D, ITD, and ILD stimulation techniques. *Brain Res. Cogn. Brain Res., 24*(3), 364-379.

Pantev, C., Okamoto, H., Ross, B., Stoll, W., Ciurlia-Guy, E., Kakigi, R., et al. (2004). Lateral inhibition and habituation of the human auditory cortex. *Eur. J. Neurosci., 19*(8), 2337-2344.

Pantev, C., Roberts, L. E., Elbert, T., Ross, B., and Wienbruch, C. (1996). Tonotopic organization of the sources of human auditory steady-state responses. *Hear Res., 101*(1-2), 62-74.

Picton, T. W., Hillyard, S. A., Krausz, H. I., and Galambos, R. (1974). Human auditory evoked potentials. I. Evaluation of components. *Electroencephalogr. Clin. Neurophysiol., 36*(2), 179-190.

Press, W. H., Teukolsky, S. A., Vetterling, W. T., and Flannery, B. P. (1992). *Numerical recipes in C: the art of scientific computing* (2nd ed.). Cambridge, UK: Cambridge University Press.

Ritter, S., Gunter Dosch, H., Specht, H. J., and Rupp, A. (2005). Neuromagnetic responses reflect the temporal pitch change of regular interval sounds. *Neuroimage, 27*(3), 533-543.

Roberts, T. P., Ferrari, P., Stufflebeam, S. M., and Poeppel, D. (2000). Latency of the auditory evoked neuromagnetic field components: stimulus dependence and insights toward perception. *J. Clin. Neurophysiol., 17*(2), 114-129.

Robinson, S. E., and Vrba, J. (1999). Functional neuroimaging by synthetic aperture magnetometry (SAM). In T. Yoshimoto, M. Kotani, S. Kuriki, H. Karibe and N. Nakasato (Eds.), *Recent advances in biomagnetism* (pp. 302-305). Sendai: Tohoku University Press.

Rojas, D. C., Bawn, S. D., Carlson, J. P., Arciniegas, D. B., Teale, P. D., and Reite, M. L. (2002). Alterations in tonotopy and auditory cerebral asymmetry in schizophrenia. *Biol Psychiatry, 52*(1), 32-39.

Romani, G. L., Williamson, S. J., and Kaufman, L. (1982). Tonotopic organization of the human auditory cortex. *Science, 216*(4552), 1339-1340.

Rosburg, T. (2003). Left hemispheric dipole locations of the neuromagnetic mismatch negativity to frequency, intensity and duration deviants. *Brain Res. Cogn. Brain Res., 16*(1), 83-90.

Rosburg, T. (2004). Effects of tone repetition on auditory evoked neuromagnetic fields. *Clin. Neurophysiol., 115*(4), 898-905.

Rosburg, T., Haueisen, J., and Sauer, H. (2002a). Habituation of the auditory evoked field component N100m and its dependence on stimulus duration. *Clin. Neurophysiol., 113*(3), 421-428.

Rosburg, T., Haueisen, J., and Sauer, H. (2002b). Stimulus duration influences the dipole location shift within the auditory evoked field component N100m. *Brain Topogr, 15*(1), 37-41.

Rosburg, T., Kreitschmann-Andermahr, I., Emmerich, E., Nowak, H., and Sauer, H. (1998). Hemispheric differences in frequency dependent dipole orientation of the human auditory evoked field component N100m. *Neurosci. Lett., 258*(2), 105-108.

Ross, B., Borgmann, C., Draganova, R., Roberts, L. E., and Pantev, C. (2000). A high-precision magnetoencephalographic study of human auditory steady-state responses to amplitude-modulated tones. *J. Acoust. Soc. Am., 108*(2), 679-691.

Ross, B., Draganova, R., Picton, T. W., and Pantev, C. (2003). Frequency specificity of 40-Hz auditory steady-state responses. *Hear Res., 186*(1-2), 57-68.

Ross, B., Herdman, A. T., and Pantev, C. (2005a). Right hemispheric laterality of human 40 Hz auditory steady-state responses. *Cereb. Cortex, 15*(12), 2029-2039.

Ross, B., Herdman, A. T., and Pantev, C. (2005b). Stimulus induced desynchronization of human auditory 40-Hz steady-state responses. *J. Neurophysiol., 94*(6), 4082-4093.

Ross, B., and Pantev, C. (2004). Auditory steady-state responses reveal amplitude modulation gap detection thresholds. *J. Acoust. Soc. Am., 115*(5 Pt 1), 2193-2206.

Ross, B., Picton, T. W., and Pantev, C. (2002). Temporal integration in the human auditory cortex as represented by the development of the steady-state magnetic field. *Hear Res., 165*(1-2), 68-84.

Rupp, A., Gutschalk, A., Hack, S., and Scherg, M. (2002). Temporal resolution of the human primary auditory cortex in gap detection. *Neuroreport, 13*(17), 2203-2207.

Rupp, A., Gutschalk, A., Uppenkamp, S., and Scherg, M. (2004). Middle latency auditory-evoked fields reflect psychoacoustic gap detection thresholds in human listeners. *J. Neurophysiol., 92*(4), 2239-2247.

Salajegheh, A., Link, A., Elster, C., Burghoff, M., Sander, T., Trahms, L., et al. (2004). Systematic latency variation of the auditory evoked M100: from average to single-trial data. *Neuroimage, 23*(1), 288-295.

Salmelin, R. (2007). Clinical neurophysiology of language: the MEG approach. *Clin. Neurophysiol, 118*(2), 237-254.

Schadow, J., Lenz, D., Thaerig, S., Busch, N. A., Frund, I. and Herrmann, C. S. (2007). Stimulus intensity affects early sensory processing: Sound intensity modulates auditory evoked gamma-band activity in human EEG. *Int. J. Psychophysiol.*, (In press).

Seither-Preisler, A., Krumbholz, K., and Lütkenhöner, B. (2003). Sensitivity of the neuromagnetic N100m deflection to spectral bandwidth: a function of the auditory periphery? *Audiol Neurootol., 8*(6), 322-337.

Seither-Preisler, A., Krumbholz, K., Patterson, R., Seither, S., and Lütkenhöner, B. (2004). Interaction between the neuromagnetic responses to sound energy onset and pitch onset suggests common generators. *Eur. J. Neurosci., 19*(11), 3073-3080.

Seither-Preisler, A., Patterson, R., Krumbholz, K., Seither, S., and Lütkenhöner, B. (2006a). Evidence of pitch processing in the N100m component of the auditory evoked field. *Hear Res., 213*(1-2), 88-98.

Seither-Preisler, A., Patterson, R. D., Krumbholz, K., Seither, S., and Lütkenhöner, B. (2006b). From noise to pitch: transient and sustained responses of the auditory evoked field. *Hear Res., 218*(1-2), 50-63.

Sieroka, N., Dosch, H. G., Specht, H. J., and Rupp, A. (2003). Additional neuromagnetic source activity outside the auditory cortex in duration discrimination correlates with behavioural ability. *Neuroimage, 20*(3), 1697-1703.

Singh, K. D., Barnes, G. R., and Hillebrand, A. (2003). Group imaging of task-related changes in cortical synchronisation using nonparametric permutation testing. *Neuroimage, 19*(4), 1589-1601.

Singh, K. D., Barnes, G. R., Hillebrand, A., Forde, E. M., and Williams, A. L. (2002). Task-related changes in cortical synchronization are spatially coincident with the hemodynamic response. *Neuroimage, 16*(1), 103-114.

Soeta, Y., Hotehama, T., Nakagawa, S., Tonoike, M., and Ando, Y. (2004). Auditory evoked magnetic fields in relation to interaural cross-correlation of band-pass noise. *Hear Res., 196*(1-2), 109-114.

Soeta, Y., Nakagawa, S., and Matsuoka, K. (2006). The effect of center frequency and bandwidth on the auditory evoked magnetic field. *Hear Res., 218*(1-2), 64-71.

Soeta, Y., Nakagawa, S., and Tonoike, M. (2005a). Auditory evoked fields to variations of interaural time delay. *Neurosci Lett, 383*(3), 311-316.

Soeta, Y., Nakagawa, S., and Tonoike, M. (2005b). Auditory evoked magnetic fields in relation to bandwidth variations of bandpass noise. *Hear Res, 202*(1-2), 47-54.

Soeta, Y., Nakagawa, S., and Tonoike, M. (2005c). Auditory evoked magnetic fields in relation to iterated rippled noise. *Hear Res., 205*(1-2), 256-261.

Stufflebeam, S. M., Poeppel, D., Rowley, H. A., and Roberts, T. P. (1998). Peri-threshold encoding of stimulus frequency and intensity in the M100 latency. *Neuroreport, 9*(1), 91-94.

Tecchio, F., Bicciolo, G., De Campora, E., Pasqualetti, P., Pizzella, V., Indovina, I., et al. (2000). Tonotopic cortical changes following stapes substitution in otosclerotic patients: a magnetoencephalographic study. *Hum. Brain Mapp., 10*(1), 28-38.

Tiitinen, H., Salminen, N. H., Palomäki, K. J., Mäkinen, V. T., Alku, P., and May, P. J. (2006). Neuromagnetic recordings reveal the temporal dynamics of auditory spatial processing in the human cortex. *Neurosci Lett., 396*(1), 17-22.

van Veen, B. D., and Buckley, K. M. (1988). Beamforming: a versatile approach to spatial filtering. *IEEE Acoustics, Speech, and Signal Processing Magazine, 5*, 4-24.

Vrba, J., and Robinson, S. E. (2001). Signal processing in magnetoencephalography. *Methods, 25*(2), 249-271.

Yost, W. A. (1996). Pitch strength of iterated rippled noise. *J. Acoust. Soc. Am., 100*(5), 3329-3335.

In: Brain Mapping Research Developments
Editor: Lars N. Bakker, pp. 43-71

ISBN 978-1-60456-007-7

Chapter II

CORTICAL ORGANIZATION OF CAT LICKING FINE TONGUE MOVEMENTS DURING CAT LICKING EXECUTED BY BILATERAL CORTICAL CONTROL

***Hisao Hiraba*[*1,2], *Takako Sato*[3] *and Koichiro Ueda*[1,2]**

[1]Department of Dysphasia Rehabilitation
[2]Division of Functional Morphology Dental Research Center
[3]Department of Oral and Maxillofacial Surgery,
Nihon University School of Dentistry, 1-8-13 Kanda-surugadai,
Chiyoda-ku, 101-8310, Tokyo, Japan

ABSTRACT

Mastication is accomplished by the cooperative movement produced by various striated muscles in the face, jaw and tongue. Their movements are generally credited with activations organized by the central pattern generator (CPG) existing in the brain stem depending on commands from the cerebral cortex.

However, studies concerning outputs from cerebral cortex generating the CPG have been rarely reported. Firstly, we explored the properties of neurons related to mastication (MRNs) using single unit recording and intracortical microstimulation (ICMS) in various areas of the cat frontal cortex. We identified the mastication-related cortical areas (MRCAs) of one orofacial SI (the facial and intraoral primary somatosensory cortex) and four motor cortical areas (area C in the anterior part of coronal sulcus, MA in the masticatory area, area M in the ventral bank of cruciate sulcus and area P in the lateral wall of presylcian sulcus). Next, we examined changes in orofacial behaviors induced by localized lesions in respective area. These results showed that the cortical control for

[*] Author for Correspondence: H. Hiraba, Department of Physiology, Nihon University School of Dentistry, 1-8-13 Kanda-surugadai, Chiyoda-ku, Tokyo 101-8310, Japan. Telephone number: +81 3 3219 8198, Fax: +81 3 3219 8203. E-mail: hiraba@dent.nihon-u.ac.jp.

appropriate feeding behaviors was organized by two distinct cortical regions for facial and masticatory (jaw and tongue) movements.

Facial movements are unilaterally controlled by the facial SI (area 3b), area C (area 3a) and area M (area 4∂), whereas masticatory movements are bilaterally controlled by the intraoral SI (areas 3b and 3a), masticatory cortex (area 43) and area P (area 6aß). Although the unilateral cortical processing for facial movements is the same as the one for the limb movement, bilateral networks for movements of jaw and tongue remain unclear. However, since the jaw movement of cats consists of jaw- opening and -closing only, we focused on the tongue movement.

We showed the characteristic change in the abnormal tongue-protrusion with the increased genioglossus muscle activities during licking after the unilateral motor cortical area (area P) lesion, and the abnormal protrusion without deviation, as well as the protrusion evoked by the ICMS.

On the other hand, the unilateral hypoglossal nerve cutting showed deviation toward the affected side (Hiraba and Sato 2004), and pyramidal neurons (PT) in the unilateral area P projected to the bilateral hypoglossal nuclei at the brain stem, as shown in anatomical data (Yasui et al., 1985b). These findings suggested that tongue muscles in the left and right sides were supplied by the hypoglossal nuclei in the left and right sides, and also that the unilateral area P contained two kinds of PTs projecting to left or right nuclei. Furthermore, we assumed the relay circuit of inhibitory interneuron between connections of both hemispheres based on the abnormal tongue protrusion after the unilateral lesion.

Keywords: mastication-related cortical areas, bilateral cortical control, tongue-protrusion, mastication, awake cats.

INTRODUCTION

The masticatory function is acquired during the weaning stage in association with the growth of the cerebral cortex. As to the central mechanisms of the masticatory movement, it is generally accepted that the command (or output) from the cortex (motor or masticatory cortex) activates the central pattern generator (CPG) in the brain stem. The activated CPG generates outputs for rhythmical (mastication-like) movements of the jaw, tongue and face as well as coordination of patterns between these movements (Nakamura and Katakura, 1995). On the other hand, since Fritsch and Hitzing (1870) discovered a contralateral muscle dominance in the dog frontal cortex, commands (or outputs) from the cerebral cortex have been explored by many investigators resulting in the drawing of many motor maps in various animals, including human (Vogt and Vogt, 1926; Penfield and Rassmussen, 1950; Woolsey, 1958; Hoffman and Luschei, 1980; Jones and Peters, 1986; Krakauer and Ghez, 2000). Furthermore, repetitive electrical stimuli of a certain area in the cerebral cortex induced rhythmical jaw movements resembling mastication in various species, including monkey (Lund and Lamarre, 1974; Huang et al., 1989a; Huang et al., 1989b), rabbit (Lund et al., 1984; Kawamura and Tukamoto, 1961; Sumi, 1969; Dellow and Lund, 1971; Enomoto et al., 1987a; Enomoto et al., 1987b; Inoue et al., 1989; Schwarts et al., 1989; Liu et al., 1993; Hidaka et al., 1997), cat (Margoun et al., 1933; Morimoto and Kawamra, 1973; Nakamura and Kubo, 1978; Iwata et al. 1985; Iwata et al., 1990; Guandalini et al., 1990; Hiraba et al.,

1993), guinea pig (Goldberg and Tal, 1978; Goldberg et al., 1982; Nozaki et al., 1986a; Nozaki et al., 1986b; Nozaki et al., 1991; Nozaki et al., 1993, Enomoto et al., 1995; Chandler et al., 1985; Chandler et al, 1985) and rat (Sasamoto et al., 1990). Thus, this area has been called the cortical masticatory area (MA, or masticatory cortex). On the other hand, bilateral lesion in the rabbit MA (Enomoto et al., 1987a; Enomoto et al, 1987b; Inoue et al., 1989) and guinea pig MA (Luschei and Goldberg, 1981; Rioch, 1934), and unilateral or bilateral lesion in the MA and/or motor cortex of the trained monkey (Luschei and Goodwin, 1975; Larson et al., 1980; Murray et al., 1991; Narita et al., 2002; Yamamura et al., 2002) evoked changes in biting or tongue protrusion task and deficits of mastication, but did not affect masticatory rhythm. These findings suggest that the cerebral cortex in various species may provide adequate information for the masticatory force or patterns of jaw and tongue movements including vertical and lateral movements, since masticatory movements change with the property and condition of food and edentulous stage. Namely, the change in movements of face, jaw and tongue may be produced by outputs from the cortex relayed to the sensory feedback.

Although the first step of the examination for mastication is the cerebral cortex, many studies of mastication have focused on the organization of the central pattern generator (CPG) in the brain stem. Thus, cortical neuronal processing linking the sensory input to the orofacial SI with the motor output from the motor cortex has not been clarified yet.

(1) Central Pattern Generator (CPG)

Lund et al. (1984) reported a rhythmical jaw movement evoked by repetitive electrical stimuli on the MA showed changes in jaw muscle activities depending on their intensities, but did not affect rhythm. The Chandler group(Chandler et al., 1985a, 1985b and 1986) reported that rhythmic jaw movements elicited by cortical stimuli changed the activity patterns of jaw muscles after the cut off in the brain stem. Furthermore, intravenous injections of various drugs changed the activity patterns of jaw movements, but did not affect rhythm. However, since the rhythm could be produced by decerebrate animals (Lund and Dellow, 1971; Bremer in Luschei and Goodwing, 1975) and anencephalic babys (Monnier and Will, 1953), the rhythm generator was thought to be located in the brain stem. Furthermore, Nozaki et al. (1986a, 1986b, 1991 and 1993) examined the detailed location and function in each nucleus in the brain stem in guinea pigs. The rhythm generator composed by multiple nucleus in the brain stem has generally been called the central pattern generator (CPG).

(2) Choice of Experimental Animals

The experimental procedures for masticatory movements at CPG have usually examined rabbits possessing lateral movements of jaw. Although rabbits are a good choice for the investigation of the trajectory of jaw movements, they are inadequate for the study of the cortical function for the control of jaw movements. Cerebral cortices in rabbits, including guinea pigs and rats, exist obviously in the overlapping between the motor and masticatory cortices (Goldberg et al., 1982; Lund et al., 1984; Sasamoto et al., 1990). On the other hand, monkeys may be the best choice for our experiment, as they are similar to humans. The exploration of somatosensory, motor, and masticatory cortices in monkey will provide us with information of the detailed organization of each area. However, since the monkey cortex is too broad to be explored by the recording of single neuronal activity, advanced comprehensive and unified measurements between various MRCAs are difficult for a limited time. This conclusion was reached based on my experience. I have studied motor and masticatory cortices in monkey with the use of the intracortical microstimulation (ICMS) and unit recording with the research group of Prof. Sessle (University of Toronto, Canada) for the past two years (Huang et al., 1988; Huang et al, 1989a; Huang et al., 1989b). Other investigators in the group have continued with the exploration in other areas, somatosensory cortex, masticatory cortex and so on (Sessle et al., 2005; Lin et al., 1993, 1994a, 1994b and 1994c; Yao et al., 2002a and 2002b; Murray et al., 1991; Narita et al., 2002; Yamamura et al., 2002).

Why did we decide to use cats to explore functional organization in the cerebral cortex of the mastication? We have three reasons: (1) their jaw movements are simple (opening and closing only without lateral movement), (2) there are a lot of anatomical data of the cortico-cortical and cortico-bulbar connections, and (3) there is somatotopic organization related to the cytoarchitecual area, such as orofacial region of the primary somatosensory cortex (orofacial SI) in areas 3b and 3a, the motor and premotor cortices in areas 4∂ and 6aß, and the masticatory cortex (MA) in area 43 according to Hassler and Mush-Clement (1964). If the jaw movement is regulated by control in cerebral cortex, pyramidal cells in the motor cortical area for jaw movement are necessary for organizations of opening, closing, lateral, backward and forward movements, and analysis of the jaw movements is very complex. On the other hand, although lingual movements are composed by movements in three dimensions, the simple vertical jaw movement of cats concentrates entirely on the analysis of tongue movements.

Woolsey (1958) reported the facial motor cortex in cats located at the anterior part of the coronal sulcus. However, according to Hassler and Mush-Clement, this area belonged to area 3a. Thus, mastication-related cortical areas (MRCAs) in awake cats firstly started from the exploration of properties of mastication-related neurons (MRNs), such as a mechanical receptive field (RF), submodality, activity patterns of MRNs during mastication, motor effects evoked by an intracortical microstimulation (ICMS) at MRN recording sites, and finally examined changes in orofacial behaviors after the lesion in each MRCA.

(3) Mastication-Related Cortical Areas (MRCA)

The surgery for head-holding apparatus and implantation of the mandibular screws for a monitor of jaw movements was performed under the surgical level of anesthesia with atropin (0.04 mg/kg), ketamine (40-50 mg/kg) and pentobarbital sodium (30-40 mg/kg). After acclimatization and training for about one month, electrodes (0.1 mm in diameter, teflon-coated stainless steel wires) for EMGs (electromyograms) were chronically implanted in the left and/or right sides of the masseter, genioglossus and anterior digastiric (or temporal) muscles. Next, a cylindrical teflon chamber was implanted under the surgical level of anesthesia.

Microelectrodes (impedance 4-6 MΩ at 1 kHz) were inserted vertically along the frontal plane through the dorsal surface of the lateral sigmoid gyrus of the cat brain. We examined the mastication-related cortical areas (MRCAs) of one orofacial SI (the facial and intraoral primary somatosensory cortex along the coronal gyrus) and four motor cortical areas (area C in the anterior part of coronal sulcus, MA in the masticatory area of the anterior part or orbital sulcus, area M in the ventral bank of cruciate sulcus and area P in the lateral wall of presylcian sulcus). Single unit recording and intracortical microstimulation for 3-4 s (C-ICMS; 200ms pulses at 50 Hz, ≤ 20 μA) were performed in the MRCAs, as shown in Figure 1. C-ICMS confirmed the ability to differentiate clearly between tetanus contractions (TC) and rhythmical jaw movements (RJM) (Figure 2B and Hiraba, 2004; Hiraba and Sato, 2004). We focused on recording MRNs showing activity related to some aspects of masticatory movements (Hiraba et al. 1997). RFs in the facial skin, teeth, tongue and other intraoral sites, as well as submodality and other properties, were determined by each isolated MRN, as described in our previous paper (Figure 2 and Hiraba et al., 1997).

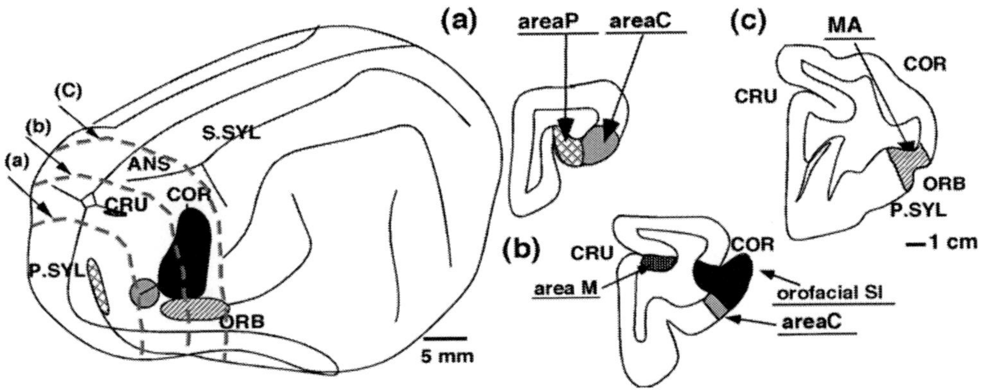

Figure 1. Cortical mastication-related areas in the cat. Broken lines on the cortical surface indicate three frontal sections (a, b and c). Orofacial SI including facial SI and intraoral SI, is the primary somatosensory cortex. MA is the masticatory cortex (or masticatory area). Other motor cortical areas are indicated as area C, area M and area P. According to Hassler and Mush-Clement (1964), facial SI and intraoral SI cytoarchitectonically belong to area 3b, and areas 3a and 3b. MA is area 43, area C is area 3a, area M is area 4∂ and area P is area 6aß.

Properties of MRNs

We used awake cats after they were acclimatized and rested comfortably in a box with their heads fixed to the apparatus, to accept mechanical stimulation to their orofacial region and to ingest and chew food without struggling. We recorded MRNs showing activity related to some aspects of masticatory movements from cats' frontal cortex (Hiraba et al., 1993, 1994, 1996 and 1997; Hiraba, 1999 and 2004; Hiraba and Sato, 2004). Based on recorded

MRNs in each MRCA, we explored properties of each MRCA (orofacial SI, area C, MA, area P and area M).

(1) Motor Effects

C-ICMS at recording sites of MRNs in each MRCA evoked the TC in the facial or intraoral region, or RJM except the facial and intraoral SI (Figure 2B). Area M belongs to area 4∂ according to Hassler and Mush-Clement (1964) and C-ICMS evokes facial twitches (facial TC) only. Area C is area 3a and C-ICMS evoked facial TC mainly, and jaw opening and tongue protrusion in rare cases. MA is area 43 and C-ICMS evokes rhythmical jaw movement (RJM) in many sites. Area P is area 6aß and C-ICMS evokes various motor effects, such as facial TC, jaw opening and jaw closing, tongue protrusion and RJM. Motor effects in each MRCA are shown in Figure 2B. From the results of motor effects evoked by C-ICMS in each MRCA, we assumed that area C and area M were organized by facial movements, and MA and area P by jaw and tongue movements.

(2) RFs

Almost all of the MRNs in each MRCA had isolated RFs in the orofacial region (Figure 2A). Orofacial SI is divided into the facial SI with the RFs in the facial region (facial MRNs) and intraoral SI with the RFs in the intraoral structures (intraoral MRNs). Almost all facial MRNs had RFs in the perioral (41%), mandibular (15%), whisker hairs (15%), maxilla (8%), vermilion bourder mucosa (6%), and nose (6%) regions, and the majority of the intraoral neurons had RFs on the tongue dorsom (53%), teeth (periodontum) (24%), palate (8%), gingival (8%) and buccul mucosa (8%), as shown in Figure 2A. Furthermore, the tendency of RF distributions in area C, area M, MA and area P is the same, although there is slight fluctuation among each MRCA (Figure 2A).

MRNs recorded in orofacial SI have shown that the facial and intraoral MRNs have contralateral (82% and 33%), ipasilateral (9% and 9%) and bilateral (9% and 58%) RFs, as shown in Figure 2C-a and Hiraba (1999). Furthermore, the tendency of RF laterality was also observed at other MRCAs and distributions of RF laterality were built by characteristic patterns among MRCAs. We reconducted an analysis on the differences of the laterality and size of RFs in perioral region based on two kinds of cortical organizations as to motor effects with the use of C-ICMS (Figure 2C-b and 2D). As shown in Figure 2C-b, the ratio of facial MRNs and intraoral MRNs with the contralateral RF in orofacial SI showed the greatest numbers, and area C and area M or MA and area P decreased in turn. On the other hand, the ratio of facial and intraoral MRNs with the bilateral RF in the orofacial SI showed the smallest numbers, and area C and area M or MA and area P increased in turn. Furthermore, we compared sizes of RFs in the perioral region of MRNs recorded at each MRCA. RF sizes of MRNs in the orofacial SI showed the smallest one, and area C and area M or MA and area P increased in turn, as shown in Figure 2D. Namely, RF sizes of MRNs recorded at facial SI, area C and area M or intraoral SI, MA and area P divided by two cortical pathways showed the hierarchical organization depending on two kinds of cortical organization.

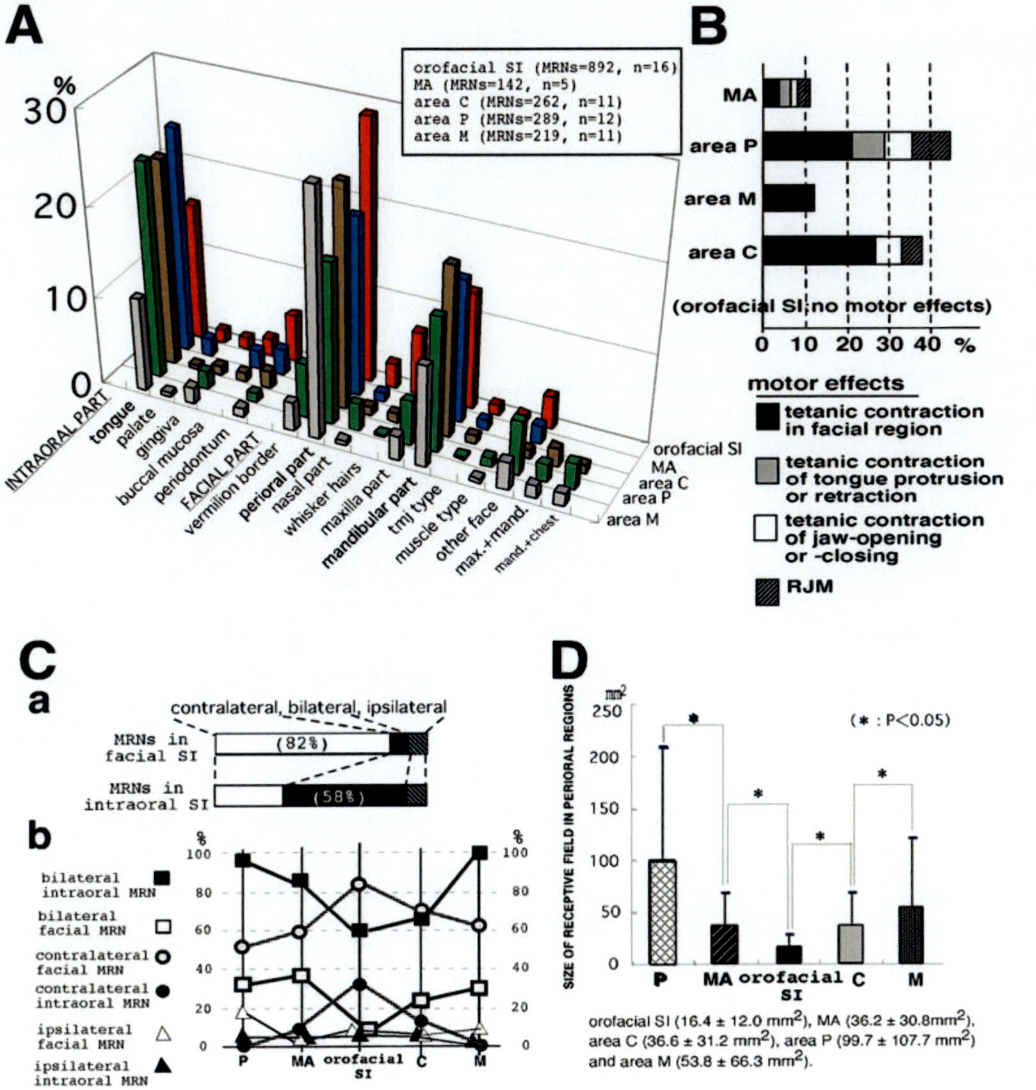

Figure 2. Distribution of RF of MRNs recorded in the masticatory-related cortical areas and motor effects evoked by C-ICMS at MRN recording site in each area. A. In inside box, MRNs: total numbers of MRNs recorded in each MRCA and n: numbers of cats. B. Motor effects evoked by C-ICMS indicate titanic contractions in face, tongue and jaw or rhythmical jaw movement (RJM). C-a. RFs' laterality of MRNs with RFs in facial or intraoral region recorded at orofacial SI. C-b. RFs' laterality of MRNs recorded in the orofacial SI, MA, area P, area C and area M. Note that many MRNs had RFs in the tongue, perioral and mandibular regions. D: Size of RFs in the perioral region of each area (*, $P < 0.05$ Student's paired t test).

These findings support two stages depending on RF sizes and laterality, as well as the hierarchical somatosensory processing (increase of RF sizes in areas 3, 1 and 2 in turn) proposed by Iwamura (Iwamura, 1998 and 2000; Iwamura and Tanaka, 1978a and 1978b) and Toda and Taoka (2002).

(3) Activity Patterns

Animals were trained to start ingestion of food when it made contact with the perioral region. We paid special attention to how the activities of MRNs changed in association with the ingestion of the fish paste, milk or small dry fish. MRNs were divided into three types by their activity patterns: the rhythmical type (RB showed rhythmical bursts in pace with the masticatory rhythm), the sustained type (SB showed a sustained type during the ingestion) and the transient type (TB showed transient intense discharges during masticatory movements) (Hiraba et al., 1997 and Hiraba and Sato, 2004). However, firings of activity evoked by various food conditions (milk, fish paste and small dry fish), were observed by MRNs recorded in each MRCA. Various activity patterns may be decided by a property of MRN, since changes in firing rates (frequency) depending on feeding various types of food (liquid, soft or hard), are modulated by hardness of food, as shown in changes in activities of RB type of MRNs recorded at orofacial SI of the previous paper (Hiraba et al. 1997). Thus, basic activity pattern of MRNs during mastication have the invariance in each activity pattern.

Furthermore, activity patterns of MRNs were classified into pre-movement and post-movement types, based on activity change preceding or following the onset of masticatory start or EMG activities. Thus, activity patterns of MRNs could be divided into the pre-SB and pre-TB, and post-RB, post-SB and post-TB types (Hiraba et al., 1997; Hiraba, 1999; Hiraba, 2004; Hiraba and Sato, 2004), as shown in Figure 3. However, in this experiment the pre-RB type was not found. In particular, the pre-TB type was based on the post-stimulus time histograms (PSTH) of neuronal activities with behavioral parameters, such as jaw movements, EMG activities of the masseter, anterior digastric and genioglossus muscles during mastication (Hiraba and Sato, 2004).

Hypothesis of Cortical Organization Based on Properties of MRNs

In Figure 3A, we show the schema of cortical processing based on the facial SI (area 3b), area C (area 3a) and area M (area 4∂) during mastication (Figure 3A-1) and the summary of typical MRN activity patterns in each MRCA (Figure 3A-2). In Figure 3B, we also show the schema of cortical processing based on the intraoral SI (areas 3b and 3a), MA (area 43) and area P (area 6aß) (Figure 3B-1) and the summary of typical MRN activity patterns in each MRCA (Figure 3B-2). Namely, the motor command from motor cortical areas in area M or in area P is firstly supplied to the facial or lingual muscles via facial or hypoglossal nucleus and the mastication kicks in. Next, somatosensory information evoked by mastication comes back to facial SI or intraoral SI, and then adequate motor command processed into each cortical organization, executes the appropriate face, jaw and tongue movements for a fine mastication. Thus, we assumed that the cortical organization for facial movements was processed by the unilateral hemisphere, and for jaw and tongue movements by the bilateral one from the anatomical data (Hiraba, 2004; Hiraba and Sato, 2004).

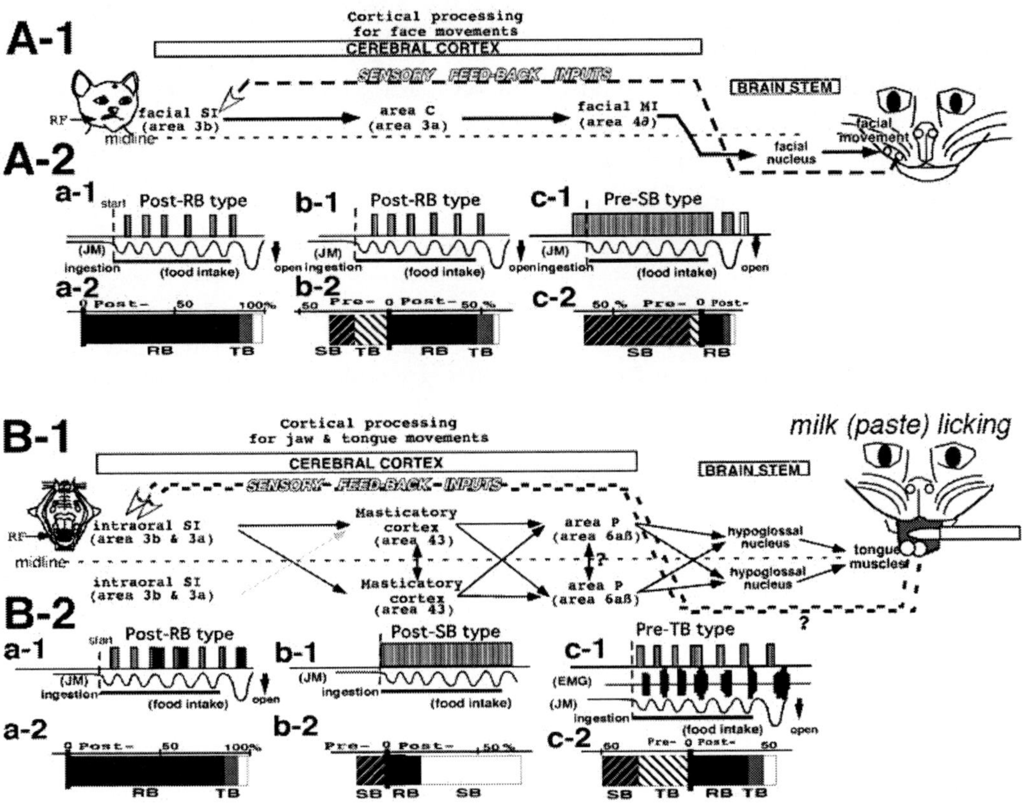

Figure 3. Ratio of activity patterns and Schemas of typical activity patterns of MRNs recorded in masticatory-related cortical areas. Motor effects are indicated by RJM (rhythmical jaw movement) and TC (tetanic contraction) in the orofacial region. MRNs recorded in the orofacial SI, show the location of RFs on the perioral and lingual region. Activity patterns in each area are indicated by Post- (post-movement) and Pre- (pre-movement) types. Furthermore, they are classified by activity changes preceding or following the onset of masticatory start, movements or EMG activities: rhythmical type (RB, showing rhythmical bursts in pace with the masticatory rhythm), transient (biting) type (TB, showing intence discharges in coincidence with biting hard food) and sustained type (SB, showing a sustained firing during the period of ingestion), as shown in previous papers (Hiraba et al., 1997; Hiraba, 2004; Hiraba and Sato, 2004).

(1) Face Movement

Our hypothesis of a cortical organization for facial movements is shown in Figure 3A. The initiation of mastication is prepared by the tension in the perioral region (around the mouth), as shown by the erection of whiskers in Figures 3A and 4. The erection of whiskers keeps the muscles' contraction around the mouth and prevents dropping of food from the mouth during ingestion period. The contraction observed by erection of whiskers is suggested by the appearance of the pre-SB type of many MRNs recorded at area M. Namely, about 60% of MRNs in area M of normal cats were the pre-SB type that showed increased firing prior to the start of mastication and tonic activity during the ingestion period, as shown in Figure 3A-2 and c. The findings are suggested from data showing that motor effect evoked by C-ICMS in area M, are facial TC only. Whereas, about 15% of MRNs recorded at area C are the pre-SB type and about 50% of MRNs are included by the post-RB type (Figure 3A-2 and b). Especially, about 80% of MRNs recorded at orofacial SI are the post-RB monitored by movements of face, jaw and tongue (Hiraba et al., 1997).

We proposed that somatosensory information in facial SI was utilized to the detailed control of facial muscles for the appropriate manipulation of food during mastication in area M, as shown in the previous paper (Hiraba, 2004). Although MRNs with orofacial RFs in each of orofacial SI, area C and area M had in common the lingual, perioral and mandibular parts, their somatosensory information were obvious different properties in each MRCA. MRNs recorded at facial SI, had a clear boundary and smaller RF size, but ones in area C and area M had unclear boundary and larger RF size, as shown in Figures 2C and 2D. Eighty percent of activity patterns of MRNs in facial SI are the post-RB type and 60% of MRNs in area M are the pre-SB type. The post-RB type of activity patterns in area C is about 50%, and the pre-SB type is about 15%. Thus, area C may show the translation toward motor outputs based on various facial sensory information, and then their motor information may narrow down localization for facial movement in area M. The findings suggest that the role of area C plays the process of transition from sensory information in facial SI to adapted motor commands in area M. We show the schema for cortical processing of face movements in Figure 3A-1. Changes in ratio of the laterality and RF sizes in facial SI, area C and area M show the hierarchy for translation toward the appropriate motor command depending on the somatosensory information, as shown in Figure 2C and 2D.

(2) Tongue Movements

Our hypothesis of a cortical organization for jaw and tongue movements is shown in Figure 3B. Food ingestion starts from jaw-opening and then is taken into the oral cavity with tongue movements. It is chewed by co-operative movements among jaw, tongue and face, and a bolus of food for swallowing is finally made. Tongue movements are divided into two components of movement, protrusion and retraction, and lateral movements. We focused on the movements of protrusion and retraction, and then added the lateral movements. Namely, we thought that tongue protrusion and retraction in cats were fundamental movements in food feeding.

Eighty percent of activity patterns of MRNs recorded at orofacial SI, were the post-RB type showing the rhythmical burst in pace with the masticatory rhythm (Figure 3B-2). Furthermore, orofacial SI was divided into the facial and intraoral areas based on the RF of MRNs (Hiraba et al., 1997; Hiraba, 1999). MRN burst activities of the post-RB type recorded in facial SI are very regular bursts during ingestion period. Ones in intraoral SI show various frequencies in each burst during ingestion period, although rhythmical bursts during ingestion period are regular, as shown in Figure 3A-2. The difference of frequency in each burst may depend on the condition of the bolus of food in the oral cavity, as shown in Figure 3B-2.

About 50% and 15% of activity patterns of MRNs recorded at MA were the post-SB and pre-SB types that showed a sustained burst during ingestion period. The motor effects by C-ICMS at MRNs recording sites mainly showed RJM, tongue protrusion and facial TC. Based on the RF of MRNs, MA in the orbiral gurus divided into the facial area projected in the posterior part and intraoral area in the anterior part (Hiraba and Sato, 2004 and 2005c). Particularly, when the electrode is inserted from the sigmoid gyrus, MRNs of MA are found after MRNs recorded in orofacial SI, since MA is located in the ventral part of orofacial SI. However, properties of MRNs between MA and orofacial SI are completely different, such as RF size, RF boundary, motor effects and so on. Thus, the discrimination between MA and orofacial SI is easy.

About 45% of MRNs in area P showed the pre-TB type showing activities prior to masticatory start or facial, masticatory or lingual EMG, and C-ICMS evoked various motor effects such as facial TC, tongue protrusion or retraction, jaw-opening or jaw-closing, and RJM (Hiraba and Sato, 2004). On the other hand, since facial MRNs and intraoral MRNs recorded at orofacial SI consist mainly of MRNs with contralateral RFs (82% of facial MRNs and 33% of intraoral MRNs in Hiraba, 1999), the construction of jaw and tongue fused with the left and right sides, may be executed depending on the integration of information of both of the MA and area P. Thus, the cortical organization in intraoral SI, MA and area P may execute the cortical processing in both hemispheres.

CHANGES IN OROFACIAL BEHAVIORS DURING MASTICATION AFTER THE LESION OF EACH MRCA

After the local confirmation of the center of each MRCA determined by MRN recordings and C-ICMS, the electrode was replaced by a stainless steel tube (0.3 mm in diameter), into which a stainless steel wire electrode (0.05 mm in diameter) coated with teflon was inserted and fixed with its tip at the opening of the tube to record multi-unit activities. Then the tube was advanced along with an electrode to the center of each MRCA that had been defined with the aid of multi-unit recording of the responses to mechanical stimulation of the orofacial regions. Kainic acid (0.1% dissolved in 0.1 M phosphate buffer) was injected into the center of each area and was injected at a rate of 0.5 μl per 30 sec from a tube connected to a Hamilton syringe (5 μl) through a polyethylene tube.

The neuronal activities and trajectory of jaw movements and ICMS-evoked masticatory movements were recorded on a 16-channel data recorder for about 30 sec. Furthermore, digital camera records were used to analyze the trajectory of jaw movements and movements of perioral and intraoral structures, such as the jaw, whiskers and tongue during mastication, as shown in Figure 4 and our previous papers (Hiraba et al.1997 and 2000; Hiraba, 2004; Hiraba and Sato, 2005b and 2005c). Based on the analysis of behaviors, EMG activities and trajectory of jaw movement as shown in Figure 4, we defined the masticatory start, ingestion period, number of swallows (Sw1, Sw2 and so on), as described in previous papers (Hiraba et al., 1997; Hiraba et al., 2000). We tested for changes in orofacial behaviors and masticatory movements for about one month after the lesion was made in each projection area.

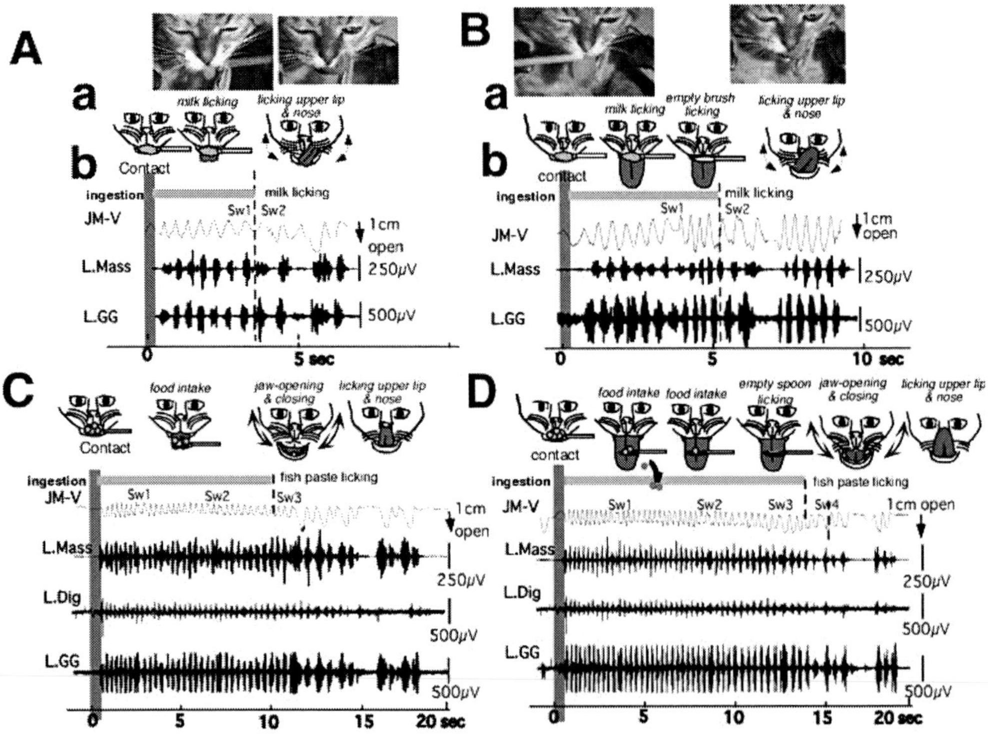

Figure 4. Sequences of milk (A) and fish paste (C) licking behaviors, trajectory of jaw movement, masticatory period, and masseter, anterior part of digastric and genioglossus EMG activities in a normal cat and in a cat after making the lesion in area P. A-a. Milk licking behavior, based on digital video analysis through a microcomputer in a normal cat. A-b. Ingestion indicates ingestion period during licking of a paintbrush soaked in milk. Trajectory of vertical jaw movement and EMG activites (L-Mass: masseter muscles in the left side, L-GG: genioglossus muscles in the left side) during milk licking. The cat started masticatory movements for licking when a paintbrush dripping with milk came into contact with the perioral hairs (contact) after a reaction time of about 0.3s. Milk licking was defined as the period during which the animal actually licked milk from the paintbrush. On the record of jaw movement trajectory, two swallows (Sw1 and Sw2) were noticed as pauses or prolongation of jaw-closing (Hiraba et al., 1997). B-a and b. An example of milk licking behavior and masticatory process at 27 days after the lesion of the cat with the area P lesion. Although the masticatory start remained normal, the cat showed abnormal tongue protrusion. During licking his upper lip and nose after ingestion, erection of whiskers on both sides was observed as in intact cats. C. fish paste licking behavior, trajectory of vertical jaw movements and EMG activities (L-Mass, L-GG and L-Dig: the anterior part of digastric muscle) in a normal cat. The cat started masticatory movements for licking when a small wooden spoon with fish paste (about 1.8 g) came into contact with the perioral hairs (contact) after a reaction time of about 0.3s. D. An example of fish paste licking behavior and masticatory process at 27 days after the lesion.

If the unilateral lesion did not induce obvious changes in orofacial behaviors, we made another lesion in the same contralateral part and examined orofacial behaviors again for about one more month. Namely, deficits were classified by the unilateral or bilateral lesion. Furthermore, since MA was divided into facial and intraoral projection areas, we made the lesions in the facial MA and intraoral MA, respectively. On the other hand, area P shows a mixture of facial MRNs and intraoral MRNs. We made cats with the entire unilateral area P lesion. In Table 1, we show changes in orofacial behaviors during mastication (or licking) after the lesion in unilateral facial SI, unilateral area C and unilateral area M, and after the lesion in unilateral intraoral SI, unilateral and bilateral MA and unilateral area P, respectively.

Table 1. Deficits caused by lesions of each area. Plus (+) and minus (-) indicate appeared deficits and no changes in masticatory behaviors, respectively. Orofacial SI: the orofacial region of the primary somasosensory cortex. MA: the masticatory cortex. Motor Cx: the motor cortex. Summary of collected data from orofacial SI in Hiraba et al. (2000), MA and area P in Hiraba and Sato (2005a, 2005b, 2005c, 2004), area M in Hiraba (2004)

cortical processing of facial movement			(-): recovered in the late phase (+): increased in the late phase	cortical processing of jaw and tongue movements			
unilateral facial SI	unilateral area C	unilateral area M	lesion site / Deficits caused in the early (late) phase / lesion site	unilateral intraoral SI	bilateral facial MA	bilateral intraoral MA	unilateral area P
+ (+)	- (-)	- (-)	delay of masticatory start	- (-)	- (-)	+ (-)	+ (-)
+ (-)	+ (-)	+ (-)	decreased food intake rate (dropping of food)	- (-)	- (-)	+ (+)	+ (+)
+ (+)	+ (+)	+ (+)	no erection of contralateral whiskers	- (-)	- (-)	- (-)	- (-)
- (+)	+ (-)	+ (-)	prolongation of ingestion period	+ (-)	+ (-)	+ (-)	+ (-)
- (-)	- (-)	- (-)	abnormal wide jaw-opening	- (-)	+ (+)	+ (+)	+ (+)
- (-)	- (-)	- (-)	abnormal tongue protrusion	- (-)	- (-)	- (-)	+ (+)
- (-)	- (-)	- (-)	rhythms of mastication and swallowing	- (-)	- (-)	- (-)	- (-)

(1) Deficits of Facial Movements

Table 1 shows the analysis based on data of cats with the unilateral lesion in the facial SI, area C and area M, respectively. Cats with the lesion in facial SI clearly showed a delay in masticaotry start after contact with the contralateral perioral hairs and dropping of food from the contralateral mouth. Furthermore, no erection of the contralateral whiskers during licking of cats with the facial SI lesion is shown by the decreased perioral tension. The deficit of no erection during licking was also observed in cats with other lesion in area C or area M. Although somatosensory information in the facial SI (area 3b) is utilized in the recognition of location depending on the perception, those in area C (area 3a) and area M (area 4∂) belonging in the motor cortical area may be translated to the motor information. Namely, area C transfers from static information in facial SI to a dynamic one, and then the information in area C is integrated with information for kinematic control in area M. Thus, a block of somatosensory information in the contralateral perioral region may be unable to produce the contraction of certain parts in the perioral region.

Cats with disorders will endeavor to recover with various strategies depending on the aspects of dyskinesia. Namely, the disorder after the facial SI lesion is not information for movement, but for localized perception, and the one after the area M is the recognition of location for activation. The disorder after the area C lesion may belong to the intermediate position between deficits in facial SI and area M. Since the deficits after the facial SI lesion are not dyskinesia, the prolongation of the ingestion period in the middle phase recovered quickly about one month after lesion, as described in Hiraba et al. (2000). However, prolongation after area C and area M lesions did not recover to the late phase. The increased masseter, digastric and genioglossus EMG activities were found after area M and area C lesions, as shown in the previous paper (Hiraba and Sato, 2005a). These findings suggest that information in area C may be confined to information for the jaw and tongue movements, and may not be separated by the local sensory information for facial movements from the somatosensory information in facial SI yet. Thus, separation from the total information in the facial region to the located information for movements may be finished in area M for exercise of the accurate motor command. We assume that the performance of cortical processing for facial movements built up with the integrated local somatosensory information in facial SI, area C and area M. Thus, facial SI recognizes the localization based on somasosensory information, area C converts it to information of localization of facial movements depending on the local recognition, and finally area M executes the adapted and detailed facial movements based on the modified information in area C, as shown by the schema in Figure 3A.

(2) Deficits of Tongue Movements

We tested for changes in orofacial behaviors and masticatory movements for about one month after the lesion was made in each projection area. If the unilateral lesion did not induce obvious changes in orofacial behaviors, we made another lesion in the same contralateral part and examined orofacial behaviors again for about one more month. Namely, we examined changes in orofacial behaviors during mastication of cats with the unilateral or bilateral lesion: the unilateral intraoral SI, bilateral facial MA of bilateral intraoral MA, and the unilateral area P.

(1) *Intraoral SI.* The deficit of the unilateral intraoral SI lesion cats showed the prolongation of ingestion period only, as shown in the previous paper (Hiraba et al., 2000). Although intraoral MRNs are divided into those with the contralateral RF (33%), bilateral RF (58%) and ipsilateral RF (9%), intraoral SI may be the contralateral dominant. In particular, the prolongation elicited in the early phase after the lesion, recovered up to the late phase (about one month), as shown in Table 1. The rapid prolongation of ingestion period produced by intraoral SI lesion cats, is the result of perceptual deficits in the tongue dorsum, since 58% have bilateral RFs. On the other hand, perceptual deficits in the tongue dorsum result in the prolongated ingestion period due to difficulty in stopping the cyclical masticatiory process. The function of intraoral SI during mastication is to control the timing for switching of continuous sensory feedback evoked by masticatory movements. Namely, somasosensory information during mastication in facial and intraoral SI may produce movements of the perceived location such as the perioral or lingual region.

(2) *Masticatory area (MA).* The unilateral facial MA or intraoral MA lesion cats showed the prolongation of ingestion period only, as well as the deficit of the intraoral SI lesion cats (Hiraba and Sato, 2005c). However, cats with lesions in the bilateral facial MA showed the prolongation of ingestion period and wide jaw-opening. Cats with the bilateral intraoral MA lesion showed disorders of decreased food intake rate due to dropping food from the mouth and delay of masticatory start, in addition to the deficits produced by the bilateral facial MA lesion cats, as shown in Table 1 and the previous paper (Hiraba and Sato, 2005c). The jaw-opening in the bilateral facial MA lesion cats might be interpreted as the lack of integrated somatosensory information. Namely, the rato of MRNs with bilateral mandibular receptive field markedly decreased after the first lesion (from 71% in normal cats before making first lesion to 30% in cats with the first lesion), as shown in the previous paper (Hiraba and Sato, 2005c). These findings suggest that sensory information in both MAs may also be processed by the callosal connection, as reported by Manzoni et al. (1989) and Iwamura (2000) in the somatosensory cortex. After recovery from the brain damage shown by the decrease of the jaw-opening, bilateral facial and intraoral MA lesion cats will became confused by the perceptions of sensory inputs that can integrate information of various parts of the facial skin or intraoral cavity in both MAs. When such cats cannot judge the magnitude or size of the bolus entering in the oral cavity following jaw-opening, they explore it with wide jaw-opening or with the increase of the space of the oral cavity. We consider that the adequate magnitude of the jaw-opening may mainly be decided by the integrated mandibular and intraoral sensory information.

(3) *Motor area (AREA P).* The unilateral area P lesion cats came into the deficit of abnormal tongue protrusion with wide jaw-opening observed by the bilateral intraoral MA lesion cats, as shown in Figure 4B and 4D. However, during licking milk in Figure 4B and licking fish paste in Figure 4D after the lesion, the degree of wide jaw-opening and abnormal tongue protrusion may be produced by different mechanisms. This is because activities of genioglossus muscles in unilateral area P lesion cats (Figure 4B and 4D) increased in comparison with them before the lesion (Figure 4A and 4C). Whereas the increase of the masseter and digastric EMGs showed negative effects, as shown in Figure 4. Thus, the wide jaw-opening after the unilateral area P lesion may be evoked by the interruption of information from bilateral MA. On the other hand, abnormal movements of jaw and tongue did not recover, although their prolongation of ingestion period and fluctuation of masticatory started to return to normal levels within one month. From these findings it is assumed that keeping the adequate tongue protrusion is regulated by bilateral area P, and applicable jaw-opening size is controlled by bilateral MA during licking, as shown in the previous paper (Hiraba and Sato, 2005c). However, since the jaw-movements of cats consists of opening and closing only without lateral movements (Hiiemae, 1987), we do not have any data related to jaw movements of cats.

For these reasons, we principally focused on the functional role of area P related to tongue movements.

Cortical Organization for Fine Tongue Movements

Tongue movements can be divided into two basal directions: the protrusion and retraction (vertical movements), and projection to the left and right (lateral movements). Namely, tongue protrusion is produced by the contraction of bilateral genioglossus muscles, and the projection to the left or right is executed by their unilateral contraction. So, we firstly organized the networks between bilateral area P for vertical movements and then the justice of networks is validated by the possible link to the lateral movements.

The detailed networks between the bilateral area P can be assumed by data from our reports: (1) The reciprocal connection between bilateral area P of both hemispheres according to anatomical researches with WGA-HRP (wheat germ agglutinin-horseradish peroxidase) was shown by Hiraba and Sato (2004). (2) Hiraba and Sato (2005b) showed characteristic changes in orofacial behaviors during mastication after the unilateral area P lesion: wide jaw-opening without the increased masseter and digastric EMG activities, and abnormal tongue protrusion with increased genioglossus EMG activities. (3) Furthermore, abnormal protrusion after the lesion is without deviation, as well as the tongue protrusion evoked by the C-ICMS (Hiraba and Sato, 2004 and 2005b). (4) On the other hand, Yasui et al. (1985b) reported that WGA-HRP injected in the unilateral trigeminal motor nucleus, projected at bilateral area P, and HRP-injection into the unilateral area P showed many positive terminals around the bilateral trigeminal motor and hypoglossal nuclei. (5) The unilateral hypoglossal nerve cutting showed deviation toward the affected side (Hiraba et al. 2002). Furthermore, we measured changes in the regional cerebral blood flow (rCBF) in the facial SI, area M and area P during trained lateral feeding (licking or chewing from the right or the left side) of milk, fish paste, and small dry fish. The rCBF in facial SI and area M showed contralateral dominance, and rCBF in area P during chewing or licking from the right or left side was almost the same value, as shown in our previous paper (Hiraba and Sato, 2005a). On the other hand, activities of genioglossus and masseter muscles in the left side showed almost the same values during ingestion of milk, fish paste, or small dry fish on the lateral feeding from the left or right side. These findings suggest that the cortical process for facial, jaw and tongue movements may be regulated by the contralateral dominance of area M and facial SI, and the bilateral one of area P.

These findings suggest that the unilateral area P is contained in L-PTs and R-PTs projected to the left or right hypoglossal nucleus at brain stem, and that the tongue will deviate to the left hand or right hand depending on the activated L-PTs or R-PTs in the bilateral area P. Thus, bilateral increased rCBF in area P is excited by the activation of L-PTs or R-PTs existing at bilateral area P.

Next, we will consider the organization for lateral (left and right hand) movements from cortical networks between area P based on vertical movements (protrusion and retraction).

(1) Cortico-Cortical and Cortico-Bulbar Connections

(1) *Facial movement.* In cats, Gosh (1997b) injected fluorescent tracers into various loci in area 4∂ in the ventral cortex of the cruciate sulcus including area M and reported that stronger labeling of cells was usually observed in area 3a, 1, 5 and insula, but labeling in area 2 was poor. Furthermore, the projection from somatosensory cortical areas in cats is topographically arranged, similar to hindlimb and forelimb areas of sensory cortex that project to different portions of postcruciate cortex concerned with the control of hindlimb and forlimb muscles, respectively (Jones and Powell, 1968; Kawamura and Otani, 1970). Furthermore, face representation is located in the rostral strip in the rostro-lateral part of precruciate area 4∂ (Yumiya and Ghez, 1984). Schwark et al. (1992) reported that there was a strong cortico-cortical connection from the central part of the coronal bank (area 3b) to the anterior part of the coronal sulcus (area 3a) in cats. These results suggested that somatosensory inputs evoked by mastication, were first projected via the ventrobasal complex (VB) of the thalamus to area 3b of the facial SI in the central part of the coronal sulcus, and then relayed to the area 4∂ of the facial motor cortex (area M) via area 3a in the anterior part of the coronal sulcus. On the other hand, it is known that the motor cortex receives one of its main inputs from the cerebellum through the ventrolateral nucleus (VL) of the thalamus (Evarts and Thach, 1969; Allem and Tsukahara, 1975; Rispal-Padel and Grangetto, 1977). Furthermore, Shinoda et al. (1992) reported that single thalamocortical axons from the cat VL project to the motor cortex located in the ventral cortex of the cruciate sulcus. Namely, the motor cortex (MI) in cats was assumed to be the localization of position for movements at the ventral cortex of the cruciate sulcus. Thus, it would appear that the MI received indirect inputs (via areas 3a and 3b in the facial SI) from the VB of the thalamus and direct inputs from the VL (Jones and Leavitt, 1973; Yumiya and Ghez, 1984; Shinoda et al, 1992). From these findings, it can also be considered that lesions in facial SI (area 3b) prevent the transfer of somatosensory information to area 4∂ (area M) via area 3a, and we reported the unilateral dominance, as shown in Figure 3A (Hiraba, 2004; Hiraba et al., 2007) and Figure 5.

(2) *Jaw and tongue movements.* We studied the distribution of projection fibers anterogradely, retrogradely and transsynaptically labelled with WGA-HRP injected into area P or MA. As shown in the summary schema of Figure 3B, WGA-HRP injected into area P or MA showed the bilateral projection (Hiraba and Sato, 2004).

Yasui et al. (1985a) reported anatomically in cats that corticoparabrachial fibers from the orbital gyrus (the region called MA by us) terminated most heavily in the medial parabrachial nucleus and less heavily in the lateral parabrachial nucleus. Furthermore, the MA in cats was found to send fibers to the rostral part of the nucleus of the solitary tract (Yasui et al. 1991). Whereas, the cortical region projecting directly to reticular regions around trigeminal motor nucleus and so on was detected into the presylvian sulcus (the region called area P by us) (Yasui et al. 1985b). Thus, the results in cats suggest that there are no connections between MA and the region around the motor nuclei in the brain stem directly.

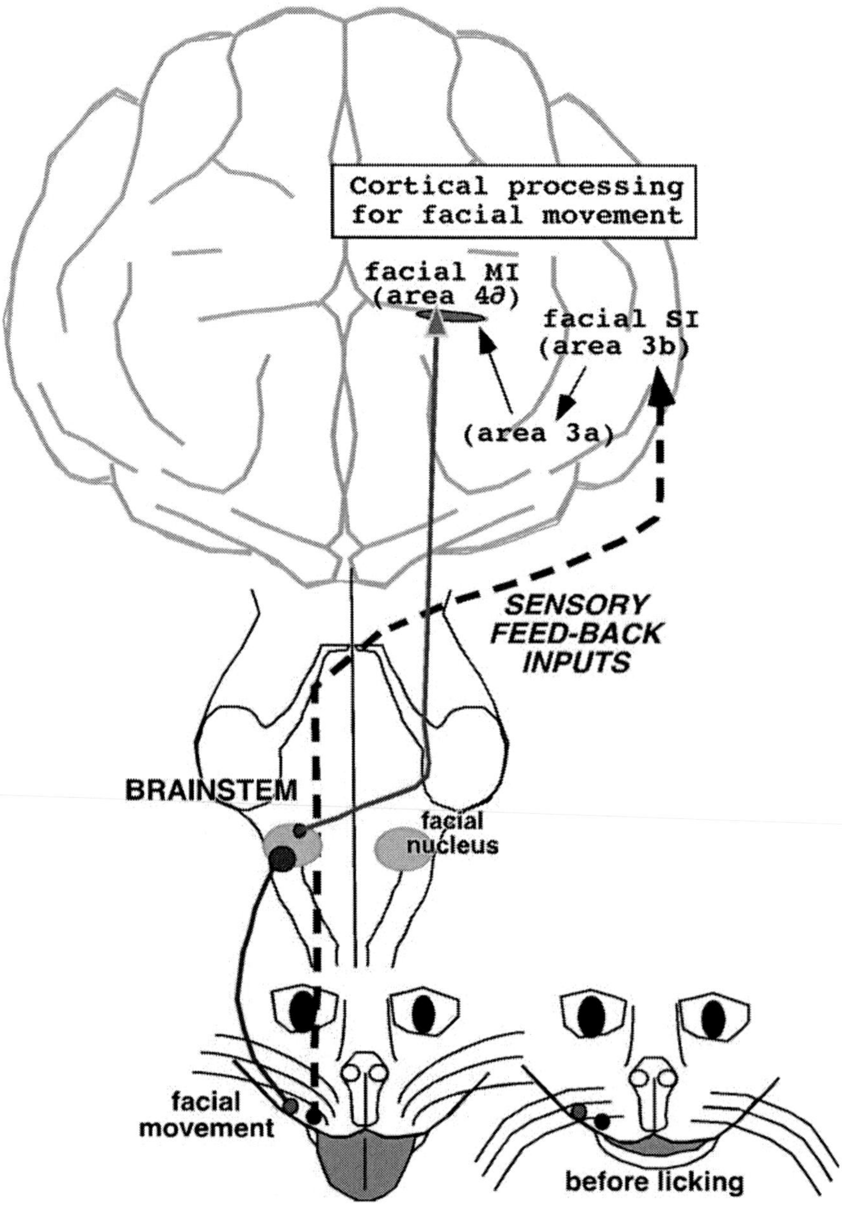

Figure 5. Schematic drawings of cortico-cortical pathway between facial SI and area M, and corticobulbar tracts for the facial movement. The details are given in the text. Note that complex projections to nuclei in the brain stem are omitted for simplification.

On the other hand, some of the cortico-fugal output from motor cortex projects directly to motor neurons in the spinal cord to activate muscle (Schwartz, 2007; Krakauer and Ghez, 2000). However, Yasui et al. (1985b) reported bilateral distribution of terminals into the reticular regions around the trigeminal motor and hypoglossal nucleus after the injection into the unilateral presylvian gyrus in cats. Although they did not state it clearly, their anatomical findings after the HRP injection into the presylvian gyrus (area P) indicated many terminals around the hypoglossal nucleus bilaterally (Yasui et al., 1985b). Thus, pyramidal neurons from area P did not show direct projection to each nucleus and a projection system of nuclei at the brain stem remains unclear. Since these complex projections to nuclei are not clear, we have shown schemas omitted for simplification of the network in the brain stem, as shown in Figures 5, 6 and 7.

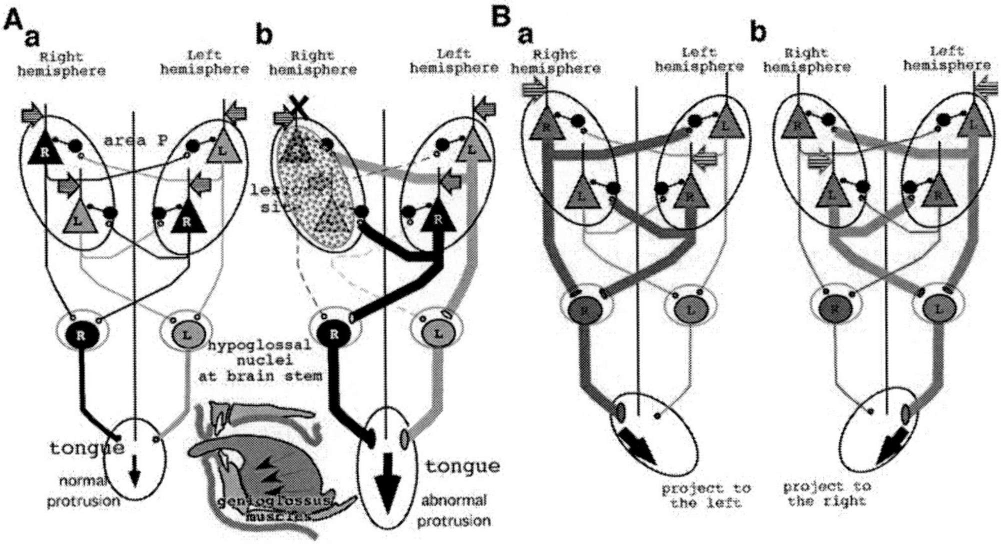

Figure 6. Schematic drawings of cortico-cortical pathway and corticobulbar tracts, and face, jaw and tongue projections. A. Area M that is related to facial movement, will be a contralateral dominance and the information will be relayed to a unilateral cortical pathway. Area P that is related to jaw and tongue movements, may include pyramidal neurons that apply to bilateral hypoglossal or trigeminal nuclei and the information will be relayed to the bilateral hemispheres. Note that complex projections to nuclei in the brainstem are omitted for simplification.

On the other hand, unilateral transcranial magnetic stimulation of the human motor cortex evoked EMGs in the tongue muscles bilaterally (Meyer et al., 1997), and functional magnetic resonance imaging (fMRI) of the lateral tongue movements in humans showed positive areas in the lateral MI (the primary motor cortex) and SI bilaterally (Wildgruber et al., 1996). A section of facial, trigeminal and hypoglossal nerves causes typical motor disorders for flaccid paralysis of the corresponding facial, jaw and tongue muscles on the side of the section: facial paralysis, chin deviation and tongue deviation (Duus, 1998; Hiraba et al., 2002). These findings suggest that each peripheral (facial, trigeminal motor and lingual) nerve is a unilateral predominance. Particularly, the unilateral tongue muscles are obviously controlled by outputs from both hemispheres (area P), based on various data (Yasui et al., 1985; Duus, 1998; Hiraba et al., 2002; Hiraba and Sato, 2005a and 2005b).

(2) Cortical Processing for Forelimb Movements

Asanuma and co-workers proposed input-output organization of neurons in the MI controlling a flexor of digits (Asanuma, 1973; Pavlides, 1993; Zarzecki et al., 1978; Asanuma et al., 1982), and Iwamura and co-workers proved the theory that the SI played an important role in the control of hand and arm movements (Hikosaka et al., 1985; Iwamura and Tanaka, 1991). Recently, Sessle et al. (2005) emphasized in their review that the intricate mastication and swallowing were executed by a close relationship between the face MI (orofacial area of MI), face SI (orofacial area of SI) and CMA (masticatory cortex) based on their extensive data (Huang et al., 1988, 1989a and 1989b; Murray et al., 1991; Narita et al., 2002; Yamamura et al., 2002; Lin et al., 1993a, 1993b, 1994a, 1994b and 1994c; Yao et al., 2002a and 2002b).

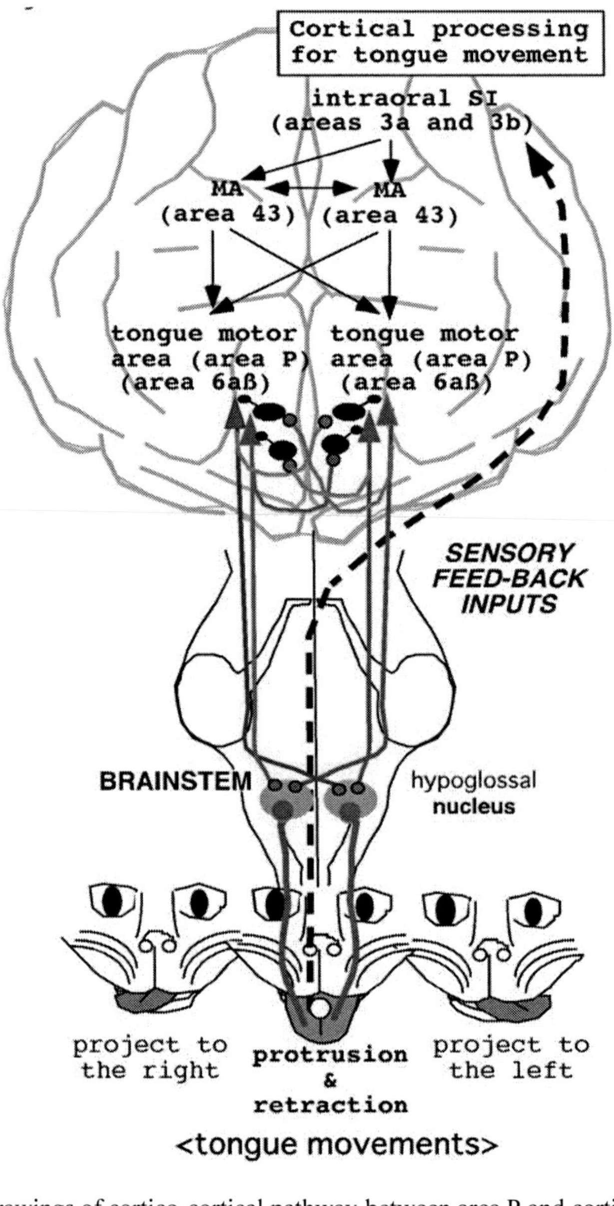

Figure 7. Schematic drawings of cortico-cortical pathway between area P and corticobulbar tracts for the tongue protrusion. Details are given in the text. Note that complex projections to nuclei in the brain stem are omitted for simplification.

Krakauer and Ghez (2000) report that the MI (Brodmann's area 4) executes movements and adapts them to new conditions, and the premotor area (PM, Brodmann's area 6) contributes to different aspects of motor planning. However, motor maps of the face and extremities can be delineated in the PM in monkeys, and unlike the MI where the stimulation typically evokes simple movements of single joint, stimulation of the PM often evoke more complex movements involving multiple joints and resembling natural coordinated hand shaping or reaching movements (Krakauer and Ghez, 2000). A detailed examination of the monkey face MI with the use of ICMS by Huang et al. (1989a) assumed that the monkey face MI had two characteristics as the MI evoking simple movements, such as facial twitch, tongue protrusion, jaw opening, and as the PM eliciting complex movements including rhythmical jaw movement. However, cortical organization for a fine separate movement in MI of the primate may not be necessary in comparison with the primates, since cat's jaw movements consist of opening and closing only, without lateral movements (Hiiemae, 1987).

(3) Cortical Organization for Tongue Movements

We showed the anatomical data between bilateral area P with the WGA-HRP method in our previous paper (Hiraba and Sato, 2004). In particular, there are reciprocal connections between bilateral area P. Furthermore, cats after the lesion in the unilateral area P produced abnormal tongue protrusion during licking. These findings are assumed to show the existence of the complex connection between bilateral area P, and between the cortex and hypoglossal nuclei, as shown in Figure 6A. Our schema of reciprocal connection between bilateral area P showed that R-PT (pyramidal cells in the area P projected to the hypoglossal nucleus in the right side of the brain stem), inhibited L-PT (pyramidal cell in the area P projected to the hypoglossal nucleus in the left side) existing in the contralateral area P. However, there are possibilities that R-PT (or L-PT) in the one side inhibits R-PT (or L-PT) in the other side. This idea may be negated by the conception of lateral movements, as shown in Figure 6B.

1) Schema Based on Tongue Protrusion

The C-ICMS in the unilateral area P evokes tongue protrusion without deviation, and tongue protrusion during mastication after the lesion is executed without deviation. On the other hand, cutting of the unilateral hypoglossal nerve produced deviation toward the affected side during the tongue protrusion. These findings suggested that motor neurons in the unilateral hypoglossal nucleus were homogeneous neurons: motor neurons in the right side of brain stem supplied the right side in the tongue, and the ones in the left side provided for the left side of the tongue. Namely, when we performed tongue protrusion, bilateral L-PTs and R-PTs within the bilateral area P projecting to the left or right hypoglossal nucleus resulted in increased activity level in bilateral area P simultaneously, as shown in Figure 6A-a. The increased activity in L-PT and R-PT of bilateral area P will be inhibited by each activity from area P in the other side, and accordingly the adequate tongue protrusion during licking will be determined.

Cats with the lesion in the unilateral area P showed the abnormal tongue protrusion with the increased activities of the genioglossus muscle (Figure 3 in Hiraba and Sato, 2005b, and Figure 4 in this paper). The lesion of unilateral area P will intercept the inhibition of the intact site, as shown in Figure 6A-b. Namely, each hypoglossal nucleus is supplied by the uninhibited real motor outputs. As a result, the abnormal tongue protrusion after unilateral lesion will be observed by the blocking of inhibitory interneurons, as shown in Figure 6A-b. Abnormal tongue protrusion after unilateral area P lesion was assumed to show the existence of the inhibitory neurons between L-PTs (or R-PTs) in one hemisphere and L-PTs (or R-PTs) in the other, or L-PTs (or R-PTs) in one side and R-PTs (or L-PTs) in the other. Namely, one schema exhibits existence of inhibitory interneuron between R-PTs in one hemisphere and L-PTs in the other one, as shown in Figure 6, and the other shows the existence of inhibitory interneurons between R-PTs in one side and contralateral R-PTs (not shown in figure). Although both schemas show the abnormal tongue protrusion during licking after the unilateral area P lesion, the latter idea has no effect on networks between area P for the lateral movements.

2) Schema Based on Lateral Movements

The balanced action of the paired genioglossal muscles is required to protrude the tongue straight out, as shown in the inside schema of Figure 6A. If one side of the genioglossal muscle is inactive, the action of the intact muscle is unopposed. The tongue then deviates toward the side of the inactive muscle (Wilson-Pauwel et al. 1988). However, when cats executed the left or right lateral movement of tongue, projection to the left or right is produced by the contraction of the ipsilateral genioglossal muscles, as shown in schema of Figure 6B-a and 6B-b. Namely, as shown in Figure 6B-a, when cats project the tongue to the left, activities of R-PTs in bilateral area P increase and they inhibit simultaneously activities of bilateral L-PTs in area P. The results produce activities of the right hypoglossal nucleus, not nucleus in the left. Finally, the tongue deviates toward the left side following the contraction of right genioglossal muscles, as shown in Figure 6B-a. The projection to the right is produced by the converse relation, as shown in Figure 6B-b. Thus, cortical organizations are based on neuronal networks of lateral movements, outputs from R-PT (or L-PT) in the right area P via fibers of the corpus callosum inhibit L-PT (or R-PT) in the left area P, as shown in the schema of Figure 6B. We proposed R-PT and L-PT connections relayed by the inhibitory interneuron between area P. On the other hand, the possibility of R-PT and R-PT or L-PT and L-PT connections was considered. From our results, connections of the same type will fail in terms of adequate lateral movements, although we have not shown this in the figure.

Thus, networks in cerebrum and brain stem can be summarized by the schema in Figure 7. Although we have drawn a projection system of somatosensory inputs from the intraoral structures to the orofacial SI, the detailed relay has been omitted.

ACKNOWLEDGEMENTS

The auther is grateful to Professor C.S. Langham for carefully reading and editing the manuscript. This work was supported in part by the Sato and Uemura Funds, Nihon University School of Dentistry, and by a grant from the Ministry of Education, Culture, Sports, Science, and Technology to promote multidisciplinary research projects.

REFERENCES

Allen, G.I. and Tukahara, N. (1975) Cerebrocerebellar communication systems. *Physiol. Rev.* 54: 957-1006.

Asanuma, H (1973) Cerebral cortical control of movement. *Physiologist* 16, 143-166.

Asanuma, H., Water, R.S. and Yumiya, H. (1982) Physiological properties of neurons projecting from area 3a to area 4 gamma of feline cerebral cortex. *J. Neurophysiol.* 48, 1048-1057.

Chandler, S.H. and Tal, M (1986) The effects of brain stem transactions on the neuronal networks responsible for rhythmical jaw muscle activity in the guinea pig. *J. Neurosci.* 6, 1831-1842.

Chandler, S.H., Goldberg, L.J. and Lamber, R.W. (1985a) The effects of orofacial input on spontaneously occurring and aponorphine-induced rhythmical jaw movements in the anesthetized guinea pig. *Neurosci. Lett.* 53, 45-49.

Chandler, S.H., Nielsen, S.A. and Goldberg, L.J. (1985b) The effects of a glycine antagonist (strychnine) on cortically induced rhythmical jaw movements in the anesthetized guinea pig. *Brain Res.* 325, 181-186.

Dellow, P.G. and Lund, J.P. (1971) Evidence for central timing of rhythmical mastication. *J. Physiol.* 215, 1-13.

Duus, P. (1998) *Topical diagnosis in neurology*. Anatomy, physiology, signs, symptom. New York, Thieme.

Enomoto, S., Katakura, N., Sunada, T., Katayama, T., Hirose, Y., Ishikawa, Y. and Nakamura, Y. (1987) Cortically induced masticatory rhythm in masseter motoneurons after blocking inhibition bu strychinie and tetamus toxin. *Neurosci. Res.*, 4, 369-412.

Enomoto, S., Kohase, H. and Nakamura, Y. (1995) Dual brain stem projection from the cortical masticatory area in guinea pig. *NeuroReport*. 6, 1573-1577.

Enomoto, S., Schwartz, G. and Lund, J.P. (1987) The effects of cortical ablation on mastication in the rabbit. *Neurosci. Lett.* 82, 162-166.

Evarts, E.V. and Thach, W.T. (1969) Motor mechanisms of the CNS: Cerebrocerebellar interactions. *Annu Rev. Physiol*. 31: 451-498.

Fritsch, G. and Hitzig, E. (1870) Über die elektrische Erregbarkeit des Grosshirns, *Archiv für Anatomie und Phyailolgie*, 37. 300-332.

Ghosh, D. (1997a) Identification of motor areas of the cat cerebral cortex based on studies of cortical stimulation and corticospinal commections. *J. Comp. Neurol.* 380, 191-214.

Ghosh, D (1997b) Comparison of the cortical connections of 4∂ in cats cerebral cortex. *J. Comp. Neurol.* 388, 371-396.

Goldberg, L.J. and Tal, M. (1978) Intracellular recording in trigeminal motoneurons of the anesthetized guinea pig during rhythmic jaw movements. *Exp. Neurol.* 58, 102-111.

Goldberg, L.J., Chandler, S.H. and Tal, M. (1982) Relationship between jaw movements and trigeminal motoneuron membrane potential fluctuations during cortically induced rhythmical jaw movements in the guinea pig. *J. Neurophysiol.* 48, 110-125.

Guandalini, P., Franchi, G. amd Spidalieri, G. (1990) Low threshold unilateral and bilateral facial movements evoked by motor cortex stimulation in cats. *Brain Res.* 508, 273-280.

Hassler, R. und Muhs-Clement, K. (1964) Architektonischer aufbau des sensomotorischen und parietalen cortex der katze. *J. Hirnforasch.* 6, 377-420.

Hidaka, O., Morimoto, T., Masuda, Y., Kato, T., Matuo, R., Inoue, T., Kobauashi, M. and Takada, K. (1997) Regulation of masticatory force during cortically induced rhythmic jaw movements in the anesthetized rabbit. *J. Neurophysiol.* 77, 3168-3179.

Hiiemae, K.M. (1987) Mammalian mastication: a review of the activity of the jaw muscles and the movements they produce in chewing. In *Development, Function and Evolution of teeth,* P.M. Butler and K.A. Jovsey, eds., pp. 359-398, Academic Press, London.

Hikosaka, O., Tanaka, M., Sakamoto, M., and Iwamura, Y. (1985) Deficits in manipulative behaviors induced by local injections of muscimol in the first somatosensory cortex of the conscious monkey. *Brain Res.* 325, 375-380.

Hiraba, H. (1999) Function of the orofacial SI during mastication in awake cats: changes in masticatory movements and activities of mastication-related neurons in motor cortices following a lesion in the orofacial SI awake cats. In: *Neurobiology and Mastication-From mokesular to System Approach,* Y Nakamura and B,J, Sessle, eds., pp.494-503, Elsevier, Amsterdam.

Hiraba, H. and Sato, T. (2005a) Cerebral control of face, jaw, and tongue movements in awake cats: Changes in regional cerebral blood flow during lateral feeding. *Somatosens. Mot. Res.* 22, 307-317.

Hiraba, H. and Sato, T. (2005b) Cortical control of mastication in cats. 2. Deficits of masticatory movements following a lesion in the motor cortex. *Somatosens. Mot. Res.* 22, 183-192.

Hiraba, H. and Sato, T. (2005c) Cortical control for mastication in cats: Changes in masticatory movements following lesions in the masticatory cortex. *Somatosens. Mot. Res.* 22, 171-181.

Hiraba, H. (2004) The function of sensory information from the first somatosensory cortex for facial movements during ingestion in cats. *Somatosens. Mot. Res.* 21, 87-97.

Hiraba, H. and Sato, T. (2004) Cortical control of mastication in the cat. –Properties of mastication-related neurons in motor and masticatory cortices. *Somatosens. Mot. Res.* 21, 217-227.

Hiraba, H., Sato, T., Manabe, K., Hori, M., Imura, S. and Tanaka, H. (2002) Changes in activities of the jaw and tongue muscles following severance of the unilateral hypoglossal nerve (medial branch) in awake cats. *Kisoshika Igakukai Zasshi*, 44,90-105 (Japanese).

Hiraba, H., Sato, T., Manabe, K., Hori, M., Imura, S. and Tanaka, H. (2002) Changes in activities of the jaw and tongue muscles following severance of the unilateral hypoglossal nerve (medial branch) in awake cats. *Kisoshika Igakukai Zasshi*, 44,90-105 (Japanese).

Hiraba, H., Yamaguchi, Y. Sato, H., Ishibashi, Y. and Iwamura, Y. (2000) Deficits of masticatory movements caused by lesions in the orofacial somatosensory cortex of the awake cat. *Somatosens. Mot. Res*. 17, 361-372.

Hiraba, H., Yamaguchi, Y. and Iwamura, Y. (1997) Mastication-related neurons in the orofacial first somatosensory cortex of awake cats. *Somatosen. Mot. Res*. 14, 126-137.

Hiraba, H., Yamaguchi, Y. Yoshida, T and Kamogawa, H. (1996) Activities of mastication-related neurons in (MRNs) the orofacial motor, sensory and masticatory cortical areas of conscious cats. *Shika Kiso Igakushi Zasshi* 38, 549-563 (in Japanese).

Hiraba, H., Yoshida, T., Yamaguchi, Y., Kamogawa, H. and Oishi, T. (1993) Neuronal activity in three oro-facial motor cortical areas of conscious cats during mastication. *Shika Kiso Igakushi Zasshi* 35, 386-401 (in Japanese).

Hiraba, H., Yoshida, T., Yamaguchi, Y., Oishi, T., Fujita, S., Kamogawa, H. and Kondo, M. (1994) Activity of mastication related neurons in the masticatory cortex of awake cats. *Shika Kiso Igakushi Zasshi* 36, 406-419 (in Japanese).

Hoffman, D.S. and Luschei E.S. (1980) Responses of monkey precentral cortical cells during a controlled jaw bite task. *J. Neurophysiol*. 44, 333-343.

Huang, C.-S., Hiraba, H., Murray, G.M. and Sessle, B.J. (1989a) Topographical distribution and functional properties of cortically induced rhythmical jaw movements in the monkey (Macava fasciularis). *J. Neurophysiol*. 61, 635-650.

Huang, D.-S., Hiraba, H. and Sessle, B.J. (1989b) Input-output relationships of the primary face motor cortex in the monkey (macaca fascicularis). *J. Neurophysiol*. 61, 350-362.

Huang, C.-S., Sirisko, M.A., Hiraba, H., Murray, G.M. and Sessle, B.J. (1988) Organization of the primate face motor cortex as revealed by intracortical microstimulatiom and electropjysiological identification of afferent inputs and corticobulbar projections. *J. Neurophysiol.* 59, 796-818.

Inoue, T., Kato, T., Masuda, Y., Nakamura, T., Kawamura, Y. and Morimoto, T. (1989) Modifications of masticatory behavior after trigeminal deafferentation in the rabbit. *Exp. Brain Res*. 74, 579-591.

Iwamura, Y. (2000) Bilateral receptive field neurons and callosal connections in the somatosensory cortex. *Phil. Trans. R. Soc*. Lond B. 355, 267-273.

Iwamura, Y. (1998) Hierachial somatosensory processing. *Curr. Opian Neurobiol*. 8, 522-528.

Iwamura, Y. and Tanaka, M. (1991) Organization of the first somatosensory cortex for manipulation of objects: an analysis of behavioral changes induced by muscimol injection into identified cortical loci of awake monkeys. In *information processing in the somatosensory system*, O. Franz and J.Westman, eds., pp.371-380, Hampshire, UK.

Iwamura, Y. and Tanaka, M. (1978) Functional organization of receptive fields in the cat somatosensory cortex. I: Integration within the coronal region. *Brain Res*. 151, 49-60.

Iwata, K., Muramatu, H., Tsuboi, Y. and Sumino, R. (1990) Input-output relationships in the jaw and orofacial motor zones of the cat cerebral cortex. *Brain Res*. 507, 337-340.

Iwata, K., Itoga, H., Ikukawa, A., Hanashima, N. and Sumino, R. (1985) Movements of the jaw and orofacial regions evoked by stimulation of two different cortical areas in cats. *Brain Res*. 418, 198-187.

Jones, E.J. and Leauvitt, L.Y. (1973) Demonstration of thalamo-cortical connectivity in the cat somato-sensory system by retrograde axonal transport of hoseradish peroxidase. *Brain Res* 63; 414-418.

Jones, E.J. and Powell, T.P.L. (1968) The ipsilateral cortical connections of the somatic sensory area in the cat. *Brain Res*. 418c: 183-187.

Jones, E.J. and Peters, A. (1986) Cerebral cortex. Vol. 5 *Sensory-Motor Areas and Aspects of cortical Connectivity*. Plenum Press, New York.

Kawamura, Y. and Tukamoto, S. (1961) Analysis of jaw movements from the cortical jaw motor area and amygdala. *Jpn. J. Physiol*. 10, 471-488.

Kawamura, K. and Otani, K. (1970) Corticocortical fiber connections in the cerebrum: the frontal region. *J Comp Neurol*. 139: 423-448.

Krakauer, J. and Ghez, C. (2000) Voluntary Movement. In: Kandel, E.R., Schwartz, J.H. and Jessell, T.M. eds., *Princeiples of neuronal science*, 4th edn, pp. 756-781,Mc Graw Hill, New York.

Larson, C.R., Byrd, E.F., Garthwaite, C.R. and Luschei, E.S. (1980) Alteration in the pattern of mastication after ablation of the lateral precentral cortex in rhesus macaques. *Exp. Neurol.* 70, 638-651.

Lin, L.-D., and Sessle, B.J. (1994a) Functional properties of single neurons in the primate face primary somatosensory cortex. III. Modulation of Responses to peripheral stimuli during trained orofacial motor behaviors. *J. Neurophysiol*. 71, 2401-2413.

Lin, L.-D., Murray, G.M. and Sessle, B.J. (1994b) Functional properties of single neurons in the primate face primary somatosensory cortex. II. Relations with different directions of trained tongue protrusion. *J. Neurophysiol*. 71, 2391-2400.

Lin, L.-D., Murray, G.M. and Sessle, B.J. (1994c) Functional properties of single neurons in the primate face primary somatosensory cortex. I. Relations with trained orofacial motor behaviors. *J. Neurophysiol*. 71, 2377-2390.

Lin, L.-D., Murray, G.M. and Sessle, B.J. (1993a) The effect of bilateral cold block of the primate face primary somatosensory cortex on the performance of trained tongue-protrusion task and biting tasks. *J. Neurophysiol*. 70, 985-996.

Liu, Z.J., Masuda, Y., Inoue, T., Fuchihata, H., Sumida, A., Takada, A. and Morimoto, T. (1993b) Coordination of cortically induced rhythmical jaw and tongue movements in the rabbit. *J. Neurophysiol*. 69, 569-584.

Lund, J.P., Sasamoto, K., Murakami, T. and Olsson, K.A. (1984) Analysis of rhythmical jaw movements produced by electrical stimulation of motor-sensory cortex of rabbits. *J. Neurophysiol.* 52, 1014-1029.

Lund, J.P. and Lamarre, Y. (1974) Activity of neurons in the lower precentral cortex during voluntary and rhythmical jaw movements in the monkey. Exp. Brain Res. 19, 289-299

Lund, J.P. and Dellow, P.G. (1971) The influence of interactive stimuli on rhythmical masticatory movements in rabbits. *Arch. Oral Biol.* 16, 325-223?.

Luschei, E.S. and Goldberg, I.J. (1981) Neural maechanisms of mandibular control: Mastication and voluntary biting. In: Brooks, V.B., editor. *Handbook of Physiology*, Sec.

1: Neurophysiology, Vol. II: Motor control. Washiongton, American Physiological society, pp 1237-1274.

Luschei, E.S. and Goodwin, G.M. (1975) Role of monkey precentral cortex in control of voluntary jaw movements. *J. Neurophysiol.* 38, 146-157.

Magoun, H.M., Ranson, S.W. and Fisher, C. (1933) Corticofugal pathways from mastication, lapping and other motor function in the cats. *Arch. Neurol. Psychiat.* (Chicago) 30, 292-308.

Meyer, B-U., Liebsch, R. and Roricht, S. (1997) Tongue motor responses following transcranial magnetic stimulation of the motor cortex and proximal hypoglossal nerve in man. *Electroencephalog. Clinical Neurophysiol.* 105, 15-23.

Monnier, M. and Will, H. (1953) Die integrative tatigkeit des nervensystems bein neso-rhombo-sponalen Anencephasius (Mittelhirnwen) 1. Physiologisch-klinischer Til. Mxchr. *Osychial. Neurol.*, 126, 239-258.

Morimoto, T and Kawamura, Y. (1973) Properties of tongue and jaw movments elicited by stimulation of the orbital gyrus of the cat. *Arch. Oral Biol.* 18, 361-372.

Murray, G.M., Lin, L.-D., Moustafa, M. and Sessle, B.J. (1991) Effects of reversible inactivation by coolng of the primate face motor cortex on the perfomance of a trained tongue-protrusion task and a trained biting task. *J. Neurophysiol.* 65, 511-530.

Nakamura, Y. and Katakura, N. (1995) Generation of masticatory rhythm in the brainstem. *Neurosci Res.* 23, 1-9.

Nakamura, Y. and Kubo, Y. (1978) Masticatory rhythm in intracellular potential of trigeminal motoneurons induced by stimulation of orbital cortex and amygdala in cats. *Brain Res.* 148, 504-509.

Nakamura, Y., Kubo, Y., Nozaki, S., and Takatori, M. (1976) Cortically induced masticatory cats. *Bull. Tokyo Med. Dent. Univ.* 23, 101-107.

Narita N., Yamamura, K., Yao, D., Martin, R.E., Masuda, Y. and Sessle, B.J. (2002) Effects on mastication of reversible bilateral inactivation of the lateral pericentral cortex in the monkey (Macaca fascicularis). *Archs. Oral Biol.* 47, 673-688.

Nozaki, S., Iriki, A., and Nakamura, Y. (1993) Trigeminal premotor neurons in the bulbar parvocellular reticular formation participating in induction of rhythmical activity of trigeminal motorneurons by repetitive stimulation of the cerebral cortex in the guinea pig. *J. Neurophysiol.* 69, 595-608.

Nozaki, S., Iriki, A., and Nakamura, Y. (1991) Brainstem commissural systems for bilateral synchronization of rhythmical jaw muscle induced by stimulation of the cortical mastictory area in the guinea pig. *Dent. Jpn.* 28, 39-43.

Nozaki, S., Iriki, A., and Nakamura, Y. (1986a) Role of corticobulbarl projection neurons in cortically induced rhythmical masticatory jaw-opening movement in the guinea pig. *J. Neurophysiol.* 55, 826-835.

Nozaki, S., Iriki, A., and Nakamura, Y. (1986b) Localization of central rhythm generator involved in cortically induced rhythmical masticatory jaw-opening movement in the guinea pig. *J. Neurophysiol.* 55, 806-825.

Pavlides, C., Miyashita, E. and Asanuma, H. (1993) Projection from the sensory to the motor cortex is important in learning motor skills in the monkey. *J. Neurophysiol.* 70, 733-741.

Penfield, J. and Rassmussen, T. (1950) *Cerebral cortex of man. A clinical study of localization of function*. pp. 77-86. Macmillan, New York.

Rioch, J.M. (1934) The neuronal mechanism of mastication. *Am. J. Physiol.* 108, 168-176.

Rispal-Padel, L. and Grangetto, A. (1977) The cerebello- thalamo-cortical pathway. Topographical investigation ar the unitary level in the cat. *Exp. Brain Res.* 28; 101-123.

Sasamoto, K., Zhang, G. and Iwasaki, M. (1990) Two types of rhythmical jaw movements evoked by stimulation of the rat cortex. *Jap. J. Physiol.* 32, 57-68.

Schwarts, G., Enomoto, S., Valiquette, C. and Lund J.P. (1989) Mastication in the rabbit: a description of movement and muscle activity. *J. Neurophysiol.* 62, 273-287.

Schwartz, A.B. (2007) Useful signals from motor cortex. *J. Physiol.* 579, 581-601.

Sessle,B.J., Yao, D., Nishiura, H., Yoshino, K., Lee, J.C., Martin, R.E. and Murray, G.M. (2005) Properties and plasticity of the primate somatosensory and motor cortex related to orofacial sensorimotor function. *Clin. Exp. Pharmacol. Physiol.* 32, 109-114.

Schwark, H.D., Estery, H. and Jones, E.D. (1992) Corticocortical connections of cat primary somatosensory cortex. *Exp. Brain Res.* 91: 425-434.

Shinoda, Y., Futami, T. and Kakei, S. (1992) Inputs from the cerebellar nuclei in the forelimb area of the motor cortex. In: Control of Arm Movement in Space. *Neurophysiological and Computational Approaches*. R. Caminitti, P.B. Johanson and Y. Burnod, eds, pp. 65-84, Springer-Verlan, Berlin.

Sumi, T. (1969) Some properties of cortically-induced swallowing and chewing in rabbits. *Brain Res.* 15, 107-120.

Toda, T. and Taoka M. (2002) Hierachial somesthetic processing of tongue inputs in the postcentral somatosensory cortec of conscious macaque monkeys. *Exp. Brain* Res. 147, 243-251.

Vogt, C. and Vogt, O. (1926) Die vergleichend-architektonische und die vergleichend-reizphysiologische felderung der grosshirnrinde unter besonderer bericksichtigung der menschlichen. *Naturalwissenschaften* 14, 1190-1194.

Wildgruber, D., Ackermann, H., Klose, U., Kardarzki, B. and Grodd, W. (1996) Functional lateralization of speech production at primary motor cortex: a fMRN study. *Neuroreport* 7, 2791-2795.

Wilson-Pauwels, L., Akesson, E.J., and Stewart P.A. (1988) XII Hypoglossal nerve. In: *Cranial nerves, anatomy and clinical comments*, L. Wilson-Pauwels, E.J. Akesson and P.A. Stewart, eds., pp148-151

Woolsey, C.N. (1958) Organization of somatic sensoru and motor areas of the cerebral cortex. In: *Biological and Biochemical bases of Behavior*, H.F. Harlow, and C.N. Woolsey, eds., pp. 63-81, Univ of Wisconsin Oress, Madison.

Yamamura, K., Narita, N., Yao, D., Martin, R.E., Masuda, Y. and Sessle, B.J. (2002) Effects of reversible bilateral inactivation of face primary motor cortex on mastication and swallowing. *Brain Res.* 944. 40-55.

Yao, D., Yamamura, K., Narita N., Murray, G.M. and Sessle, B.J. (2002a) Effects of reversible cold block of face primary somatosensory cortex on orofacial movements and related face primary motor cortex neuronal activity. *Somatosen. Mot. Res.* 19, 261-271.

Yao, D., Yamamura, K., Narita, N., Martin, R.E., Murray, G.M. and Sessle, B.J. (2002b) Neuronal activity patterns in primate primary motor cortex related to trained or semiautomatic jaw and tongue movements. *J. Neurophysiol.* 87, 2531-2541.

Yasui Y, Ito K, Kaneko T, Shigenoto R, Mizuno N (1991) Topographical projection from the cerebral cortex in the nucleus of the solitary tract in cat. *Exp. Brain Res.* 85; 75-84.

Yasui Y, Ito K, Takada M, Mitani A, Kaneko T, Mizuno N (1985a) Direct cortical projection in the parabracjial nucleus in the cat. *J. Comp. Neurol.* 234; 77-86.

Yasui, Y., Ito, K., Mirani, A., Takada, M. and Mizuno, N. (1985b) Cerebral cortex projections to the reticular regions around the trigeminal motor nucleus in the cat. *J. Com. Neurol.* 241, 348-356.

Yumiya, H. and Ghez, C. (1984) Specialization subregions in the cortx: anatomical demonstration of differential projections and cusal sections. *Exp. Brain Res.* 53: 259-276.

Zarzecki, P., Shinoda, Y. and Asanuma, H. (1978) Projection from area 3a to the motor cortex by neurons activated from group I muscle afferents. *Exp. Brain Res.* 13, 269-282.

In: Brain Mapping Research Developments
Editor: Lars N. Bakker, pp. 73-100

ISBN 978-1-60456-007-7

Chapter III

ROLE OF THE CORPUS CALLOSUM IN THE INTERHEMISPHERIC TRANSFER OF SOMATOSENSORY INFORMATION: AN FMRI STUDY

Mara Fabri* and Gabriele Polonara [#]

*Dipartimento di Neuroscienze, Sezione di Fisiologia and
[#]Istituto di Radiologia;
Facoltà di Medicina, Università Politecnica delle Marche,
Via Tronto 10/A, 60020 Ancona, Italy.

ABSTRACT

This chapter reviews the functional magnetic resonance imaging (fMRI) studies carried out by the authors' group in the past 10 years to elucidate the role of the human corpus callosum (CC) in the interhemispheric transfer of somatosensory information.

Functional studies using various techniques (somatosensory evoked potentials, magneto-encephalography, positron emission tomography) have shown that unilateral tactile stimulation evokes bilateral activation in two cortical regions involved in the processing of tactile stimuli: the posterior parietal (PP) cortex in the postcentral gyrus, containing the first somatic sensory area, and the parietal operculum in the upper bank of the Sylvian sulcus, containing the second somatic sensory area (SII).

The pathways by which sensory afferents reach the ipsilateral cortices are still unknown. It is a widely held view that the CC transfers sensory information by relaying it to the somatic sensory areas of the contralateral hemisphere. The "callosal recrossing" hypothesis is supported by experiments on the callosal connectivity of homologous cortical regions of non-human primates and other mammals.

The fMRI researches described here were organized as follows:

1. a "normal" activation pattern was established by investigating cortical somatic sensory areas in normal volunteers, who received unilateral moving tactile stimulation of the hand and fingers or of the ventral trunk surface;
2. the "callosal recrossing" hypothesis was tested by performing the same studies in patients subjected to surgical resection of the CC to control medically intractable epilepsy;
3. the possible role of the CC in mediating pain-related ipsilateral cortical activation was investigated by analyzing the pattern of cortical activation evoked by painful mechanical stimulation in normal volunteers and in three patients with complete CC resection.

Results point to the following conclusions: the CC is mainly responsible for somatic sensory cortex bilateral activation evoked by unilateral tactile stimulation of the hand and fingers. Callosal fibres carrying activation to the ipsilateral PP cortex and SII cross in the posterior third of the body of the commissure, anterior to the splenium. By contrast, ipsilateral activation evoked by tactile trunk and painful hand stimulation is at least partially independent of callosal transmission, being probably mediated by extracallosal pathways: uncrossed subcortical pathways, subcortical commissures, or both.

INTRODUCTION

One of the major and as yet unexplained features of the organization of the central nervous system is that each brain hemisphere receives afferents mainly from the contralateral, i.e. opposite side of the body (Amaral, 2000). One consequence is that each somatic sensory cortical area in each hemisphere contains the peripheral representation of the contralateral hemibody (Kaas, 1983; Kaas et al., 2002), and discontinuities may occur in processing of stimuli that move from one side of the sensory space to the other. Some body regions, i.e. the midline territories, are represented in both hemispheres. Such bilateral representation could be a way to ensure anatomical and functional continuity.

In animals with bilateral symmetry, the midline is the imaginary line dividing the body into two mirror halves. In sensory physiology, midline territories are the cutaneous regions straddling the midsagittal plane and forming a central strip of somatosensory space lacking lateralization, found close to the geometric midline (Manzoni et al., 1989). Sensory midline regions are represented in the first somatic sensory cortex (SI) of both hemispheres in cats (Manzoni et al., 1980), macaque monkeys (Conti et al., 1986; Taoka et al., 1998; Iwamura et al., 2001), and man (Fabri et al., 2005b). In humans, tactile stimulation of ventral midline territories also evokes bilateral activation of the second somatic sensory cortex (SII; Fabri at al., 2005b).

The pathways by which tactile stimuli from the trunk region reach the ipsilateral postcentral gyrus (PCG) are unknown. Neuroanatomical animal studies combining electrophysiological recording and neuronal tracing have shown that in the trunk representation zone both axon terminals and cell bodies of callosal projecting neurons are concentrated in SI, in areas where bilateral receptive field (RF) cells are especially numerous, namely on the borders of cytoarchitectonic areas 3a-3b, 3b-1 and 1-2 in monkeys (Conti et al., 1986) and in areas 3b and 2 in cats (Manzoni et al., 1980). These findings suggested that the ipsilateral component of bilateral RFs might have a callosal origin (for a review see Manzoni et al., 1989, 1997), a hypothesis that has subsequently been confirmed in animal studies also of non-human primates (Iwamura et al., 1994; see Manzoni, 1997, and Iwamura et al., 2001, for a review), although a direct demonstration has not yet been provided in these species.

Other observations are consistent with the alternative hypothesis of an extracallosal origin of bilateral RFs. Neurons with bilateral RFs straddling the trunk midline have been described in the cat thalamic ventrobasal nucleus (Barbaresi et al., 1984) and dorsal column nuclei (Cheema et al., 1983) and in the rat spinal cord (Smith, 1986), suggesting a subcortical contribution to ipsilateral RFs, at least in these species.

In primates the hands, in addition to midline territories, are often activated together during daily activities, suggesting a possible bilateral representation also for these regions. In humans, several studies performed with somatosensory evoked potentials (SEP; Lüders et al., 1985; Allison et al., 1989; Hämäläinen et al., 1990; Kany and Treede, 1997; Mima et al., 1997; Frot and Mauguière, 1999; Kagiki et a., 2000), magneto-encephalography (MEG; Hari et al., 1983, 1990, 1993; Kaukoranta et al., 1986; Forss et al,. 1994a,b; Schnitzler et al., 1995; Hoshiyama et al,. 1997; Mima et al., 1997; Forss and Jousmaki, 1998; Hari and Forss, 1999; Kovernoja et al., 1999), positron emission tomography (PET; Burton et al., 1993, 1997; Ledberg et al., 1995) and functional magnetic resonance imaging (fMRI; Boecker et al., 1995; Lin et al., 1996; Davis et al., 1998; Disbrow et al., 1998; Gelnar et al., 1998; Maldjian et al., 1999; Polonara et al., 1999) have shown that unilateral tactile stimulation of the hand evokes bilateral activation in two main cortical regions involved in processing tactile stimuli, one in the posterior parietal cortex (PPC) and the other in the parietal operculum (PO; Polonara et al., 1999; for a review, see Manzoni, 1997). The former region lies in the PCG around the postcentral sulcus (PCS), posterior and medial to the anterior parietal cortex (APC) forming the posterior bank of the central sulcus (CS) and containing area SI; the PPC probably includes cytoarchitectonic areas 2 and 5-7. The second region lies in the PO in the cortex forming the upper bank of the Sylvian sulcus (SS) and is commonly identified with area SII (Burton, 1986, 2002).

The pathways by which sensory afferents reach ipsilateral PO and PPC are still largely unknown. A widely held view is that they do so via the corpus callosum (CC) after relaying in the somatic sensory areas of the contralateral hemisphere. Indeed, latency studies showed that ipsilateral activation is delayed in both cortical fields compared with that of contralateral homotopic regions by a time-lag compatible with interhemispheric transmission time (Allison et al., 1989; Hari et al., 1993; Coghill et al., 1994; Forss et al., 1994a). Experiments on the callosal connectivity of homologous cortical regions of non-human primates and other mammals support the callosal recrossing hypothesis (see Manzoni, 1997).

Bilateral cortical activation of human area SII in PO is also evoked by painful stimulation, as shown by PET, MEG, laser evoked potentials (LEP), and, recently, fMRI studies. In normal subjects unilateral painful stimulation generally induced activation of SII in both hemispheres (Casey et al., 1994; Kitamura et al., 1995; Xu et al., 1997; Disbrow et al., 1998; Gelnar et al., 1999; see Treede et al., 1999, for a review). In some investigations area SII was activated in parallel with SI (Svensson et al., 1997; Ploner et al., 1999), while in others activation occurred also in absence of SI recruitment (Lenz et al., 1998; Frot et al.,

1999); moreover, the latencies of activation of contralateral SI and SII and of ipsilateral SII were very similar. Such pain-induced simultaneous activation of contralateral and ipsilateral SII, likely by means of extracallosal pathways (Frot and Mauguière, 1999; Kanda et al., 2000; Ploner et al., 2000), and the fact that patients with lesions involving the PO report altered pain sensitivity (Greenspan and Winfield, 1992; Potagas et al., 1997; Greenspan et al., 1999) suggest that area SII may have a primary role in pain processing.

The area also participates in tactile information processing. Animal studies have suggested its involvement in tactile learning and retention (Garcha and Ettlinger, 1980) as well as in the integration of afferents from the two body halves (see Hari and Forss, 1999, for a review). For all these reasons it is interesting to explore whether the somatosensory modalities of touch and pain may share a common mechanism of SII activation in the two hemispheres.

Functional MRI studies carried out by our group in the last 10 years have investigated the neural mechanism of the bilateral activation of the hand and trunk zones, particularly the role of the human CC. Functional MRI is a safe and non-invasive method to study brain function *in vivo*. Particular attention was devoted to the bilateral activation of somatic sensory areas evoked by tactile stimulation of body regions with different anatomical and functional characteristics (hand and trunk), to assess the role of the commissure in the interhemispheric transfer of somatosensory inputs. The corpus callosum links the hemispheres and provides for interhemispheric integration and transfer of information (Gazzaniga, 2000). Post-mortem human studies and data from non-human primates suggest that the CC is topographically organized. This organization seems to result in modality-specific regions: the anterior fibres, which connect the frontal lobes, transfer motor information, whereas the posterior fibres, which connect the temporal, parietal and occipital lobes, are involved in the integration of somatosensory (posterior midbody), auditory (isthmus), and visual (splenium) information (see data and literature in Fabri et al., 2005a).

We first investigated the neural mechanisms underpinning the bilateral activation of somatic sensory cortices elicited by unilateral tactile stimulation of the hand. This activation pattern was then compared with the activation evoked by unilateral painful stimulation of the hand. We then recorded the bilateral activation induced by tactile stimulation of tactile trunk receptors close to the ventral midline, and finally compared this activation pattern with that evoked by hand tactile receptor stimulation. The choice of the hand and trunk regions was based on their anatomo-functional characteristics. The trunk midline is the territory where the two halves of the body join and whose cortical representation shifts from one hemisphere to the other (anatomical midline); in contrast, the hands are far removed from one another, but since they are often mobilized together they need to be coordinated (functional midline). The studies described here emphasize the results obtained in a special type of subjects, a group of callosotomized patients, who provide a valuable model to investigate human brain function in living "experimental" preparations. The fMRI studies were organized as follows:

(1) cortical somatic sensory areas were investigated in normal volunteers, who received unilateral moving tactile stimuli on hand and fingers to obtain a "normal activation pattern",

(2) to verify the callosal recrossing hypothesis, the study was also performed in a group of patients subjected to surgical resection of the CC to control medically intractable epilepsy. Subsequently, a patient requiring a second callosotomy accepted to be studied before and after the operation, where the posterior part of the trunk and the splenium of the CC were resected; this patient thus served both as a "control" and as an "experimental" subject;

(3) to establish whether the CC contribution depends on the sensory modality, i.e., whether ipsilateral pain-related cortical activation might be mediated by the CC, the pattern of cortical activation evoked by painful mechanical stimulation of the hand was investigated in a group of normal volunteers and in three patients with complete CC resection;

(4) to evaluate whether the CC contribution might depend on body regions within the same sensory modality, the activation pattern of cortical somatic sensory areas was investigated in normal volunteers and in a group of callosotomized patients who received unilateral moving tactile stimuli on ventral trunk surfaces;

(5) finally, a group of callosotomized patients underwent specific neuropsychological tests evaluating interhemispheric tactile transfer to compare functional with behavioural data.

SUBJECTS

Each part of the research involved control subjects and callosotomized patients. Some patients participated in a single study and others in two or three. The data of all patients are reported in Table I.

Touch Studies - Hand

This part of the research was performed on 12 healthy volunteers (7 F, 5 M aged 21 to 59 years; control group) and on 12 callosotomized patients (5 F, 7 M aged 19 to 49 years) with total or partial callosal resection (Quattrini et al., 1989, 1997). Three patients had complete resection of the callosum; in one the caudalmost part of the splenium was intact; in 7 the entire splenium and, to a variable extent, the posterior part of the body were spared, while in the last patient, the splenium and the posterior part of the body had been resected. Patients were studied 1 to 11 years from callosotomy. All subjects but three (2 controls and 1 patient) were right-handed as determined by the Edinburgh handedness inventory (Oldfield, 1971). In this patient group, post-operative IQ scores to Wechsler Adult Inteligence Scale (WAIS) testing ranged from 70 to 93. The study was also performed in a 40-year old male patient who underwent CC resection in two stages: the anterior two thirds of the body were resected in the first operation and the posterior third of the body and the splenium were resected 15 months later. This patient was tested one week before, and 6 and 12 months after the second surgical session (see Fabri et al., 2001).

Table I. Characteristics of the callosotomized patients and studies in which participated

Subject	Gender	Handedness (Oldfield score)	Age at surgery§	IQ	Callosal resection	Hand touch*	Hand pain*	Trunk touch*	Transfer tests*
L.P.	F	right (10)	20	70	anterior	3		9	5
P.M.	M	right (10)	21	70	anterior	3		9	5
A.P.	M	right (10)	28	87	anterior	4		11	6
R.V.	M	left (46)	19	70	anterior	8		14	
R.F.	M	right (12)	38	70	anterior	8			
C.Q.	M	left (45)	21	82	anterior	5			
G.B.	M	right (14)	46	80	anterior	3			
M.C.	M	right (10)	40	88	posterior	1		4	1
M.R.	F	right (10)	25	70	posterior#	1			
D.B.	F	right (10)	31	92	subtotal	10			
D.D.C.	M	right (14)	19	83	total		2	9	4
D.D.V.	M	right (10)	22	81	total	11	13	14	12
R.N.	F	right (10)	31	93	total	6	7		7
F.B.	F	right (14)	16	70	total	3		8	

§years.
*years from surgery.
#M.R. required a second callosotomy and now has total CC resection.

Pain Study – Hand

We studied 6 healthy volunteers (3 F, 3 M aged 34 to 44 years; control group) and 3 patients (1 F, 2 M aged 21 to 38 years) who had undergone complete CC resection 3 to 13 years previously. All subjects were right-handed. Patients' post-operative IQ scores (WAIS test) ranged from 81 to 93.

Touch Studies - Trunk

For this part of the research the control group was made up of 10 healthy volunteers (6 F, 4 M aged 22 to 29 years); patients were 2 females and 6 males (age 28 to 42 years) with complete or partial CC resection performed 4 to 14 years earlier. Callosal resection was complete in 3 patients, partial posterior in 1, and partial anterior in the remaining 4; in 2 of the latter patients only the splenium was spared and in the other two both the splenium and the posterior third of the callosal body. Details on the clinical history and extent of callosal resection have been reported previously (Quattrini et al., 1989, 1997). All subjects but one (a patient) were right-handed. Patients' post-operative IQ scores (WAIS test) ranged from 70 to 88. All these patients also participated in the touch studies with hand stimulation.

Neuropsychological Study

This part of the investigation involved 20 healthy subjects (13 F, 7 M aged 22 to 40 years) and 7 patients (2 females; aged 24 to 40 years) who were studied 1 to 12 years from callosotomy. Three patients had partial anterior callosal resection, three had complete callosal resection and one patient was studied before and after posterior callosotomy. All patients were right-handed; their post-operative IQ scores (WAIS test) ranged from 70 to 93. All these patients also participated in the functional hand touch study.

Control subjects and patients gave their informed consent to participate in the studies. The experimental protocols were approved by the Ethical Committee of Università Politecnica delle Marche (Ancona, Italy) and complied with the Code of Ethics of the World Medical Association (Declaration of Helsinki).

Imaging Protocols

Subjects participating in hand touch and pain studies were placed in a 1.0-Tesla (T) scanner (Signa Horizon, General Electric Medical System, Milwaukee, WI, USA) equipped with 23 mT/m gradients. Their head was restrained within a standard polarized head coil.

The experimental procedure consisted of three steps: the first involved the acquisition of an anatomical sagittal localizer (SPGR, scan time 31 s) to inspect the callosal resection and select section levels; during the second step the acquisition of functional MR images was performed using a single-shot T2*-weighted gradient-echo EPI sequence (scan time 2:30

min) in coronal planes orthogonal to the sagittal plane and parallel to the floor of the IV ventricle. Coronal sections allow clear recognition of the SS and the PO cortex containing SII. Five hundred coronal functional images were acquired during the stimulation cycle from 10 contiguous 7-mm-thick coronal sections (50 images *per* section, 1 image/3 s). Activation maps were obtained from functional images with the blood oxygenation level-dependent contrast (BOLD) method. The third step consisted of the acquisition of high-resolution anatomical images (SPGR, scan time 3:17 min for 10 images) in the same coronal plane so that the functional images could be superimposed on the anatomical images; the latter also allow visualization of blood vessels, which are possible sources of BOLD signal. The second and third steps were repeated to acquire functional images from axial sections, which allowed to identify the CS and PCG. The axial planes were orthogonal to both the sagittal and the coronal planes.

Participants in the trunk touch study were placed in a 1.5-T scanner (Signa LX NV/i, General Electric Medical System) equipped with 50 mT/m gradients. Their head was restrained within a circularly polarized head coil. The experimental procedure consisted of the three steps described above. In addition, a 3D data set (IR Prep Fast SPGR, slice thickness 0.7 mm, scan time 12 min) was also acquired. In this study 1000 functional images were acquired during the stimulation cycle (scan time 5:12 min; 100 images *per* section, 1 image/3 s) from the 10 contiguous 5-mm-thick axial sections selected under the first step.

STIMULATION PARADIGM

Tactile stimulation of the hand consisted of brushing the subject's palm and fingers with a rough sponge at a frequency of about 1 Hz. In 8 of the 12 patients, stimulation was applied first to the right and then to the left hand during different scans; in control subjects and in the remaining 4 patients, the stimuli were applied only to the right hand. The experimental paradigm lasted 2:30 min and consisted of 5 alternating 30-s periods of rest and stimulation (see Polonara et al., 1999; Fabri et al., 1999, 2001).

Painful stimulation of the hand was obtained by pricking the palm skin with a sharp wooden probe (tip diameter 0.4-0.5 mm) at 1-s intervals to evoke pinprick pain. This kind of stimulus has been shown to be effective in activating both high-threshold mechanoreceptors with myelinated fibres (Aδ) and polymodal nociceptors with unmyelinated fibres (C; Perl, 1984, 2007). In 2 of the 3 patients and in 4 of the 6 controls, stimulation was applied first to the right and then to the left hand during different scans; in the remaining patient and the 2 controls only the right hand was stimulated. This paradigm consisted of 5 alternating 30-s periods of rest and stimulation (Fabri et al., 2002).

Tactile stimulation of the trunk consisted of gently rubbing 20 x 10 cm skin areas of the ventral medial trunk surface, close to the midline but not reaching or abutting on it, between two imaginary horizontal lines crossing the umbilicus and the nipples, respectively. Stimulation of this skin area likely involves cutaneous receptors of dermatomes from Th4 to Th10. The stimulus was applied with a soft cotton pad (frequency 1 Hz) using a block-design experimental paradigm lasting 5 min and consisting of 10 alternating 30-s periods of rest and stimulation. In 7 of the 8 patients the stimulus was applied first to the left and then to the right side of the ventral trunk in two different scans; in the remaining patients and in control subjects it was applied only to the left side (Fabri et al., 2005b, 2006). Owing to the subjects' position in the magnet, the stimulus was applied only to the ventral, not the dorsal trunk surface.

In all studies, the experimenter made the same movements 10-15 cm above the patient's body also during rest periods as a control for stimulus-related signal intensity changes (Yetkin et al., 1996).

Neuropsychological Tests

Some of the patients were administered three tests devised to evaluate the interhemispheric transfer of somatosensory information: Tactile Naming Test (TNT), Same-Different Recognition Test (S-DRT), and intra- and intermanual Tactile Finger Localization Test (TFLT). They were studied 1-12 years after surgery. The tests were administered in a quiet room with the subjects seated in front of the experimenter. Objects were presented out of view and placed on a soft board to avoid possible cross-cueing from noise. Chance-level performance was calculated based on the number of stimulus alternatives.

The TNT evaluates the ability to name tactile stimuli presented only to the right hemisphere (left hand; for a detailed description of the procedure see Fabri et al., 1999, 2001, 2005a). The S-DRT indicates whether the patient can cross-compare tactile stimuli separately presented to the two hemispheres. Patients are required to simultaneously explore manually two common objects held in each hand and to say whether they are the same or different objects. This decision requires the interhemispheric transfer of tactile information (Myers and Sperry, 1985; Geffen et al., 1985; Aglioti et al., 1998; Fabri et al., 2001, 2005a). The TFLT assesses the ability to localize tactile stimuli applied to the proximal or distal phalanx of the fingers of one hand and to transfer the information to the opposite hand (Aglioti et al., 1998; Fabri et al., 2001, 2005a).

Data Analysis

At the end of the experimental sessions, the images were transferred to a Unix workstation (General Electric Advantage Windows 1.2 for hand studies, 4.4 for trunk studies). Data were analyzed with different softwares: Functool (a custom-designed General Electric software), BrainVoyager package (BV; Brain Innovation, QX, Maastricht, The Netherlands) and Statistical Parametric Mapping software (SPM2; Wellcome Department of Imaging Neuroscience, Institute of Neurology, University College London, UK).

In brief, the first two images of each functional series were discarded. Data from each subject were processed to remove noise and artefacts. In BV analysis, the functional images of each patient were overlaid on the 2D anatomical images and incorporated into their 3D data sets through trilinear interpolation. Data were then transformed into Talairach space (Talairach and Tournoux, 1988). Preprocessing of functional scans included 3D motion correction. SPM2 analysis included preprocessing to remove movement artefacts (spatial realignment of images), to co-register coplanar and echoplanar images to the high-resolution image. Data were then resampled into 2-mm isotropic voxels and warped into a standardized atlas space (normalization; Talairach and Tournoux, 1988). Individual scans were adjusted to the Talairach coordinate system to identify the position of activated areas.

Somatic sensory areas were identified by analyzing their localization according to standard anatomical landmarks (e.g. the omega-shaped CS in axial views) and reference atlases (Duvernoy, 1991; Mai et al., 1997). For each subject, a maximum intensity projection (MIP) was displayed on a glass brain in three orthogonal planes and normalized to the Talairach template.

When the signal increase in the selected regions of interest (ROIs) - lying in areas corresponding anatomically to SI (in PCG) and the second somatic sensory area (SII; in PO) in the upper bank of the Sylvian sulcus (SS) - correlated temporally with the stimulation pattern, activation was assumed to be evoked by the tactile or painful stimulus. Averaged time courses were calculated within each ROI in order to show the mean BOLD signal change due to the stimulus. The BOLD signal change was expressed as a percentage of baseline. Mean signal increases in patients and controls were compared using a two-tailed t test (a P value > 0.05 was considered not significant).

Neuropsychological test scores were expressed as proportion of correct answers. The results of the intramanual TFLT task were considered as control scores and the values of the two hands pooled in a single mean value. Results were divided into control, total and partial callosotomy group. Differences in the performances of groups were analyzed using the chi-square test for independent data and the t-test.

Results from Touch Studies: Hand Stimulation

Control Subjects

In all control subjects, cortical activation due to unilateral tactile stimulation of the hand was consistently observed in the following somatic sensory areas (for a detailed description, see Polonara et al., 1999):

- in the contralateral APC, anteriorly in the PCG, just posterior to the CS. This focus likely corresponds to the hand representation zone of SI (Figure 1A, 1, focus 1);
- in the PPC of both hemispheres, posteriorly in the PCG, just anterior to the PCS, a region likely corresponding to cytoarchitectonic areas 2 and 5-7 (Figure 1A, 1, foci 2, contralateral, and 3, ipsilateral);
- in the PO cortex of both hemispheres, in a cortical region of the upper bank of the SS, which contains SII (Figure 1B, 1, foci 6, contralateral, and 7, ipsilateral).

TABLE II. Functional MRI data and neuropsychological test results of callosotomized patients

Subject	Hand touch stimulation		Hand pain stimulation		Trunk touch stimulation		Neuropsychological tests*		
	PCG activation	PO activation	PCG activation	PO activation	PCG activation	PO activation	TNT left hand	S-DRT	TFLT intermanual°
L.P.	contralateral	bilateral			bilateral	bilateral	100	95	98
P.M.	bilateral	bilateral			bilateral	bilateral	93	100	98
A.P.	contralateral	contralateral			bilateral	bilateral	100	100	100
R.V.	contralateral	contralateral			bilateral	bilateral			
R.F.	contralateral	contralateral							
C.Q.	contralateral	contralateral							
G.B.	contralateral	contralateral							
M.C.	contralateral	contralateral			bilateral	bilateral	16	24	18
M.R.	contralateral	contralateral							
D.B.	contralateral	contralateral							
D.D.C.	contralateral	contralateral	contralateral	bilateral	bilateral	bilateral	60	100	76
D.D.V.	contralateral	contralateral	bilateral	bilateral	bilateral	bilateral	15	55	80
R.N.	contralateral	contralateral	contralateral	bilateral			14	50	85
F.B.	contralateral	contralateral			bilateral	bilateral			

*proportion of correct answers.

°mean of right and left hand responses.

These results confirmed those obtained in previous functional studies (Allison et al., 1989; Burton et al., 1997; Kovernoja et al., 1999; see also the literature in Fabri et al., 1999).

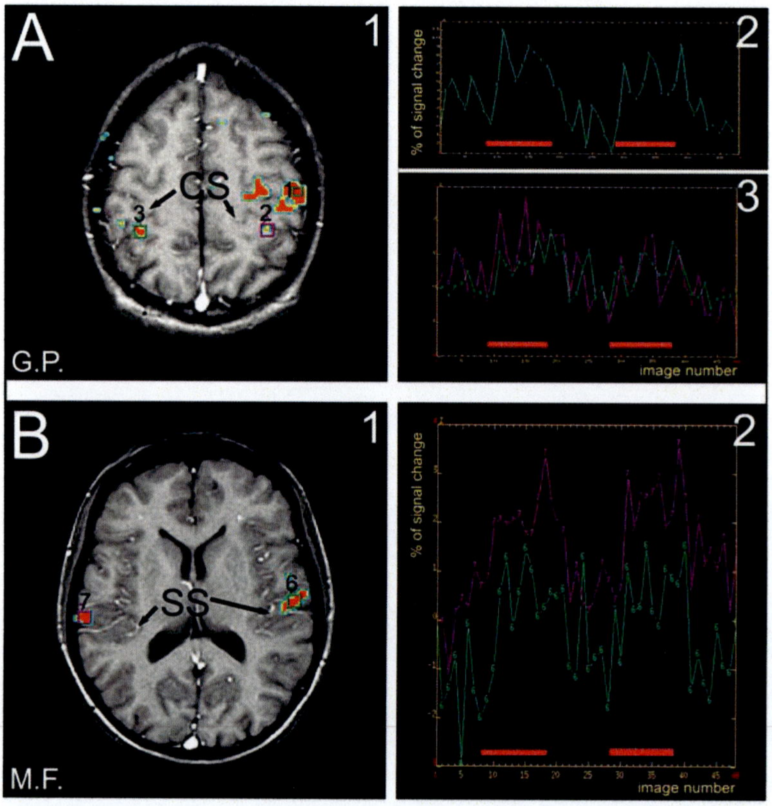

Figure 1. Cortical activation by unilateral tactile stimulation of one hand obtained in representative control subjects. Left hemisphere on the right. *A1,* Axial image obtained from a SPGR T1-weighted sequence on which regions activated during tactile stimulation have been superimposed. A region of interest (ROI) was placed on an activated region in the anterior parietal cortex presumably corresponding to SI hand representation (box 1). Two ROIs were placed on two activated cortical regions of the posterior parietal cortex, one in the contralateral (box 2) and one in the ipsilateral (box 3) hemisphere. *A2*, graph illustrating the signal increase in the ROI shown in A1. The X axis reports the progressive number of the images acquired (one image/3 s) and therefore represents a time scale in s; the Y axis is a scale where signal changes are expressed as the percentage of the signal obtained from the brain during the rest periods. Usually, the first value recorded was taken as 0%. In the two 30-s stimulation periods (images 8-18 and 28-38 on the X axis), the signal increased by about 5% above the baseline. Red bars indicate the stimulation periods. *A3*, graphs illustrating the signal increase in ROIs 2 and 3 shown in A1. *B1*, axial image from a different control subject showing activation foci in the parietal operculum, in a region likely corresponding to SII. ROIs indicated by boxes 6 and 7 are from the contralateral and the ipsilateral hemisphere, respectively. *B2*, graphs 6 (green) and 7 (red) show the signal changes in corresponding ROIs 6 and 7 selected in B1. CS, central sulcus; SS Sylvian sulcus. Modified from Polonara et al., 1999.

Callosotomized Subjects

Midsagittal MR slices from the 12 callosotomized subjects showed CC surgical resection to be complete in 3 patients and partial in the other 9. Accordingly, subjects were assigned to the *total* and the *partial callosotomy* subgroups, respectively. The activation and neuropsychological data of the patients participating in the different studies are reported in Table II.

Total Callosotomy

In these 3 patients, the activation pattern in the hemisphere contralateral to the hand receiving the stimulus was similar to that obtained in control subjects, activation foci being consistently observed in the APC, PPC and PO and, occasionally, in the precentral and medial frontal cortices. Conversely, tactile stimulation of the hand failed to elicit activation foci in the ipsilateral hemisphere, unlike the pattern observed in control subjects (Figure 2A, 2). The cortical activation pattern obtained in these subjects during stimulation of one hand was the mirror image of the pattern induced by stimulation of the other hand (see Fabri et al., 1999).

Partial Callosotomy

In all 9 patients of this subgroup, stimulation of one hand resulted in a pattern of contralateral activation that was similar to the one obtained in control and callosotomized subjects. Contralateral activation foci were consistently observed in the APC, PPC and PO.

Ipsilateral activation was absent in 7 patients, while it was observed in the PO cortex in one subject and in the PO and PPC in the ninth.

Of the 7 patients lacking ipsilateral activation, one still retained a small portion of the splenium, one the rostral 2/3 of the CC and 2 the entire splenium. In the remaining 3 subjects the posterior region of the CC had been spared. However, since the borders between the different portions of the CC cannot be established with certainty, it is unclear whether in the last 3 subjects a part of the posterior body of the CC was also extant, besides the splenium. In the 2 patients in whom unilateral hand tactile stimulation did induce ipsilateral activation in PO or PO and PPC, the spared portion of the CC included the entire splenium and probably also the posterior part of the body (Figure 2B, 1). The data from one of these patients, showing activation in the ipsilateral PO cortex, are reported in Figures 2B, 2,3 (see Fabri et al., 1999).

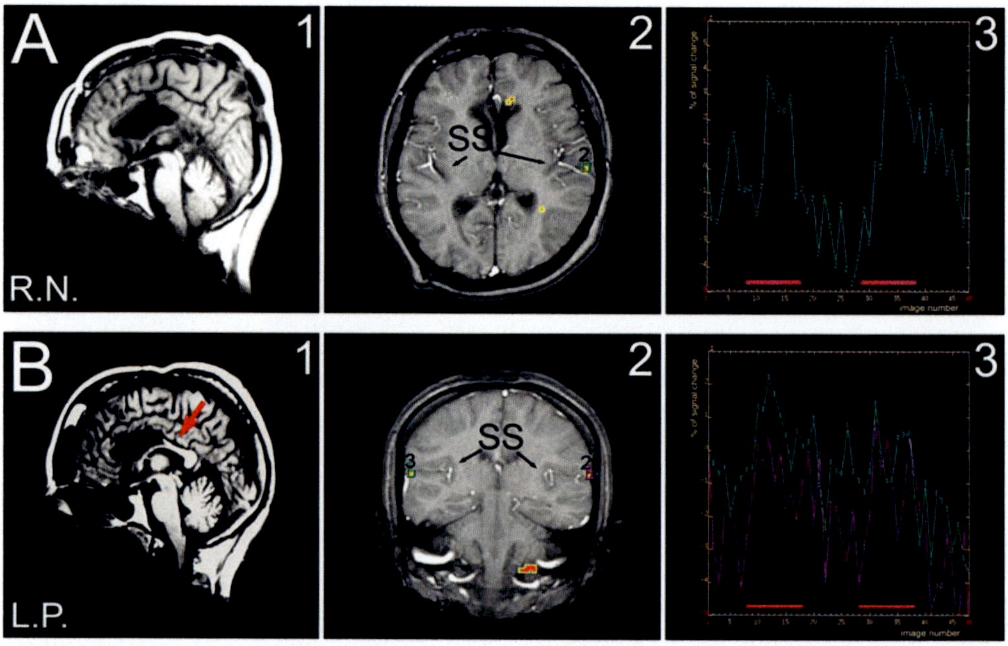

Figure 2. Cortical activation by unilateral tactile stimulation of one hand obtained in two callosotomized patients with total (A) and partial (B) callosal resection, respectively. Left hemisphere on the right. *A1*, MR images of midsagittal brain slices obtained from T1-weighted spin-echo sequences showing the absence of CC in patient R.N. *A2,* axial image showing activation in the contralateral PO (box 2). *A3*, graph showing the signal increase in ROI 2 of B2. *B1*, MR images of midsagittal brain slices showing the extent of callosal resection in patient L.P. Red arrow points to the spared posterior body. *B2*, coronal image showing an activation focus in contralateral (box 2) and ipsilateral (box 3) PO. *B3*, graphs showing the signal increase in ROIs 2 (graph 2) and 3 (graph 3) of C2. In this and in the adjacent sections no activation was detected in the ipsilateral PO. CS, central sulcus; SS, Sylvian sulcus. Modified from Fabri et al., 1999.

Also in these patients, the cortical activation pattern obtained during stimulation of one hand was the mirror image of the pattern induced by stimulation of the other. During our investigations, a patient requiring a second callosotomy due to drug-refractory epilepsy accepted to be studied before and after surgery. Activation due to unilateral tactile stimulation of the hand was explored with fMRI one week before the second operation and 6 months and one year afterwards. Before this operation, tactile stimulation of either hand activated the contralateral PPC and areas SI and SII as well as ipsilateral PPC and SII (Figure 3A, 2, 3). In both postoperative sessions, somatosensory activation was detected in contralateral SI, SII and the PPC, but failed to be recorded in ipsilateral SII and PPC (Figure 3B, 2,3). This case provides direct demonstration of the hypothesis that the posterior third of the body of the CC is crucial for interhemispheric transfer of hand somatosensory information, as strongly suggested by previous data (for a detailed description, see Fabri et al., 2001).

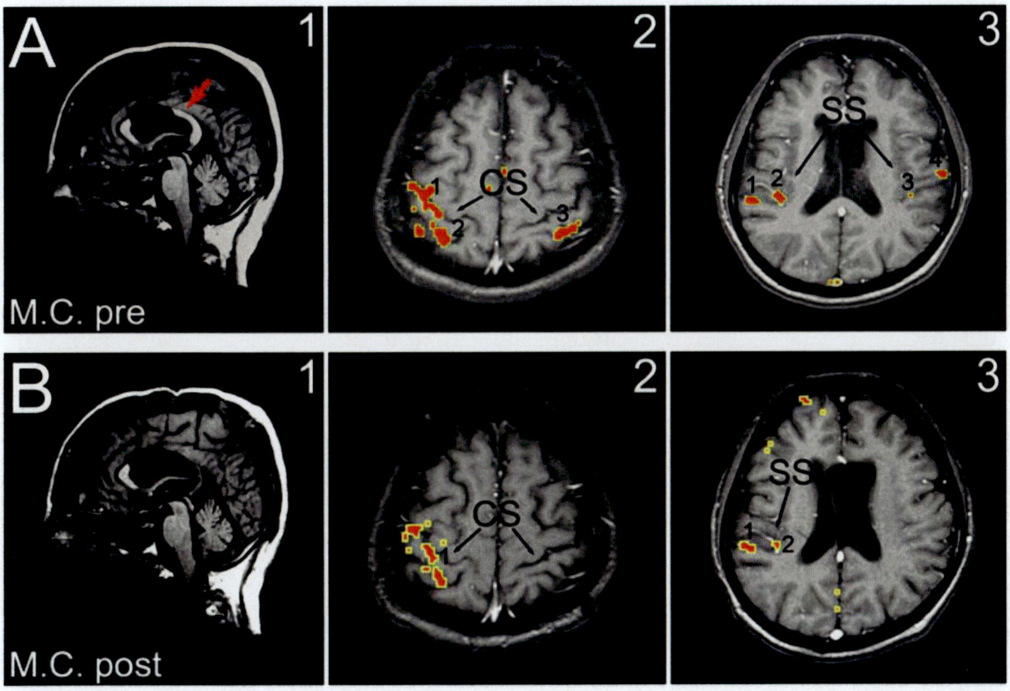

Figure 3. Cortical activation by unilateral tactile stimulation of left hand obtained in patient M.C. before and after posterior callosotomy. Left hemisphere on the right. *A1*, MR image of a midsagittal brain slice obtained with a T1-weighted spin-echo sequence showing the extent of callosal resection before the second operation. Red arrow marks the extant posterior body of the commissure. *A2*, axial image obtained from a SPGR T1-weighted sequence on which the regions activated during tactile stimulation (obtained from a gradient-echo T2*-weighted single-shot EPI sequence) have been superimposed. Main activation foci were in the contralateral APC (1) and in the contralateral (2) and ipsilateral (3) PPC. *A3*: axial image obtained as in A2 from a more ventral level, showing activation foci in contralateral (1, 2) and ipsilateral (3, 4) PO. *B1*, MR image obtained as in A1, showing the extent of callosal resection after the second operation. *B2*, axial image obtained as in A2, on which the regions activated during tactile stimulation have been superimposed. Main activation foci were in the contralateral APC (1) and PPC (2). In this and in the adjacent sections no activation was detected in the ipsilateral PPC. *B3*, axial image obtained as in A3 on which the regions activated during tactile stimulation have been superimposed. The same, main activation foci were identified in the contralateral PO (1, 2) only. CS, central sulcus; SS, Sylvian sulcus. Modified from Fabri et al., 2001.

Results from Pain Studies: Hand Stimulation

Control Subjects

Cortical activation due to painful mechanical stimulation of one hand was in line with previous studies and was consistently observed in the following areas (Frot and Mauguière, 1999; Ploner et al., 2000):

- in the contralateral APC, anteriorly in the PCG, just posterior to the CS;
- in the PPC of both hemispheres, posteriorly in the PCG, just anterior to the PCS;
- in the PO cortex of both hemispheres, in a cortical region in the upper bank of the SS, which contains SII (Figure 4A,2);
- in the cingulate (Cin) cortex of the contralateral (5 cases) and ipsilateral (2 cases) hemispheres;
- in the insular cortex of the contralateral (4 cases) and ipsilateral (2 cases) hemispheres.

Callosotomized Patients

Contralateral activation was observed in the PO in all patients (Figure 4B,2, foci 1,2), in the APC in 2 cases and in the PPC in 1 case; the insular cortex was activated in 1 patient. The ipsilateral PO was also activated in all patients (Figure 4B,2, focus 3), the insular cortex in 1 and the PP in another, whereas the APC and the cingulate cortex were never activated.

A preliminary analysis of these data indicates that painful stimulation of either hand activated similar regions of the PO in both hemispheres, and generally evoked activation foci in PO regions more anterior and/or more medial than those activated by tactile stimulation (compare, for example, pain-evoked focus 2 in Figure 4A,2 and touch-evoked focus 1 in Figure 4A,1).

This study indicates that the activation evoked by painful stimulation of the hand in ipsilateral SII is at least partially independent of the CC, suggesting that painful and tactile stimuli might use different pathways to reach the same PO target area (Fabri et al., 2002).

Results from Touch Studies: Trunk Stimulation

Control Subjects

Cortical activation due to tactile stimulation of the trunk surface was consistently observed:

- in the APC of both hemispheres, anteriorly in the PCG, just posterior to the CS, when the ventromedial surface was stimulated, and solely in the contralateral hemisphere when the lateral surface was stimulated. This focus likely corresponds to the trunk representation zone of SI (Figure 5A,2, foci 1, contralateral, and 2, ipsilateral). These results agree with data from non-human primates (Manzoni et al., 1989);
- in the PO cortex of both hemispheres, in a cortical region in the upper bank of the SS, which contains SII (Figure 5A,3, foci 1 contralateral, and 2, ipsilateral).

These data showed for the first time that in man, as in non-human primates, the trunk regions close to the midline are represented bilaterally in SI.

Callosotomized Subjects

In the patient with an intact splenium and posterior callosal body and in the two with partial anterior resection sparing only the callosal splenium, unilateral stimulation of medial ventral trunk evoked cortical activation in the PCG (Figure 5B,2) and PO of both hemispheres (Figure 5B,3), as in control subjects.

The patient with partial posterior callosotomy displayed bilateral cortical activation in area SI when stimulation was applied to the right ventral trunk and contralateral activation when it was applied to the left side.

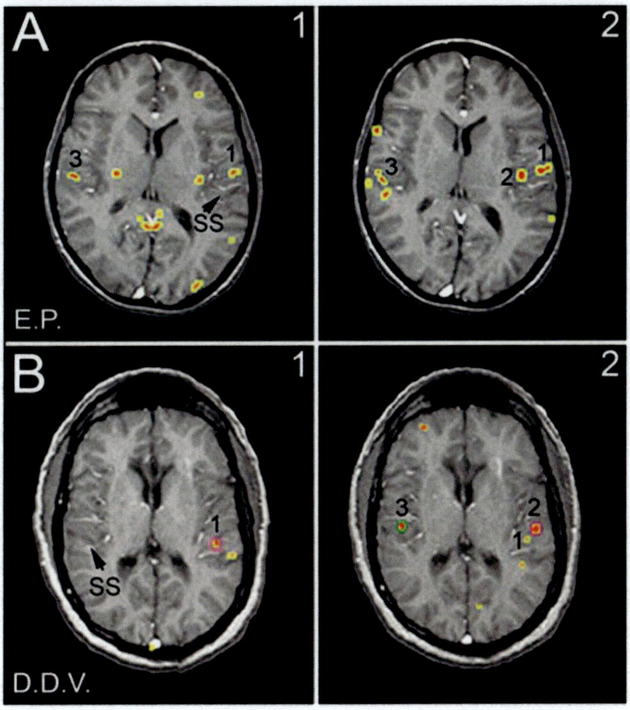

Figure 4. Cortical activation during tactile and painful stimulation of the right hand in a representative control subject (E.P.) and in a patient with total CC resection (D.D.V.), representative of the patients group. Left hemisphere on the right. *A1*, axial image obtained from a SPGR T1-weighted gradient echo EPI sequence showing the cortical areas activated in the PO by tactile stimulation of the right hand. Numbers 1 and 3 indicate the contralateral and ipsilateral activation foci, respectively. *A2*, axial image obtained as in A showing the cortical areas activated in the PO by painful stimulation of the right hand. 1,2, contralateral foci; 3,4, ipsilateral foci. *B1*, axial image obtained as in A, showing activation in the contralateral PO (focus 1) by tactile stimulation of the right hand. No activation was detected in the ipsilateral PO in this and in adjacent sections. *B2*, axial image showing PO activation by painful stimulation of the right hand. Activation is found both in the contralateral (1 and 2) and the ipsilateral (3) PO. SS, Sylvian sulcus. Modified from Fabri et al., 2002.

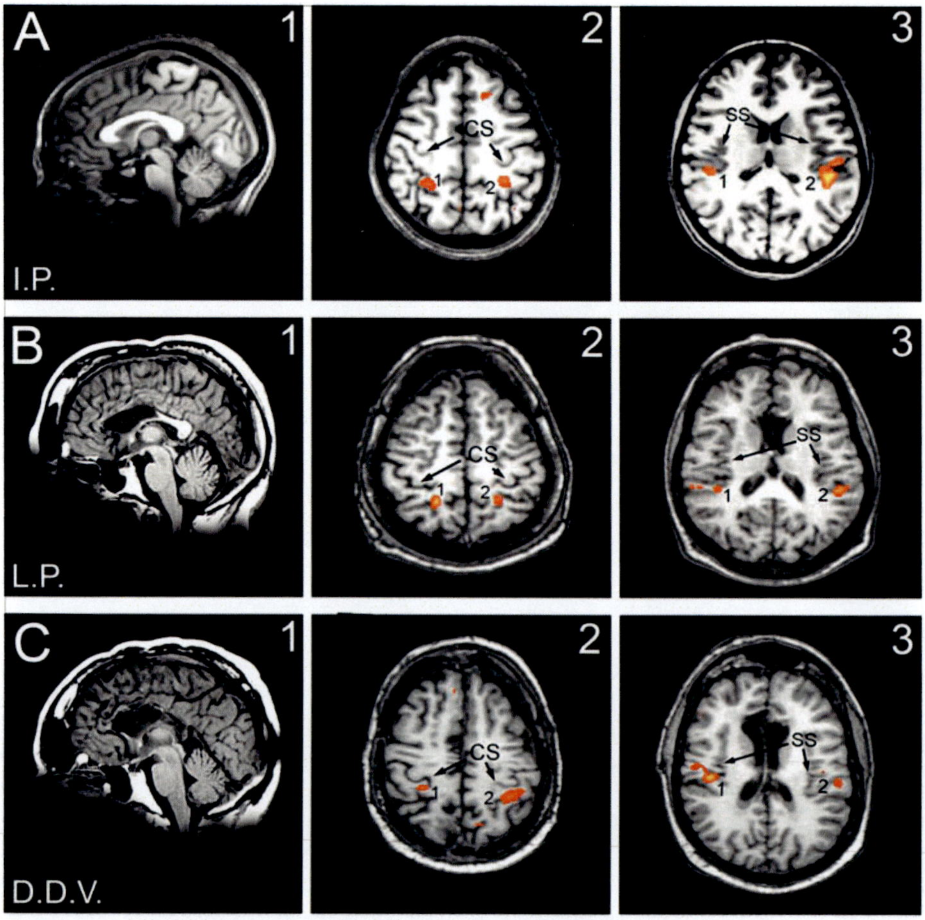

Figure 5. Cortical activation obtained during tactile stimulation of the left midline trunk surface in a control subject and two callosotomized patients. Left hemisphere on the right. *A1*, MR image of midsagittal brain slice obtained with a T1-weighted spin-echo sequence showing the intact callosal commissure in a control subject (I.P.). *A2*, Stimulus-related activation was observed in the PCG of both hemispheres (focus 1, contralateral, and 2 ipsilateral). *A3*, Cortical activation was also evoked bilaterally in the PO, in the upper bank of the SS (focus 1, contralateral, and 2 ipsilateral). *B1*, MR image of midsagittal brain slice obtained with a T1-weighted spin-echo sequence showing the extent of callosal resection in patient L.P. *B2*, Stimulus-related activation was observed in the PCG of the contralateral hemisphere (focus 1), in the trunk representation zone of SI, and in a corresponding ipsilateral region (focus 2). *B3*, Cortical activation was also evoked in PO, bilaterally in area SII (focus 1, contralateral, and 2 ipsilateral). *C1*, MR image of midsagittal brain slice obtained with a T1-weighted spin-echo sequence showing complete resection of the corpus callosum in patient D.D.V. *C2*, Stimulus-related activation was observed in the PCG of the contralateral hemisphere (focus 1), in the trunk representation zone of SI, and in a corresponding ipsilateral region (focus 2). *C3,* Cortical activation was also evoked in PO, bilaterally in area SII (focus 1, contralateral, and 2 ipsilateral). CS, central sulcus; SS, Sylvian sulcus. A, modified from Fabri et al., 2005b; B and C, modified from Fabri et al., 2006.

The 3 patients with complete callosal resection had activation patterns similar to those of the last two groups: in two patients left and right tactile stimulation of the trunk ventral surface close to the midline caused bilateral activation in the PCG (Figure 5C2) and PO

(Figure 5C3); in the other patient bilateral activation was detected after left side stimulation, and contralateral activation after right side stimulation. Data from callosotomized patients indicate that the activation evoked in ipsilateral SI by ventral midline stimulation is at least partially independent of the CC (for a detailed description see Fabri et al., 2006).

RESULTS FROM THE NEUROPSYCHOLOGICAL STUDY

Control Subjects

This group performed well with both hands in the TNT and S-DRT tests (mean 99% of correct answers), and obtained high scores in the intermanual TFLT task with both hands (mean proportion of correct answers: 95% and 96% with the right and left hand, respectively).

Callosotomized Subjects

Patients with Partial Anterior Callosotomy

All these subjects performed well with both hands in the TNT (mean 93% and 95% of correct responses for the right and the left hand, respectively). One had an intact splenium and PCB, while in the other two the splenium and possibly also part of the trunk of the CC were extant. These data indicate that somatosensory information from the left hand reached the speaking hemisphere (very likely the left, all patients having high right-handedness scores), probably along the fibres crossing through the posterior region of the callosal body.

These patients also provided 95-100% of correct answers in the S-DRT and 77% to 100% in the intra- and intermanual TFLT tasks with both hands, denoting interhemispheric exchange of tactile information.

Patient with Partial Posterior Callosotomy

Before posterior callosotomy, in 100% of trials, he was able to name the familiar objects explored with either hand (TNT), to state whether the object explored with one hand was the same or a different object from that explored with the other hand (SDRT), and to localise with the thumb the points on fingers 2-5 that had been touched by the experimenter in the same (TLFT, intramanual mode) or in the contralateral (TLFT, intermanual mode) hand. The patient's postoperative performance in the TNT was as correct as preoperatively with the right hand, whereas he failed to name correctly the objects explored with the left hand in 89% and 84% of trials after six months and one year, respectively. His performance in the SDRT was also very poor, with correct responses well below chance in both postoperative sessions. In the TFL, performance was as high as preoperatively in the intramanual mode: with both hands he could localise with the thumb the points touched on fingers 2-5 of the same hand without errors six months from surgery, and with few errors after one year. Conversely, in the intermanual mode he made errors in 82% of trials in the right-to-left transfer and in 83% in the opposite direction after six month; after one year errors were 85% and 79%, respectively. This case provides the direct demonstration that activation of SII and PPC to stimulation of the ipsilateral hand requires the integrity of the posterior body of the CC.

Patients with Total Callosotomy

Patients with total resections performed well in the TNT with the right hand (93% of correct responses), but poorly with the left (mean: 30% of correct responses). Left hand performances were significantly different in patients with total callosotomy compared with those with partial resection, whereas their right hand performances were similar. Performance in the S-DRT was highly variable, with correct responses ranging from 50% to 100%. Two of the three patients with complete resection obtained chance level scores (55% and 50%, respectively) and failed the TNT with the left hand, while surprisingly the third patient performed well in this test. However, the results from this group were overall significantly poorer than those of the partial callosotomy group. In the TFLT, the three complete callosotomy patients gave 100% of correct answers with both hands in the intramanual task; in the intermanual task correct responses were 78% to 93% with the right hand and 67% to 90% with the left. Although these values are above chance (12.5%), differences from the results of partially callosotomized patients are statistically significant.

Conclusion

The results of the fMRI studies described above can be summarized as follows:

1. unilateral tactile stimulation of the hand and fingers evoked bilateral activation of the PPC and area SII in control subjects; in patients with complete or partial callosotomy sparing only the splenium activation was only in contralateral PPC and area SII. Bilateral activation was also recorded in patients with an extant posterior callosal body and preoperatively in the patient who underwent a second (posterior) callosotomy. Lack of ipsilateral somatosensory cortex activation in callosotomized patients shows that stimulus transmission is mediated by the corpus callosum. The disappearance of ipsilateral SI and SII activation in the patient who was evaluated before and after posterior callosotomy indicates that the fibres carrying activation to ipsilateral SI and SII run in the posterior body of the CC;
2. unilateral painful stimulation of the hand evoked bilateral activation of area SII both in control subjects and in patients with complete callosotomy, suggesting that the two modalities (touch and pain) may use different mechanisms, and that activation of ipsilateral SII by painful stimuli could be elicited by extracallosal pathways, likely subcortical fibres;

3. unilateral tactile stimulation of receptors on trunk regions close to the ventral midline evoked bilateral activation of areas SI and SII in healthy subjects and patients, indicating that afferents from different body regions reach the ipsilateral hemisphere by different ways, likely through a direct subcortical uncrossed pathway;

Comparison of neuropsychological results with fMRI data provides further evidence that the interhemispheric transfer of tactile afferents from hand receptors is likely mediated by the fibres running in the posterior part of the callosal body, confirming that the posterior midbody of the CC is the "tactual" channel.

In the patients participating in the various studies, different kinds of stimulation (i.e., tactile *versus* painful) and different sites of application of the tactile stimulus (i.e., hand *versus* trunk midline) resulted in different patterns of bilateral activation of somatic sensory areas. It can be hypothesized that the bilateral cortical representation of peripheral inputs might, in principle, be subserved by different mechanisms, according to the nature and functional significance of the incoming stimulus. Tactile afferents from proximal body regions (e.g. trunk midline) may reach the ipsilateral hemisphere by a direct subcortical uncrossed pathway, independent of the CC *(subcortical)*, to ensure anatomical continuity of the cortical representation of the sensory periphery. It has recently been shown that oral structures are represented in SI of both hemispheres and that the ipsilateral representation is at least partially independent of the commissure, since differences in the latency of cortical activation between the hemispheres are not significant (Disbrow et al., 2003). A recent fMRI mapping study showed that some body regions other than the midline territories are represented bilaterally in SI: unilateral tactile stimulation of shoulder, arm and thigh regions evoked activation foci in PCG of both hemispheres (Polonara et al., 2007), but the neural mechanism of this bilateral representation has not yet been investigated. Alternatively, tactile afferents from distal body regions (e.g. hand) may reach the ipsilateral hemisphere by an indirect cortico-cortical recrossed pathway, dependent on the CC *(callosal),* to ensure functional continuity. Finally, pain afferents from distal body regions (hands) reach the ipsilateral hemisphere by a direct subcortical uncrossed pathway, independent of the CC (subcortical), probably to ensure prompt stimulus processing and appropriate reaction to potentially harmful situations. The callosally dependent mechanism, related to a more complex behaviour, likely appeared late in mammal evolution. Indeed, the corpus callosum is first found in the brain of Eutherian mammals (Lent and Schmidt, 1993; Mihrshahi, 2006), possibly "as a more efficient commissural system" (Mihrshahi, 2006) connecting increasingly distant sensory cortical areas in the expanding brain, or, more likely, as a consequence of the evolution of a separate motor cortex in Eutherian brains (Kaas, 2004; Mihrshahi, 2006) and the emerging ability to perform complex or skilled motor tasks. It is therefore conceivable that the callosal commissure is necessary to connect and integrate effectors of complex behaviour (the hands), and not for fusing the left and right sensory periphery, or to alert the nervous system in case of danger, all functions that are found in lower mammals (Prototherians and Metatherians), and that in callosal mammals are accomplished, at least in part, by alternative commissure and/or mechanisms.

The analysis of the hand touch and pain, trunk touch and neuropsychological studies performed on patients with various degree of callosal resection prompts the following considerations:

1. activation of ipsilateral PPC and area SII by unilateral tactile stimulation of the hand is mediated by somatic sensory areas in the contralateral hemisphere, through the CC;
2. the callosal fibres carrying activation to the ipsilateral PP cortex, SI and SII pass through the posterior third of the body of the commissure, anterior to the splenium;
3. activation of ipsilateral area SII by unilateral painful stimulation of the hand is at least partially independent of callosal transmission; nociceptive inputs reach area SII likely via uncrossed ipsilateral subcortical pathways;
4. activation of ipsilateral areas SI and SII by unilateral tactile stimulation of the ventral trunk midline is at least partially independent of the CC;
5. in the last two cases, extracallosal pathways are probably involved: uncrossed subcortical pathways, subcortical commissures, or both.

The contribution of the corpus callosum to the bilateral cortical representation of peripheral sensory inputs is thus critical for tactile afferents from the hands, probably to integrate and coordinate sensory and motor activity of both hands in performing complex tasks. It is not crucial for more primitive functions, i.e., processing tactile afferent stimuli from midline trunk regions or painful stimuli from the hands. In these two cases the corpus callosum could, however, have a general modulatory role: callosal projections may exert a facilitatory action, combining the excitatory signals from the two hemispheres to yield bilateral RFs, and/or a synchronizing action, enabling activation of adjacent regions at the same time, or even an inhibitory action, as suggested by the finding that cooling area 3 in monkey SI cortex results in augmented activity and enlargement of the RFs of neurons in the homotopic cortical area of the contralateral hemisphere (Clarey et al., 1996), and by the presence of callosally projecting GAD-immunoreactive neurons in rat and cat somatic sensory areas (Fabri and Manzoni, 2004).

Acknowledgements

The authors wish to thank Profs Tullio Manzoni and Ugo Salvolini for helpful criticism and support during the research; Drs Angelo Quattrini and Aldo Paggi for encouraging callosotomized patients to participate in the studies; Dr Giulia Mascioli for her great fMRI processing work; Ms Gabriella Venanzi for scheduling patient exams; the technical staff of the Istituto di Radiologia for their invaluable assistance during the scan acquisition; the patients and their families, all the volunteers who participated in the research, and Dr Silvia Modena for language revision.

REFERENCES

Aglioti, S., Beltramello, A., Tassinari, G., and Berlucchi, G. (1998). Paradoxically greater interhemispheric transfer deficits in partial than complete callosal agenesis. *Neuropsychologia, 36,* 1015-1024.

Allison, T, McCarthy, G., Wood, C.C., Williamson, P.D., and Spencer, D.D. (1989). Human cortical potentials evoked by stimulation of median nerve. II. Cytoarchitectonic areas generating long-latency activity. *J. Neurophysiol., 62*, 711-722.

Amaral, D.G. (2000). The anatomical organization of the central nervous system. In E.R. Kandel, J.H. Schwartz, and T.M. Jessel (Eds.), *Principles of neural science* (edition, pp. 00-00). New York, USA: McGraw-Hill.

Barbaresi, P., Conti, F., and Manzoni, T. (1984). Topography and receptive field organization of the body midline representation in the ventrobasal complex of the cat. *Exp. Brain Res., 54*, 327-336.

Boecker, H., Khorram-Sefat, D., Kleinschmidt, A., Merboldt, K.-D., Häanicke, W., Requardt, M. and Frahm, J. (1995) High-resolution functional magnetic resonance imaging of cortical activation during tactile exploration. *Human Brain Mapp., 3,* 236-244.

Burton, H. (1986). Second somatosensory cortex and related areas. In E.G. Jones, and A. Peters (Eds.), *Cerebral Cortex, Vol 5* (edition, pp. 31-98). New York, USA: Plenum Press.

Burton, H. (2002). Cerebral cortex regions devoted to somatosensory system: results from brain imaging studies in humans. In R. Nelson (Ed.) *The Somatosensory System: Deciphering the Brain's Own Body Image.* (edition, pp. 27-72). Boca Raton, USA: CRC.

Burton, H., Mac Leod, A.M., Videen, T.O., and Raichle, M.E. (1997). Multiple foci in parietal and frontal cortex by rubbing embossed grating pattern across fingerpads: a positron emission tomography study in humans. *Cerebral Cortex, 7,* 3-17.

Burton, H., Videen, T.O., and Raichle, M.E. (1993). Tactile-vibration activated foci in insular and parietal-opercular cortex studied with positron emission tomography: mapping the second somatosensory area in humans. *Somatosens. Motor Res., 10,* 297-308.

Casey, L.K., Minoshima, S., Berger, K.L., Koeppe, R.A., Morrow, T.J., and Frey, K.A. (1994). Positron emission tomographic analysis of cerebral structures activated specifically by repetitive noxious heat stimuli. *J. Neurophysiol., 71*, 802-807.

Cheema, S.S., Whitsel, B.L. and Rustioni, A. (1983). The cortico-cuneate pathway in the cat: relations among terminal distribution pattern, cytoarchitecture, and single neuron functional properties. *Somatosens. Res., 1*, 169-205.

Clarey, J.C., Tweedale, R., and Calford, M.B. (1996). Interhemispheric modulation of somatosensory receptive fields: evidence for plasticity in primary somatosensory cortex. *Cerebral Cortex, 6,* 196-206.

Coghill, R.C., Talbot, J.D., Evans, A.C., Meyer, E., Gjedde, A., Bushnell, M.C., and Duncan, G.H. (1994). Distributed processing of pain and vibration by the human brain. *J. Neurosci. 14*, 4095-4108.

Conti, F., Fabri, M., and Manzoni, T. (1986). Bilateral receptive fields and callosal connectivity of the body midline representation in the first somatosensory area of Primates. *Somatosensory Res*., 3, 273-289.

Davis, K.D., Kwan, C.L., Crawley, A.P., and Mikulis, D.J. (1998). Functional MRI study of thalamic and cortical activation evoked by cutaneous heat, cold, and tactile stimuli. *J. Neurophysiol., 80,* 1533-1546.

Disbrow, E., Buonocore, M., Antognini, J., Carstens, E., and Rowley, H.A. (1998). Somatosensory cortex: a comparison of the response to noxious thermal, mechanical, and electrical stimuli using functional magnetic resonance imaging. *Hum. Brain Mapp., 6,* 150-159.

Disbrow, E.A., Hinkley, L.B.N., and Roberts, T.P.L. (2003). Ipsilateral representation of oral structures in human anterior parietal somatosensory cortex and integration of inputs across the midline. *J. Comp. Neurol., 467*, 487-495.

Duvernoy, H.M. (1991). *The Human Brain. Surface, Tridimentional Sectional Anatomy and MRI.* Wien: Springer-Verlag.

Fabri, M., Del Pesce, M., Paggi, A., Polonara, G., Bartolini, M., Salvolini, U., and Manzoni, T. (2005a). Contribution of posterior corpus callosum to the interhemispheric transfer of tactile information. *Cogn. Brain Res., 24,* 73-80.

Fabri, M., and Manzoni, T. (2004). GAD immunoreactivity in callosal projecting neurons of cat and rat somatic sensory areas. *Neuroscience, 123*, 557-566.

Fabri, M., Polonara, G., Del Pesce, M., Quattrini, A., Salvolini, U., and Manzoni, T. (2001). Posterior corpus callosum and interhemispheric transfer of somatosensory information: an fMRI and neuropsychological study of a partially callosotomized patient. *J. Cogn. Neurosci., 13,* 1071-1079.

Fabri, M., Polonara, G., Mascioli, G., Paggi, A., Salvolini, U., and Manzoni, T. (2006). Contribution of the corpus callosum to bilateral representation of the trunk midline in the human brain: a fMRI study of callosotomized patients. *Eur. J. Neurosci., 23,* 3139-3148.

Fabri, M., Polonara, G., Quattrini, A., and Salvolini, U. (2002). Mechanical noxious stimuli cause bilateral activation of parietal operculum in callosotomized subjects. *Cerebral Cortex, 1,* 446-451.

Fabri, M., Polonara, G., Quattrini, A., Salvolini, U., Del Pesce, M. and, Manzoni, T. (1999). Role of the corpus callosum in the somatosensory activation of the ipsilateral cerebral cortex: an fMRI study of callosotomized patients. *Eur. J. Neurosci., 11,* 3983-3994.

Fabri, M., Polonara, G., Salvolini, U., and Manzoni, T. (2005b). Bilateral cortical representation of the trunk midline in human first somatic sensory area. *Hum. Brain Map.,* 25, 287-296.

Forss, N., Hari, R., Salmelin, R., Ahonen, A., Hämäläinen, M., Kajola, M., Knuutila, J., and Simola, J. (1994a). Activation of the human posterior parietal cortex by median nerve stimulation. *Exp. Brain Res., 99*, 309-315.

Forss, N., and Jousmäki, V. (1998). Sensorimotor integration in human primary and secondary somatosensory cortices. *Brain Res., 781*, 259-267.

Forss, N., Salmelin, R., and Hari, R. (1994b.) Comparison of somatosensory evoked fields to aipuff and electric stimuli. *Electroencephalogr. Clin. Neurophysiol., 92,* 510-517.

Frot, M., and Mauguière, F. (1999). Operculo-insular responses to nociceptive skin stimulation in humans. A review of the literature. *Neurophysiol. Clin.,* 29, 401-410.

Frot, M., Rambaud, L., Guénot, M., and Mauguière, F. (1999). Intracortical recordings of early pain-related CO_2-laser evoked potentials in the human second somatosensory (SII) area. *Clin. Neurophysiol.,* 110, 133-145.

Garcha, H.S. and Ettlinger, G. (1980). Tactile discrimination learning in the monkey: the effects of unilateral or bilateral removals of the second somatosensory cortex (area SII). *Cortex, 16,* 397-412.

Gazzaniga, M.S. (2000). Cerebral specialization and interhemispheric communication: does the corpus callosum enable the human condition? *Brain, 123,* 1293-1326.

Geffen, G., Nilsson, J., and Quinn, K. (1985). The effect of lesions of the corpus callosum on finger localization. *Neuropsychologia, 23,* 497-514.

Gelnar, P.A., Krauss, B.R., Szeverenyi, N.M. and Apkarian, A.V. (1998) Fingertip representation in the human somatosensory cortex: an fMRI study. *Neuroimage, 7,* 261-283.

Greenspan, J.D., Lee, R.R., and Lenz, F.A. (1999). Pain sensitivity alterations as a function of lesion location in the parasylvian cortex. *Pain, 81,* 273-282.

Greenspan, J.D., and Winfield, J.A. (1992). Reversible pain and tactile deficits associated with a cerebral tumor compressing the posterior insula and parietal operculum. *Pain, 50,* 29-39.

Hämäläinen, H., Kekoni, J., Sams, M., Reinikainen, K., and Näätänen, R. (1990). Human somatosensory evoked potentials to mechanical pulses and vibration: contribution of SI and SII somatosensory cortices P50 and P100 components. *Electroencephalogr. Clin. Neurophysiol., 75,* 13-21.

Hari, R., Hämäläinen, H., Hämäläinen, M., Kekoni, J., Sams, M., and Tiihonen, J. (1990). Separate finger representations at the human second somatosensory cortex. *Neuroscience, 37,* 245-249.

Hari, R., Hämäläinen, M., Kaukoranta, E., Reinikainen, K., and Teszner, D. (1983). Neuromagnetic responses from the second somatosensory cortex in man. *Acta Neurol. Scand., 68,* 207-212.

Hari, R., Karhu, J., Hämäläinen, M., Salonen, O., Sams, M., and Vilkman, V. (1993). Functional organization of the first and second somatosensory cortices: a neuromagnetic study. *Eur. J. Neurosci., 5,* 724-734.

Hari, R., and Forss, N. (1999). Magnetoencephalography in the study of human somatosensory cortical processing. *Phil. Trans. of the Royal Soc. of London, Series B, 354,* 1145-1154.

Hoshiyama, M., Kakigi, R., Koyama, S., Watanabe, S. and Shimojo, M. (1997) Activity in the posterior parietal cortex following somatosensory stimulation in man: magnetoelectroencephalographic study using spatio-temporal source analysis. *Brain Topogr., 10,* 23-30.

Iwamura, Y., Iriki, A., and Tanaka, M. (1994). Bilateral hand representation in the postcentral somato-sensory cortex. *Nature, 369,* 554-556.

Iwamura, Y., Taoka, M., and Iriki, A. (2001). Bilateral activity and callosal connections in the somatosensory cortex. *Neuroscientist, 7,* 419-429.

Kaas, J.H. (1983). What, if anything, is SI? Organization of first somatosensory area of cortex. *Physiol. Rev.,* 63, 206-230.

Kaas, J.H. (2004) Evolution of somatosensory and motor cortex in primates. *Anat. Rec. A, 281,* 1148-1156.

Kaas, J.H., Jain, N., and Qi, H.-X. (2002). The organization of somatosensory system in primates. In R. Nelson (Ed.), *The Somatosensory System: Deciphering the Brain's Own Body Image* (pp. 1-25) . Boca Raton: CRC. p 1-25.

Kagiki, R., Hoshiyama, M., Shimojo, M., Naka, D., Yamasaki, H., Watanabe, S., Xiang, J., Maeda, K., Lam, K., Itomi, K., and Nakamura, A. (2000), The somatosensory evoked magnetic field. *Prog. Neurobiol., 61,* 495-523.

Kany, C. and Treede, R.D. (1997). Median and tibial nerve somatosensory evoked potentials: middle-latency components from the vicinity of the secondary somatosensory cortex in humans. *Electroencephalogr. Clin. Neurophysiol., 104*, 402-410.

Kanda, M., Nagamine, T, Ikeda, A., Ohara, S., Kunieda, T., Fujiwara, N., Yazawa, S., Sawamoto, N., Matsumoto, R., Taki, W., and Shibasaki, H. (2000). Primary somatosensory cortex is actively involved in pain processing in human. Brain Res., 853, 282-289.

Kaukoranta, E., Hari, R., Hämäläinen, M. and Huttunen, J. (1986) Cerebral magnetic fields evoked by peroneal nerve stimulation. *Somatosens. Res*., *3*, 309-321.

Kim, S.-G., and Urgubil, K. (1997). Functional magnetic resonance imaging of the human brain. *J. Neurosci. Methods, 74*, 229-243.

Kitamura, Y., Kagiki, R., Hoshiyama, M., Koyama, S., Watanabe, S., and Shimojo, M. (1997). Pain-related somatosensory evoked magnetic fields following lower limb stimulation. *J. Neurol. Sci., 145,* 187-194.

Kovernoja, A., Huttunen, J., Salli, E., Pohjonen, H., Martinkauppi, S., Palva, J.M., Lauronen, L., Virtanen, J., Ilmoniemi, R.J., and Aronen, H.J. (1999). Activation of multiple cortical areas in response to somatosensoty stimulation: combined magnetoencephalographic and functional magnetic resonance imaging. *Hum. Brain Mapp., 8,* 13-27.

Ledberg, A., Brendan, T., O'Sullivan, T., Kinomura, S. and Roland, P.E. (1995) Somatosensory activations of the parietal operculum of man. A PET study. *Eur. J. Neurosci*., *7*, 1934-1941.

Lent, R., and Schmidt, S.L. (1993). The ontogenesis of the forebrain comissures and the determination of brain asymmetries. *Progr. Neurobiol., 40,* 249-276.

Lenz, F.A., Rios, M., Chau, D., Krauss, G.L., Zirh, T.A., and Lesser, R.P. (1998). Painful stimuli evoke potentials recorded from the parasylvian cortex in humans. *J. Neurophysiol., 80,* 2077-2088, 1998.

Lin, W., Kuppusamy, K., Haacke, E.M., and Burton, H. (1996). Functional MRI in human somatosensory cortex activated by touching textured surfaces. *J. Magn. Res. Imag., 6,* 565-572.

Lüders, H., Lesser, R., Dinner, D.S., Hahn, J.F., Salanga, V. and Morris, H.H. (1985). The second sensory area in humans: evoked potentials and electrical stimulation studies. *Ann. Neurol*., *17*, 177-184.

Mai, J.K., Assheuer, J., and Paxinos, G. (1997). *Atlas of the human brain.* S. Diego: Academic Press.

Maldjian, J.A., Gottschalk, A., Patel, R.S., Pincus, D., Detre, J. and Alsop, D.C. (1999). Mapping of secondary somatosensory cortex activation induced by vibrational stimulation: an fMRI study. *Brain Res., 824*, 291-295.

Manzoni, T. (1997). The callosal connections of the hierarchically organized somatosensory areas of primates. *J. Neurosurg. Scie., 41,* 1-22.

Manzoni, T., Barbaresi, P., Bellardinelli, E., and Caminiti, R. (1980). Callosal projections from the two body midlines. *Exp. Brain Res., 39,* 1-19.

Manzoni, T., Barbaresi, P., Conti, F., and Fabri, M. (1989). The callosal connections of the primary somatosensory cortex and the neural bases of midline fusion. *Exp. Brain Res., 76,* 251-266.

Mihrshahi, R. (2006). The corpus callosum as an evolutionary innovation. *J. Exp.Zool., 306B,* 8-17.

Mima, T., Ikeda, A., Nagamine, T., Yazawa, S., Kunieda, T., Mikuni, N., Taki, W., Kimura, J. and Shibasaki, H. (1997). Human second somatosensory area: subdural and magnetoencephalo-graphy recording of somatosensory evoked responses. *J. Neurol. Neurosurg. Psychiatry, 63*, 501-505.

Myers, J.J., and Sperry, R.W. (1985). Interhemispheric communication after section of the forebrain commissures. *Cortex, 21*, 249-260.

Oldfield, R.C. (1971). The assessment and analysis of handedness: the Edinburgh inventory. *Neuropsychologia, 9*, 97-113.

Perl, E.R. (1984). Pain and nociception. In J.M. Brookhart, V.B. Mountcastle, I. Darian-Smith, and S.R. Geiger (Eds.), *Handbook of Physiology, Section I: The nervous system, Vol. III. Sensory processes, part 2* (edition, pp. 00-00). City, Country: Publisher.

Perl, E.R. (2007). Ideas about pain, a historical view. *Nat. Rev. Neurosci., 8,* 71-80.

Ploner, M., Schmitz, F., Freund, H.-J., and Schnitzler, A. (2000). Differential organisation of touch and pain in human primary somatosensory cortex. *J. Neurophysiol., 83*, 1770-1776.

Polonara, G., Fabri, M., Manzoni, T., and Salvolini, U. (1999). Localization of the first (SI) and second (SII) somatic sensory areas in human cerebral cortex with fMRI. *AJNR, Am. J. NeuroRadiol., 20*, 199-205.

Polonara, G., Mascioli, G., Salvolini, U., Manzoni, T., and Fabri, M. (2007). Representation of cutaneous receptors in human anterior parietal cortex: a functional imaging study. *Hum. Brain Mapp., submitted.*

Potagas, C., Avdelidis, D., Singounas, E., Missir, O., and Aessopos, A. (1997). Episodic pain associated with a tumor in the parietal operculum: a case report and literature review. *Pain, 77,* 201-208.

Quattrini, A., Papo, I., Cesarano, R., Fioravanti, P., Paggi, A., Ortensi, A., Foschi, N., Rychlicky, F., Del Pesce, M., Pistoli, E., and Marinelli, M. (1997). EEG patterns after callosotomy. *J. Neurosurg. Scie., 41,* 85-92.

Quattrini, A., Papo, I., Paggi, A., Ortensi, A., Rychlicki, F., Fronzoni, M., Recchioni, M.A., Marchioro, R., Pauri, G.L., Bonaparte, A., and Mancini, S. (1989). Anterior callosotomy in drug-resistant epilepsy. *Adv. Epileptol., 17*, 4245.

Schnitzler, A., Salmelin, R., Salenius, S., Jousmäki, V. and Hari, R. (1995). Tactile information from the human hand reaches the ipsilateral primary somatosensory cortex. *Neurosci. Lett., 200,* 25-28.

Smith, C.L,. (1986). Sensory neurons supplying touch domes near the body midlines project bilaterally in the thoracic spinal cord of rats. *J. Comp. Neurol., 245,* 541-552.

Svensson, P., Minoshima, S., Beydoun, A., Morrow, T., and Casey, K.L. (1997). Cerebral processing of acute skin and muscle pain in humans. *J. Neurophysiol., 78,* 450-460.

Talairach, J., and Tournoux, P. (1988). *Co-planar stereotaxic atlas of the human brain.* Stuttgart: Thieme.

Taoka, M. Toda, T., and Iwamura, I. (1998). Representation of the midline trunk, bilateral arms, and shoulders in the monkey postcentral somatosensory cortex. *Exp. Brain Res., 123,* 315-322.

Treede, R.-D., Kenshalo, D.R., Gracely, R.H., and Jones, A.KP. (1999). The cortical representation of pain. *Pain, 79,* 105-111.

Xu, X., Fukuyama, H., Yazawa, S., Mima, T., Hanakawa, T., Magata, Y., Kanda, M., Fujiwara, N., Shindo, K., Nagamine, T., Shibasaki, H. (1997). Functional localisation of pain perception in the human brain studied by PET. *NeuroReport, 8,* 555-559.

Yetkin, F.Z., Haughton, V.M., Cox, R.W., Hyde, J., Birn, R.M., Wong, E.C., and Prost, R. (1996). Effect of motion outside the field of view on functional MR. *AJNR, Am. J. NeuroRadiol., 17,* 1005-1009.

In: Brain Mapping Research Developments
Editor: Lars N. Bakker, pp. 101-127

ISBN 978-1-60456-007-7

Chapter IV

Laboratory Memory Tasks and Autobiographical Recollection: Cognitive and Neurofunctional Evidence for Differential Forms of Episodic Memory

Martina Piefke*
Physiological Psychology,
Department of Psychology and Sports Sciences,
University of Bielefeld, Germany

Abstract

The classic model of episodic memory refers to both laboratory tasks requiring the conscious recall or recognition of experimental materials and autobiographical recollection of one's personal past experiences. Recent research in cognitive neuroscience, however, showed evidence that laboratory and autobiographical memory may share aspects of conscious retrieval and reference to the temporal and spatial context at the time of encoding of information, but are different from each other in some important respects. The autobiographical memory domain is characterized by self-referential information processing, subjective emotional evaluation of memories, and the accompanying autonoetic conscious awareness. In contrast, laboratory episodic memory requires the effortful search for impersonal target information and the intentional use of retrieval strategies. Subregions of the prefrontal, medial temporal, and retrosplenial cortices appear to be differentially involved in the neural processing of each type of episodic memory, thus suggesting that they are supported by anatomically and

* Correspondence to: Martina Piefke, Physiological Psychology, Department of Psychology and Sports Sciences, University of Bielefeld, Universitätsstr. 25, 33615 Bielefeld, Germany. Tel.: ++49-521-106-4484. Fax : ++49-521-106-6049. E-mail: martina.piefke@uni-bielefeld.de

functionally overlapping, but also segregated neural circuits. The empirical data reviewed here support the view that laboratory and autobiographical episodic memory can at least in part be distinguished on the cognitive-behavioral and the neurofunctional levels. Accordingly, the review proposes an integrated view of laboratory and autobiographical forms of episodic memory which accounts for an overlap, but also emphasizes the unique features distinguishing the two memory types.

Keywords: fMRI, memory, cognition, self, hippocampus, prefrontal cortex.

1. Introduction

The classic episodic memory model introduced by Tulving (1972, 1983) is currently applied to depict both laboratory (i.e., experimental) episodic memory and autobiographical recollection. Experimental episodic memory deals with the conscious recall or recognition of items learned in a laboratory setting while episodic autobiographical recollection provides a direct link into *one's own past*. It allows for the awareness of the time course of one's life history, and is closely interconnected with an individual's sense of self-coherence and self-continuity, as well as emotion processing (Markowitsch, 2003; Piefke et al., 2003). Episodic autobiographical memory builds up the basis of our ability to reconstruct an individual and personally meaningful past (Tulving, 1995; Tulving and Markowitsch, 1998). For both types of episodic memory, the current model requires that the retrieval of information is conscious and includes the spatial and temporal context of information at encoding.

I here review evidence for both commonalities and differences between laboratory and autobiographical episodic memory with regard to behavioral performance and the underlying brain mechanisms. The autobiographical memory domain is uniquely associated with automatic self-referential information processing, subjective emotional evaluation of memory contents, and "mental time travel" (Tulving, 1995). In contrast, the effortful search for impersonal target information and the intentional use of retrieval strategies predominate in laboratory episodic memory. Besides these differences, both memory types are associated with conscious retrieval and include context information (see above). Neuropsychological and functional neuroimaging data support the notion that laboratory and autobiographical episodic memory are at least in part supported by differential brain mechanisms. In particular, there appears to be a functional segregation of regions in the prefrontal, medial temporal, and posterior cingulate cortices related to the neural processing of each memory type (Cabeza et al., 2004; Nyberg et al., 2002; Piefke and Fink, 2005). It is thus conceivable that experimental and autobiographical episodic memories are processed by at least in part functionally and anatomically segregated neural circuits which together constitute a broader episodic memory network.

2. Subdivisions of Long-Term Memory

Tulving (1972) introduced a concept for the partition of human long-term memory which has now become a basic model for the understanding of human memory (Tulving, 1995; Tulving and Markowitsch, 1998): the *multiple memory systems* view. The model proposes two memory systems which act at the implicit, that is, unconscious level of information processing (*procedural memory* and the *priming system*), one memory system acting at the explicit, that is, conscious level of processing (*episodic memory*), and one being involved in both implicit and explicit memory (*semantic memory*). *Figure 1* summarizes this multiple memory systems account of human long-term memory and specifies the kind of information processed by each system.

Episodic and semantic memory are sometimes subsumed under the notion of "declarative memory" (e.g., Squire and Zola, 1996) to describe explicit memory which can be observed in rodents, non-human primates, as well as humans. It is supposed to rely on an intact function of the hippocampal formation. In contrast, non-declarative memory comprises implicit forms of memory which are independent of the hippocampal complex (Squire, 1992; Squire and Zola, 1996; Squire, 1998).

The Multiple Memory Systems View (Tulving, 1995)

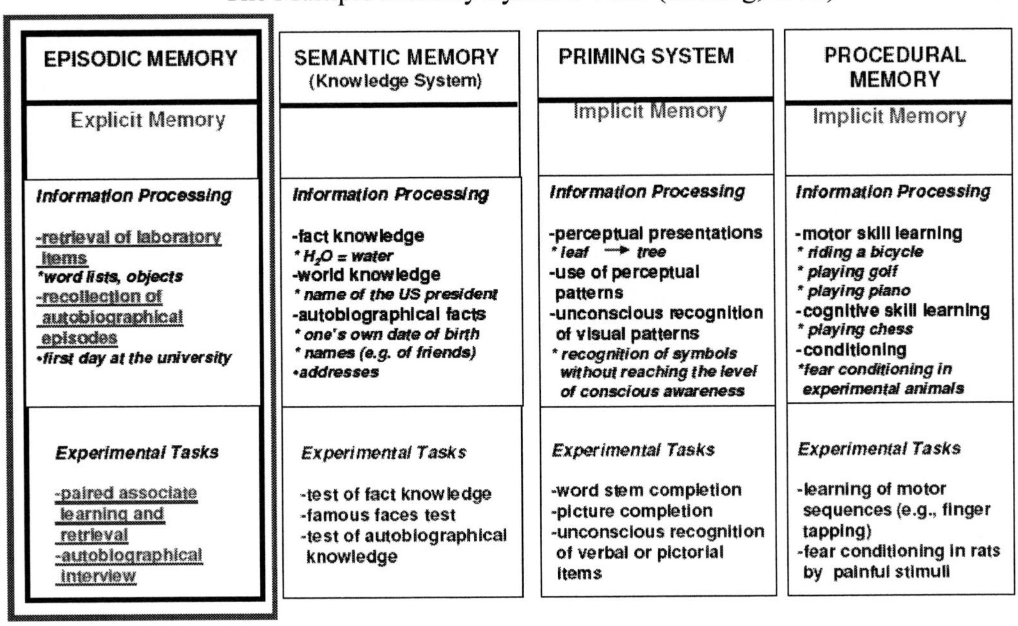

Figure 1. According to the classic multiple memory systems view (Tulving, 1995), human long-term memory comprises at least four memory systems: episodic memory, semantic memory (the knowledge system), the priming system, and procedural memory. The figure specifies the distinct memory types by the categories of information processed by each system and the tasks used to selectively investigate each memory system experimentally. *Both laboratory episodic memory and autobiographical recollection are included the episodic memory system* (highlighted in red). Learning and retrieval of fact knowledge (also autobiographical facts) belong to the domain of semantic memory. Unconscious forms of memory are mediated by the priming system (e.g., perceptual representations) and procedural memory (e.g., skill learning).

Basic and clinical studies on human brain function, however, suggest that episodic and semantic memory represent separate forms of declarative memory. According to the multiple memory systems view (Tulving, 1995), semantic memory does not refer to the context of information encoding. It implies "noetic" awareness, that is, the awareness of retrieving pieces of knowledge (such as "London is the capital of Great Britain") detached from the situational context of information encoding. Episodic memory, in contrast, provides context information and is associated with "autonoetic" awareness. The notion of autonoetic awareness depicts conscious recollection with contextual detail related to time and space of information encoding.

3. The Episodic Memory Account

The initial concept of episodic memory (Tulving, 1972) referred to the free recall and recognition of items within their temporal and spatial context of presentation in a given laboratory setting. It is widely used in behavioral and neuroimaging experiments on human memory (e.g., Burgess et al., 2001; Dalla Barba et al., 1997). However, the concept has also been adapted to studies of conscious memory encoding and retrieval (e.g., of a word list or a series of pictures) without controlling for the inclusion of contextual aspects into the information retrieved (e.g., Henson et al., 2000). Even animal studies of learning and memory in rodents sometimes refer to the episodic memory model (e.g., Meilandt et al., 2004; Remondes and Schuman, 2004), in particular, when tasks are applied which include some kind of declarative spatial, conceptual, or contextual memory (e.g., Morris water maze). Other investigators have retained the broad episodic memory concept, but also developed the model into a framework which allows, at least in part, for the specification of autobiographical recollection (Tulving, 1995; Tulving and Markowitsch, 1998; Piefke et al., 2003). According to this account, laboratory and autobiographical episodic memory share basic similarities which allow for the inclusion of the two forms of memory into one episodic memory model.

The extended use of the episodic memory model calls for a revisit of issues concerning the characteristics of this form of human memory and, in particular, a reconsideration of overlapping and distinct features of autobiographical and laboratory episodic memory.

4. Laboratory and Autobiographical Episodic Memory

4.1. Cognitive Neuropsychology of Episodic Memory

The introduction of "remember-know paradigms" aimed at identifying autonoetic awareness in laboratory experiments of episodic memory (Gardiner and Java, 1993; Knowlton and Squire, 1995; Dalla Barba et al., 1997). Typically, a remember-know paradigm includes a learning phase and a subsequent testing phase requiring the recognition of studied items out of a set of new and learned stimuli. For each item recognized, participants additionally indicate whether they "remember" having seen the item in the study phase including the respective temporo-spatial context information (e.g., that it was displayed in the upper left of the screen), or rather "know" that it was one of the studied items (in the sense of a "feeling of familiarity") but are unable to provide information about the specific context of the item's presentation. In terms of this approach, only "remember-responses" are indicators of autonoetic conscious awareness and thus for episodic memory of an item. The remember-know account claims to show evidence for the coherence of laboratory and autobiographical forms of episodic memory: it refers to the presentation of experimental stimuli in a laboratory context as "mini-events" in the autobiographical sense (Tulving, 1972, 1983). However, laboratory "remember responses" differ from episodic autobiographical recollections at least with respect to the following aspects:

(i) the *time-window* of memory-related information processing which is restricted to the experimental setting in the laboratory type of episodic memory but potentially covers one's entire life history during autobiographical recollection,
(ii) the (often emotional) *re-experience* of an autobiographical event during its recollection which is usually absent in laboratory episodic memory,
(iii) the (emotionally and cognitively determined) *personal significance* of autobiographical recollections which cannot be attributed to laboratory episodic memories,
(iv) the *self-referential perspective* naturally associated with autobiographical recollection but not with laboratory episodic memory tasks,
(v) processes of *mental time travel* associated with autobiographical recollection which are absent or marginal during non-autobiographical episodic memory,
(vi) *reconstructive mechanisms* of autobiographical memory which enable us to reconstruct our personally meaningful past, but are absent (or at least widely reduced) in laboratory episodic memory tasks.

The same is true for the "source memory paradigms" developed some time later (e.g., Cansino et al., 2002). A standard laboratory source memory task requires that a subject learns items (e.g., objects or abstract figures) and their spatial position on the screen (context information). In the following recognition memory test, the participant has to decide whether each shown item was one of the studied items (old/new judgment). If yes, the paradigm requires the localization of the item's position on the screen at encoding. Although source memory paradigms are well applicable for a measure of experimental episodic memory (as are remember-know paradigms), they are no surrogate of a study of episodic autobiographical memory. *Figure 2* illustrates the source memory paradigm used by Cansino et al. (2002).

It is in good accordance with this view that the philosophical perspective of Gallagher (2000) associates autonoetic consciousness with the senses of *self-ownership* (i.e., that I am the one who is undergoing an experience) and *self-agency* (i.e., that I am the source or the initiator of an action). In the non-pathological case, we are therefore sure to have episodic autobiographical memories of our *own* personal past (Fink et al., 1996). Both senses are "naturally" involved in episodic autobiographical memory, but unlikely to emerge during recall of a word list within a laboratory experiment, even if reference to the context at encoding of information is required.

Laboratory tests developed in experimental psychology are the tools used intentionally as simplifications of real life to allow for the controlled assessment of a relevant cognitive process. Although these tests represent valuable approaches that yielded a wealth of knowledge on episodic memory and other brain functions, I would like to argue for the abovementioned reasons that laboratory episodic memory tasks lack crucial aspects of the cognitive and emotional characteristics of autobiographical recollection.

Source Memory Paradigm (Cansino et al. 2002)

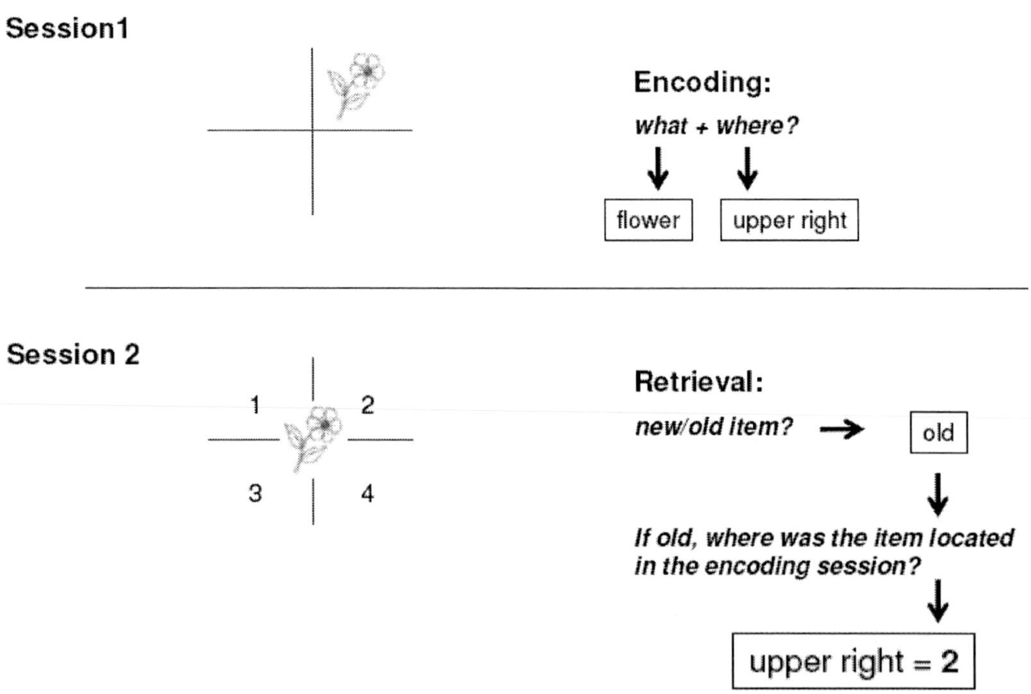

Figure 2. Source memory paradigm which requires the learning (session 1; upper part of the figure) and retrieval (session 2; lower part of the figure) of objects and their position on the screen (four positions are possible). In session 1, participants are asked to learn what is presented and where it is located on the screen (here: flower in the upper right part of the screen). In session two, subjects see the learned objects in their positions and additional new objects located in one of the four positions on the screen. Participants are initially asked to decide whether the item is one of the learned objects or a new one. If it is regarded as one of the learned items, they then have to indicate where it was located in the learning session (here: upper right part of the screen, i.e., quadrant 2). Source memory paradigms allow for the assessment of laboratory episodic memory.

Conway and Pleydell-Pearce (2000) aimed at modeling the specificity of autobiographical memory by the introduction of a "self-memory system" which operates on distinct types of autobiographical information (e.g., knowledge of specific events and lifetime periods). The approach is based on the argument that finally all memories are autobiographical in nature and that "episodic memory" represents a general system which provides sensory and perceptual information on recent events (retention interval: minutes to hours) which has to be integrated into the "autobiographical knowledge base" (Conway, 2001). Therefore, experimental and autobiographical episodic memory cannot be differentiated by this account.

4.2. Brain Correlates of Episodic Memory

Studies of brain damage and neuropsychological performance of amnesic patients suggest that the hippocampus and adjacent medial temporal brain structures, prefrontal, posterior cingulate, and retrosplenial regions all support both laboratory and autobiographical episodic memory. Importantly, however, the studies also indicate that these brain areas may at least in part be differentially involved in the two forms of episodic memory (Aggleton et al., 2000; Bowers et al., 1988; Gaffan et al., 2001; Gainotti et al., 1998; Markowitsch, 1995; Mayes and Downes, 1997; Mayes and Montaldi, 2001; Valenstein et al., 1987). Functional neuroimaging studies of healthy human subjects support these patient data (e.g., Maddock and Buonocore, 1997; Nyberg et al. 2002; Piefke et al., 2003). Moreover, they have shown some evidence for differences in hemispheric lateralization of the two types of episodic memory (Maguire and Frith, 2003a; Piefke et al., 2003; Ranganath et al., 2000).

4.2.1. The Prefrontal Cortex

The "Hemispheric-Encoding-Retrieval-Asymmetry" (HERA) account (Tulving et al., 1994; Habib et al., 2003) assumes that the left prefrontal cortex (PFC) is predominantly involved in episodic encoding, and that right prefrontal regions are mainly recruited during episodic retrieval. According to the model encoding deficits should predominate in patients with episodic memory impairments resulting from left prefrontal lesions, and dysfunctions of episodic retrieval should occur in patients with right prefrontal brain damage. In particular for verbal materials, there is some evidence in support of the HERA account (e.g., Incisa della Rocchetta and Milner, 1993; Stuss et al., 1994; Schacter et al., 1996a). Note, however, that encoding and retrieval deficits can hardly be isolated from each other by studies of laboratory episodic memory in amnesic patients. The application of episodic non-autobiographical memory tests in a laboratory setting is restricted to the investigation of *anterograde memory*, that is, memory of information encoded and retrieved after the occurrence of brain damage. Clues are thus unavailable which may help to decide whether the patient failed to successfully encode the respective information or suffers from a retrieval deficit. In tests of autobiographical recollection, retrograde and anterograde memory deficits can selectively be detected. With regard to anterograde autobiographical memory, however, the problem of the differentiation between encoding and retrieval deficits is the same as in tests of laboratory episodic memory. Given that there is a corresponding lateralization of prefrontal involvement in laboratory and autobiographical episodic memory processing, combined assessment of the experimental and autobiographical forms of episodic memory may nevertheless help to elucidate the validity of the HERA account. Functional neuroimaging studies of normal volunteers cannot directly contribute to the issue since autobiographical encoding may hardly be assessed in a magnetic resonance imaging (MRI) or positron emission tomography (PET) scanner. Moreover, data on prefrontal lateralization during autobiographical memory retrieval are currently rare and inconsistent (Fink et al., 1996; Piefke et al., 2003, 2005). The study of Piefke et al. (2005) suggests that differences in the hemispheric lateralization of autobiographical memory retrieval may also depend on a gender-specific variation in the laterality of brain functions.

No consensus has yet been achieved with regard to the issue of hemispheric lateralization of episodic autobiographical and non-autobiographical memory processes. Recent functional neuroimaging data suggest that laterality effects in the neural activation patterns associated with laboratory tasks of episodic memory encoding and retrieval may depend upon *distinct stimulus characteristics, the complexity of stimulus materials and information to be retrieved, and specific task demands rather than a clear functional hemispheric specialization for memory encoding and retrieval* (as suggested by the HERA account; for a review, see Lee et al., 2003). In fMRI studies of Nolde et al. (1998a, b), laboratory episodic memory tasks with low complexity yielded right prefrontal activations, but the left PFC became activated only with *increasing complexity of retrieval demands* (see also Hunkin et al., 2000). *It is thus conceivable that working memory and executive control processes contribute to the varying laterality of prefrontal activation patterns related to laboratory episodic memory tasks* (Lee et al., 2003; Wager and Smith, 2003). Ranganath et al. (2000) reported a further putative determinant of hemispheric lateralization: in their study, demands of laboratory episodic retrieval of *specific perceptual information* increased neural activity in the left PFC.

In general, these data converge with recent functional neuroimaging studies of autobiographical recollection which provide evidence for a left hemisphere predominance of PFC activations during the retrieval of *complex autobiographical episodes with highly specific perceptual details* (Addis et al., 2004; Maguire and Frith, 2003a, Piefke et al., 2003; but see Fink et al., 1996). The findings suggest that the degree of lateralization of PFC activity associated with both laboratory and autobiographical episodic memory is at least in part determined by a non-linear function of perceptual and cognitive complexity of information processing. With regard to the assumption that there may also exist neurofunctional differences in the brain mechanisms of laboratory and autobiographical episodic memory, it is important to note that laterality effects were mainly *restricted to the PFC in laboratory episodic memory* (Nolde et al., 1998a, b; Ranganath et al., 2000) while *additional medial temporal and parieto-occipital brain regions showed left lateralized activity in autobiographical recollection* (Addis et al., 2004; Maguire and Frith, 2003a; Piefke et al., 2003).

With respect to laboratory episodic memory, evidence has been shown for a high degree of functional segregation within the PFC (for reviews, see Aron et al., 2004; Wager and Smith, 2003). However, the data are inconsistent: right PFC regions have been implicated in "retrieval mode" (Kapur et al., 1995; Nyberg et al., 1995; Tulving, 1983), "retrieval effort" (Schacter et al., 1996b), and "post-retrieval monitoring" (Rugg et al., 1996; Shallice et al., 1994). Fletcher et al. (1998) proposed a dorsolateral/ventrolateral functional segregation within the right PFC, with dorsolateral regions being recruited by increasing monitoring demands and ventrolateral mediating retrieval mode. An alternative view relates differential patterns of PFC involvement in laboratory episodic memory to a neurofunctional differentiation between "retrieval attempt" and "retrieval success" (e.g., Kapur et al., 1995;

Nyberg et al., 1995; Rugg et al., 1996; Buckner et al., 1998a, b). The differentiation between memory processes and other cognitive functions that may correspond to ventrolateral and dorsolateral activations, however, has turned out to be difficult. Both regions subserve executive functions such as working memory, cognitive control, and strategic planning (for reviews, see Aron et al., 2004; Wager and Smith, 2003). Any of these processes may be involved in laboratory episodic memory tasks. Accordingly, one cannot easily determine the extent to which PFC activations are directly related to memory functions or rather subserve executive control (e.g., monitoring of retrieved information). In addition to the ventrolateral and dorsolateral PFC, laboratory episodic memory tasks may sometimes recruit orbitofrontal and frontal polar regions. Involvement of these PFC areas in laboratory episodic memory has been related to high context memory demands (Fujii et al., 2004; Nyberg et al., 2002) and emotional aspects (e.g., Smith et al., 2004) of a given task.

The ventrolateral and dorsolateral PFC is also implicated in the executive control of autobiographical episodic recollection (e.g., Maguire et al., 2001a, Piefke et al., 2003; Vanderkerckhove et al., 2005). However, orbitofrontal and medial PFC regions play a predominating role in remembering the personal past. They are involved in self-referential (Vogeley et al., 2001) and social cognition (e.g., theory of mind: Gallagher et al., 2000), as well as emotion and its control (e.g., empathy: Geday et al., 2003; emotional memory: Piefke et al., 2003; Smith et al., 2004). These cognitive and emotional abilities build up major components of autobiographical recollection.

In a review of functional neuroimaging data on corresponding and differential PFC activations associated with laboratory and autobiographical episodic memory, Gilboa (2004) proposed that the right mid-dorsolateral PFC is primarily involved in experimental episodic memor. In contrast, the left ventromedial PFC would predominate in autobiographical recollection. The author interprets the observed prefrontal functional segregation in terms of *distinct modes of post-retrieval verification and monitoring of episodic non-autobiographical and autobiographical memories*. According to this account, autobiographical memories are monitored by a subjective "feeling of rightness" related to a "self-schema" which recruits the left ventromedial PFC. In contrast, experimental episodic memory requires more elaborate monitoring and control strategies to avoid errors such as omissions and repetitions. Therefore, the laboratory type of episodic memory engages the right mid-dorsolateral PFC. It seems conceivable that the monitoring of retrieved information is built upon differential cognitive strategies in laboratory and autobiographical episodic memory. However, it is unlikely that PFC involvement in either type of episodic memory can be reduced to differences in monitoring demands. Distinct aspects concerning the quality of context memory, self-referential information processing, emotional evaluation, and autonoetic conscious awareness which may directly be mediated by functionally segregated prefrontal areas need to be considered, as well.

4.2.2. The Hippocampus

In both animals and humans, the hippocampus plays a key role in declarative memory processing (Markowitsch, 2003; Squire, 1992; Squire and Knowlton, 2000). There is a longstanding debate, however, on the time-window of hippocampal functions in the consolidation, storage, and retrieval of declarative memories. The consolidation theory

(Squire, 1992) assumes that memory functions of the hippocampus are time-limited such that older (consolidated) memories which have already been transferred to neocortical storage sites become independent of the hippocampal complex. By contrast, the "multiple trace theory" (MTT; Nadel and Moscovitch, 1997) argues that at least episodic (but not necessarily semantic) memories always depend on the hippocampus. To date, neither model fully accounts for the various forms of amnesia resulting from hippocampal lesions in humans and animals. Differences in the location and the extent of hippocampal lesions, and the application of a wide range of differential tasks in studies of retrograde amnesia may contribute to the inconsistent data reported from studies on memory impairments following damage of the hippocampus (Barr et al., 1990; Bolhuis et al., 1994; Kapur et al., 1992, 1994; Kim and Fanselow, 1992; McDonald and White, 1993; Rempel-Clower, et al., 1996; Scoville and Milner, 1957; Walker, 1957; Zola-Morgan et al., 1986). *Figure 3* depicts the assumptions of the consolidation theory and the MTT, respectively.

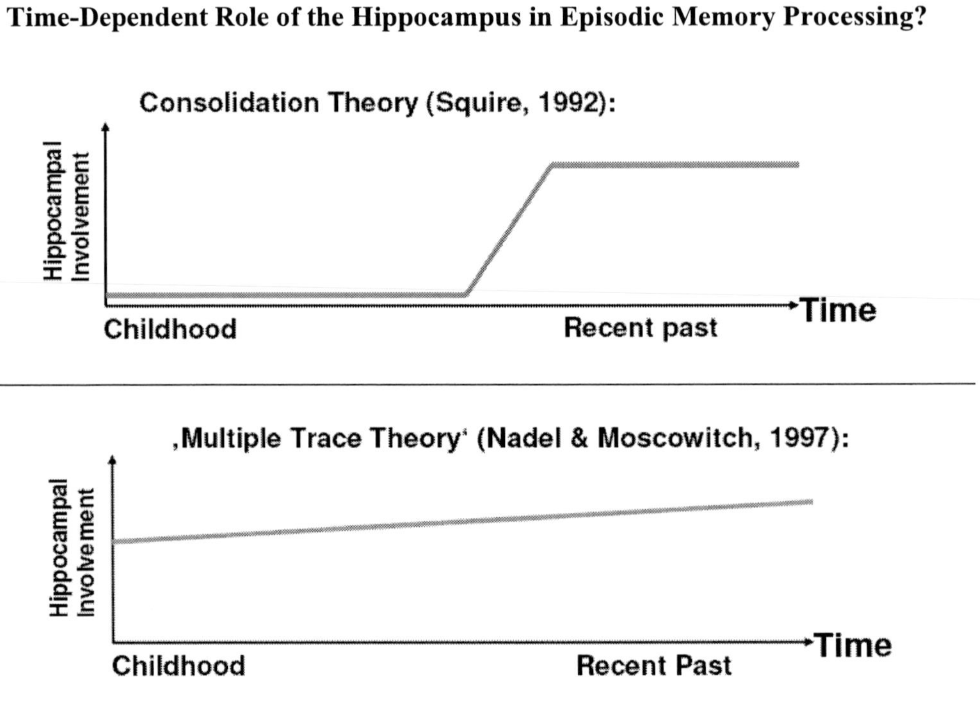

Figure 3. Assumptions of the consolidation theory and the multiple trace theory (MTT) concerning involvement of the hippocampus in episodic memory retrieval. The classic consolidation model (upper part of the figure) presumes a time-limited involvement of the hippocampus in the retrieval of recent episodic memories during the consolidation period. Later, upon long-term storage of information in the neocortex, retrieval processes become independent of the hippocampus. In contrast, the MTT (lower part of the figure) suggests that the hippocampus is always needed for the retrieval of episodic memories, irrespective of the length of the time-period which has passed since the encoding of information. It predicts a flat gradient of hippocampal involvement in retrieval processes as time passes (with remote information requiring less engagement of the hippocampus) which can be due, for example, to the association-related stabilization of information. It is still a matter of debate which of the two theories might better account for the currently available clinical and neuroimaging data on hippocampal memory functions.

When considering the consolidation theory with respect to the assumption of neuropsychological and neurofunctional differences between laboratory and autobiographical episodic memory, it is important to note that the two forms of episodic memory *differ from each other with regard to the time-window defining recent and remote memories*. Laboratory episodic memory tasks normally bear upon time intervals ranging from minutes to hours while the time-window of autobiographical recollection covers one's whole life history.

It remains to be investigated whether temporally graded autobiographical memory loss following hippocampal damage may be paralleled by a corresponding pattern of experimental episodic memory impairment on much shorter time scales. The time-window of experimental declarative memory appears to be sufficient for the assessment of temporally graded retrograde amnesia in animals. In rats with hippocampal lesions induced *after* the learning of target information, temporally graded retrograde amnesia sometimes covered days to weeks (for a review, see Squire, 1992). Reference to the concept of declarative memory in experimental animals, however, does not necessarily contribute to the issue of behavioral and neurofunctional differences between laboratory and autobiographical episodic memory in humans.

Neuropsychological assessment of patients with hippocampal damage suggests that the hippocampus is involved in both laboratory and autobiographical episodic memory (Cohen and Eichenbaum, 1993; Scoville and Milner, 1957; Squire and Zola-Morgan, 1991; Vargha Khadem et al., 1997). Surprisingly, however, functional neuroimaging studies of laboratory episodic memory in healthy volunteers do not consistently reveal hippocampal activations (for a preliminary discussion, see Maguire and Frith, 2003b). In contrast, the hippocampus was activated in most functional neuroimaging investigations of autobiographical recollection (Addis et al., 2004; Fink et al., 1996; Gilboa et al., 2004; Maguire and Frith, 2003b; Maguire et al., 2001a; Niki and Luo, 2002; Piefke et al., 2003). These functional neuroimaging findings suggest that the hippocampus and perhaps adjacent structures of the medial temporal lobe are more sensitive to the characteristics of episodic autobiographical memories (e.g., their complex spatial, temporal, and self-referential contexts, and their emotional significance) than laboratory episodic memory tasks. *It is reasonable to assume that the autobiographical life-time context and the associated processes of mental time travel and self-referential emotional cognition act as modulators of hippocampal memory functions. The degree to which these characteristics of autobiographical memory can be elicited during laboratory episodic memory tasks most likely influences hippocampal involvement in a given experimental task.*

In the autobiographical memory domain, the hippocampus has differentially been implicated in recent (relative to remote) memories by some, but not all functional neuroimaging experiments (Addis et al., 2004; Niki and Luo, 2002; Piefke et al., 2003; but see Maguire et al., 2001a; Ryan et al., 2001; Viard et al., 2007; Cabeza and St. Jacques, 2007). *Figure 4* displays fMRI evidence for differential activations of the hippocampus in the recollection of recent (relative to remote) emotional autobiographical episodes (Piefke et al., 2003).

The finding of differential hippocampal engagement in the recollection of recent (relative to remote) episodic autobiographical information supports the consolidation theory (Squire, 1992; see above). In this regard, the lack of consistent functional neuroimaging evidence for hippocampal activation during laboratory episodic memory tasks is even more intriguing since the processes of encoding and retrieval of "laboratory events" belong to the category of recent memory per se.

Differential Hippocampal Activity Associated with Recent Relative to Remote Emotional Autobiographical Memory Retrieval

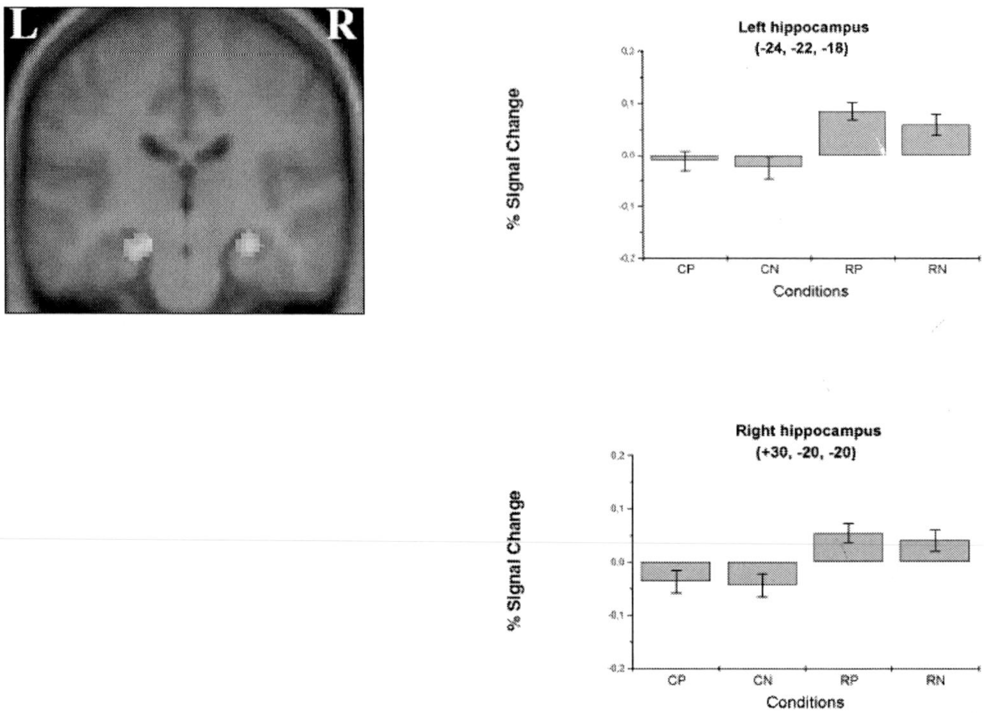

Figure 4. Relative increases in hippocampal activity associated with the recollection of recent compared to remote emotional autobiographical episodes (irrespective of positive or negative valence) of memories reported by Piefke et al. (2003). The histograms display the percentage BOLD signal change for the maxima of significantly increased hippocampal activity as a function of the respective experimental condition. The reverse contrast (remote relative to recent memories) did not yield any statistically significant activations.

R = right; L = left; A = anterior, P = posterior. CP = positive childhood events, CN = negative childhood events, RP = positive recent events, RN = negative recent events.

Functional neuroimaging data suggesting a time-limited hippocampal involvement in recent autobiographical episodic memory is corroborated by the sequential development of memory deficits in patients with Alzheimer's disease (AD) (for a review, see Piefke and Fink, 2005). The loss of recent memories appears during Braak stages III-IV, when conspicuous neurofibrillary changes are mainly restricted to the hippocampal and parahippocampal regions (Braak et al., 1996). Only during later stages of AD, (Braak stages V-VI), as the neurofibrillary changes spread out to the association areas of the neocortex, memories of remote autobiographical events also become impaired. *Figure 5* illustrates the progression of brain pathology and autobiographical memory loss typically associated with AD.

Clinical evidence for AD-related laboratory episodic memory deficits in the anterograde (and thus per se recent) domain (Backman et al., 2001; Eustache et al., 2001; for a review, see Buckner, 2004) may also support of the consolidation theory.

Progression of Brain Pathology in Alzheimer's Disease

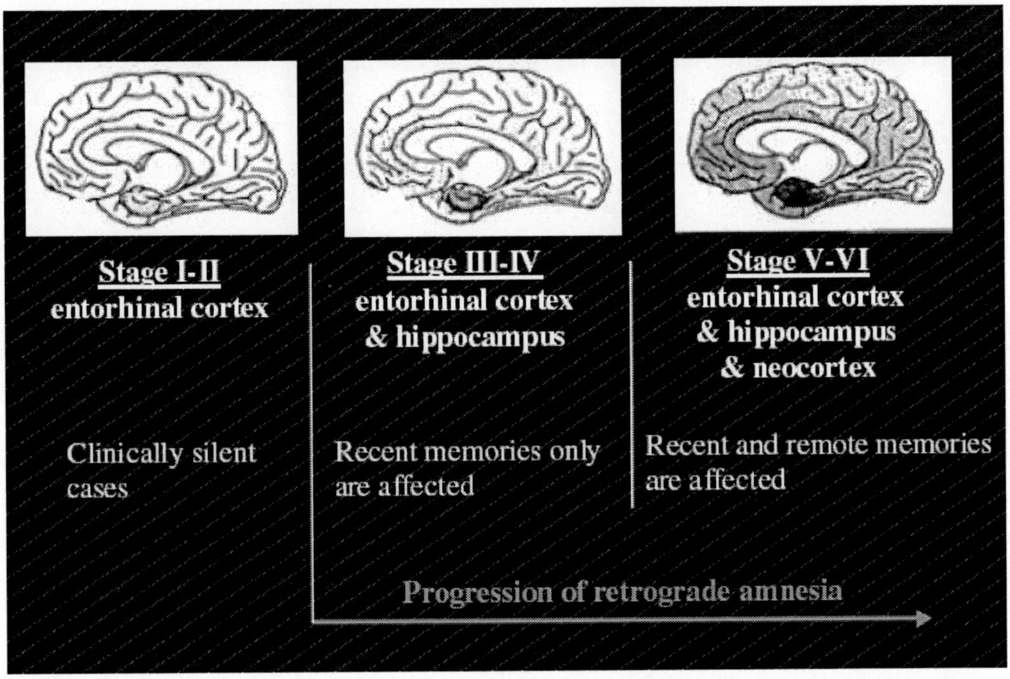

Figure 5. Progression of memory disturbances in patients with Alzheimer's disease (AD) according to Braak et al. (1996). Braak stages I and II depict clinically silent cases where minor changes of the entorhinal cortex can frequently be observed. The sequential development of memory decline is characterized by the early loss of recent memories appearing in the course of Braak stages III-IV during which conspicuous neurofibrillary alterations are typically restricted to hippocampal and entorhinal regions. As the neurofibrillary changes spread out into association areas of the neocortex during the later Braak stages V-VI, remote memory also becomes impaired.

However, other clinical data showing that MTL atrophy in AD patients may result in retrograde amnesia covering both recent and remote episodic autobiographical memories to a similar degree rather support the MTT (see, e.g., Gilboa et al., 2005). Issues concerning the time-window of hippocampal involvement in laboratory and autobiographical memory thus need to be further investigated.

4.2.3. The Posterior Cingulate and Retrosplenial Cortices

The retrosplenial cortex lies adjacent to the retrocommissural hippocampus, a small tissue stripe extending around the posterior end of the corpus callosum. It is interconnected with the entorhinal, the parahippocampal, and the perirhinal cortices and thus closely associated with the hippocampal formation and other structures of the medial temporal lobe subserving memory functions and emotion processing (Insausti et al., 1987). The retrosplenial cortex and its multiple anatomical connections could provide a basis for the typical interplay of emotion and cognition in autobiographical recollections.

Clinical studies reported severe and lasting amnesia for both laboratory and autobiographical materials following selective retrosplenial damage (Bowers et al., 1988; Gainotti et al., 1998; Heilman et al., 1990). Functional neuroimaging studies relate the retrosplenial and posterior cingulate cortices to *emotional* memory in the non-autobiographical (Maddock and Buonocore, 1997; Maratos et al., 2001) and the autobiographical episodic memory domain (Fink et al., 1996; Piefke et al., 2003; Markowitsch et al., 2003). Moreover, the retrosplenial cortex has been related to emotion processing in a more general sense (for a review, see Maddock, 1999).

However, there is also some evidence in support of a specific retrosplenial engagement in autobiographical recollection. Neuropsychological and neuroimaging data converge on the view that autobiographical memory decline associated with normal cognitive aging as well as dementia may be related to pathology of the hippocampal-retrosplenial circuits (for a review, see Piefke and Fink, 2005). Most functional neuroimaging studies on normal volunteers are in good accordance with these clinical data (Fink et al., 1996; Maguire et al., 2001b; Piefke et al. 2003; Shah et al., 2001; Sugiura et al., 2005; but see Maddock, 1999). Piefke et al. (2003) reported increased neural activity in the retrosplenial cortex in combination with bilateral hippocampal activation during the retrieval of recent (relative to remote) emotional autobiographical memories (see also Fink et al., 1996). This finding corroborates the view that the retrosplenial region closely interacts with the hippocampus, and that this interaction may be this interaction may be crucial for the recall of emotionally salient and familiar autobiographical episodes of one's recent past.

Retrosplenial areas have further been implicated in the recognition of personally familiar faces and voices (Shah et al., 2001) as well as objects and places (Sugiura et al., 2005). Although the two latter studies did not directly assess autobiographical recollection, the autobiographically familiar stimulus materials employed in these experiments are likely to have triggered the recall of personal past episodes. Sugiura et al. (2005) argued that the retrosplenial and posterior cingulate cortices are composed of a number of functionally segregated subdivisions. Based on a meta-analysis of functional neuroimaging data on retrosplenial/posterior cingulate involvement in episodic retrieval, they proposed a functional differentiation between the caudal posterior cingulate cortex (cPPC), middorsal PCC (mPCC), posterodorsal PCC (pPCC), and the retrosplenial cortex.

According to this account, the pPCC and the retrosplenial cortex are selectively activated during tasks requiring the retrieval of "real life information", including autobiographical episodes (e.g., Maguire and Frith, 2003b; Piefke et al., 2003), familiar people, and other self-related real world entities (e.g., Leveroni et al., 2000; Kircher et al., 2002; Zysset et al., 2003), and the mental imagery of moving around in a personally familiar environment (Mellet et al., 2000). Activations associated with the retrieval of materials learned in a laboratory context, by contrast, were predominantly located in the mPCC (e.g., Buckner et al., 1996; Henson et al., 1999; Konishi et al., 2000). Finally, the cPCC has been implicated in memory-related navigation in large-scale space (for a review, see Maguire, 2001) and effortful episodic retrieval (Sugiura et al., 2005). The meta-analysis of Sugiura et al. (2005) supports the view suggesting a retrosplenial/posterior cingulate neurofunctional segregation between laboratory and autobiographical episodic memory. *Figure 6* illustrates activation of the retrosplenial area during the recollection of real life information.

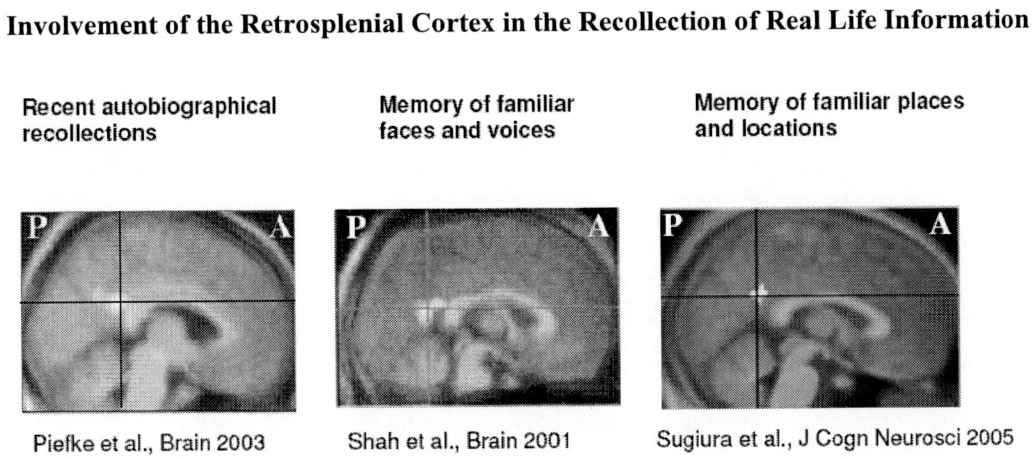

Figure 6. FMRI evidence for retrosplenial activation during the retrieval of real life information. Piefke et al. (2003) demonstrated increased neural activity in the retrosplenial cortex (in combination with bilateral hippocampal activation) during the retrieval of recent (relative to remote) emotional autobiographical memories, suggesting that this brain region is specifically involved in the *recall of emotionally salient and familiar autobiographical episodes of one's recent past* (*a*) (see also Markowitsch et al., 2003). Shah et al. (2001) implicated a corresponding retrosplenial area in the retrieval of personally familiar faces and voices (*b*), and Sugiura et al. (2005) reported activation of the retrosplenial cortex associated with memories of familiar places (*c*). The two latter studies did not directly assess autobiographical recollection. However, the autobiographically familiar stimulus materials used have presumably triggered the recall of personal past episodes.

5. Direct Functional Neuroimaging Comparison of Labortory and Autobiographical Episodic Memory

The studies reviewed above provide evidence that prefrontal, hippocampal and adjacent medial temporal areas, as well as retrosplenial/posterior cingulate brain regions may support both episodic non-autobiographical and autobiographical memory. Parts of these brain structures, however, appear to be differentially engaged in laboratory episodic memory tasks and autobiographical recollection, thus suggesting a *neurofunctional segregation of specific functions involved in each memory type*.

There are some previous neuroimaging experiments which contrasted the brain activations related to autobiographical event memory with those underlying the retrieval of autobiographical facts, public event memory, and the retrieval of general knowledge (Maguire and Mummery, 1999; Maguire and Frith, 2003a, b; Maguire et al., 2001a). However, these do not directly differentiate between laboratory and autobiographical episodic memory: they are based on the distinctions between (i) episodic and semantic memory and (ii) self-referential and impersonal information processing using a 2 x 2 factorial design. Only two functional neuroimaging studies have been published which *directly compared the neural correlates of laboratory episodic memory and autobiographical recollection* using a within-subject design (Cabeza et al., 2004; Nyberg et al., 2002). Nyberg et al. (2002) used a Crovitz cueing technique (Crovitz and Schiffman, 1974) to trigger autobiographical memories across each individual's whole life span and memories of items learned in a recent laboratory context. The types of episodic memories investigated in that study necessarily differed from each other with regard to the main parameters discussed above. These are *memory age* (recent to remote retrograde memory in the autobiographical condition, recent anterograde memory in the laboratory condition), the degree of *self-referential* information processing, the memories' *emotional significance*, the *recollective experience* associated with memory retrieval (which were all high in the autobiographical condition and lacking or at least low in the laboratory condition), and the differential degree and quality of *executive control* (see Gilboa, 2004). Differential neural activations associated with the two memory types were observed in medial and lateral prefrontal as well as parietal brain regions. This finding may indicate the operation of differential brain mechanisms underlying laboratory and autobiographical episodic memory. However, the above confounding between-condition differences have to be taken into consideration when interpreting the data.

Cabeza et al. (2004) a priori defined dimensions determining differences between laboratory and autobiographical episodic memory which were used for the control for confounding variables. Dimensions comprised (i) the proportion of retrieval processes (production and monitoring), (ii) age of memories, (iii) emotional content, (iv) retrieval success, (v) self-referential information processing, (vi) visual/spatial memory, and (vii) recollection. A photo paradigm was used which included photos of (pre-selected) places *taken by the subjects themselves* ("controlled autobiographical condition") and photos of the same places taken by others, but *shown to the subjects in the laboratory* ("laboratory condition"). During the fMRI measurement, participants viewed both types of photos, as well as new ones. They indicated by button press whether each photo had been taken by themselves, shown to them in the laboratory context, or was a new photo. Differential activations related to the controlled autobiographical (relative to the laboratory) condition were observed in the medial prefrontal cortex (an area engaged in self-referential information processing), visual areas and the parahippocampal gyrus (regions involved in visuo-spatial memory), and the hippocampus (a structure implicated in recollective experience). The fMRI data of Cabeza et al. (2004) are in good accordance with the here proposed view of a neurofunctional segregation of laboratory and autobiographical episodic memory in the prefrontal, medial temporal, and retrosplenial/posterior cingulate cortices.

Further investigations are needed, however, in order to evaluate whether the experimental design employed by Cabeza et al. (2004) sufficiently assessed the characteristic attributes of autobiographical memory. Even if the subjects remembered the "real-life" photo-taking episodes during "autobiographical photo recognition", *these episodes remain experimental events*, that is, events which did not occur in the "natural" context of each participant's life history. The attempt to match laboratory and "real life autobiographical" episodic memory for some major dimensions of putative differences between them may have raised the problem that the experimental "real life events" lost some basic attributes of autobiographical episodes. Moreover, the recognition task could well have engaged subjects in the recognition and categorization (own versus others' photo) of photo materials by button presses, but not in the episodic recollection of each respective event. Similar recognition paradigms had been applied in previous functional neuroimaging experiments on autobiographical memory (e.g., Maguire and Frith 2003a, b; Maguire et al., 2001; Ryan et al., 2001). This approach, however, should be treated with caution: one cannot be sure to which degree a neurofunctional measure of recognition memory may give information on *autobiographical recollective re-experience* during memory retrieval.

The photo paradigm employed by Cabeza et al. (2004) meets the requirements of an autobiographical memory study to a higher degree than, for example, fMRI virtual reality (VR) experiments in which VR events were used as a "surrogate" of autobiographical episodes (e.g., Burgess et al., 2001). VR events lack the characteristic features of real life experiences. Rather, they represent experimental events in the sense of an encounter with any kind of stimulus materials which implies visuo-spatial context information. The criteria used by Cabeza et al. (2004) for the identification of differences between autobiographical recollection and laboratory episodic memory are well applicable to the purpose of an up-to-date differentiation between laboratory and autobiographical episodic memory model. Two further aspects could be added: (i) the normal processes and changes of subjective autobiographical reconstruction across time and (ii) the emotional and cognitive evaluation of autobiographical episodes which allow for their integration into a meaningful personal past.

6. Implications of the Present Review

Based on the evidence provided by behavioral, clinical, and neuroimaging studies of laboratory and autobiographical episodic memory reviewed above, I here aim at providing a first step towards a view of episodic memory which accounts for both the commonalities and differences between laboratory and real life autobiographical episodic memory. The classic episodic memory model of the multiple memory systems account (Tulving, 1972, 1983; Tulving and Markowitsch, 1998) represents a well elaborated starting point for a specification of the relationship between laboratory and autobiographical episodic memory. Before the main criterions differentiating laboratory and autobiographical memory will be extracted from the studies reviewed in this article, some important points made by the classic episodic memory model should be summarized. According to the model, common characteristics of laboratory and autobiographical episodic memory concern (i) conscious memory retrieval (but not necessarily conscious encoding, see below) and (ii) reference to the spatial and temporal context of the situation of information encoding. *Laboratory memory tasks which do not explicitly require the conscious processing of spatio-temporal context information during retrieval would therefore not be considered as episodic memory tasks by this account.* In contrast, laboratory tasks relying on remember-know (e.g., Dalla Barba et al., 1997) or source memory paradigms (e.g., Cansino et al., 2002) can be assumed appropriate measures of experimental episodic memory as they require the conscious retrieval of the spatial and/or temporal context of information encoding.

A measure of autobiographical episodic memory can be achieved only by referring to an individual's whole real life context. It always deals with the conscious episodic retrieval of one's own personal past experiences. This point has not always been emphasized by the classic model of episodic memory. The main cognitive-behavioral differences between laboratory and autobiographical episodic memory can be defined along the following criteria:

(1) The requirements of encoding of laboratory and autobiographical episodic information (and the underlying neural mechanisms) differ from each other. Laboratory episodic learning is characterized by an experimentally induced (i.e., artificial) conscious awareness of information processing. This aspect does not need to include the intentional learning of target materials. For example, the semantic categorization of verbal items ("deep encoding") or detection of a particular letter in words or pseudo-words ("shallow encoding") have also been used as episodic memory encoding tasks (e.g., Fletcher et al., 2003; Otten et al., 2001). Autobiographical memory encoding differs from experimental learning in an important respect: the encoding of autobiographical episodes occurs automatically and depending on the subjective relevance of an event such that it does not require any artificial task instruction. To my knowledge, these encoding differences between experimental and autobiographical episodic memory have not explicitly been considered by any neuropsychological or functional neuroimaging study on human memory, yet. In the study of Cabeza et al. (2004), subjects were instructed to learn and intentionally memorize each picture taking episode as an individual event including physical (e.g., light) and psychological (e.g., mental associations) context information. Most likely, the intentional and thus artificial learning of the photo taking events implicates that the "controlled autobiographical events" departed from being autobiographical in nature.
(2) Autonoetic conscious awareness is uniquely associated with autobiographical recollection. Consciousness during laboratory episodic memory retrieval is restricted to an individual's conscious awareness of being engaged in contextual memory retrieval. It needs to be further investigated whether the autonoetic consciousness emerging during autobiographical recollections may at least in part be built upon the processes of automatic encoding of episodic autobiographical information.
(3) The extension of a self-referential context across an individual's whole life history and its association with social-cultural norms during autobiographical information processing may operate as key factors in both the (unconsciously) relevance-oriented automatic encoding of autobiographical episodes and the appearance of autonoetic conscious awareness during autobiographical recollection. The absence of these aspects in laboratory episodic memory tasks most likely requires one's engagement in a conscious and intentional effort to achieve successful encoding and retention of target information.

The neuropsychological and behavioral commonalities and differences of laboratory and autobiographical episodic memory are reflected by a partial integration and segregation of brain mechanisms underlying the two memory types. The prefrontal, temporal, and retrosplenial/posterior cingulate cortices are involved in both laboratory and autobiographical episodic memory, however, with subregions showing a differential engagement in the two memory types. The common aspects include basic neuronal interactions between prefrontal, temporal, and posterior brain regions underlying conjoint conscious item *and* context memory and the monitoring of information retrieval. A segregation of laboratory and autobiographical memory functions occurs at diverse levels of processing. This neurofunctional differentiation can be defined by the following criteria:

(1) The neural mechanisms of the two memory types differ from each other in respect of PFC subregions involved in the executive control of retrieval processes (see also Gilboa, 2004). The dorsolateral and ventrolateral PFC predominate in the support of retrieval effort and post-retrieval monitoring during laboratory episodic memory tasks (e.g., Fletcher et al., 1998). In contrast, the medial PFC is a key player in the self-referential and emotional control of autobiographical recollections (e.g., Cabeza et al., 2004; Piefke et al., 2003). Since the dorsolateral and ventrolateral PFC also mediate strategic aspects of information retrieval, these areas have sometimes also been implicated in autobiographical memory (Gilboa, 2004; Maguire et al., 2001a, Piefke et al., 2003, 2005). Moreover, these PFC regions are involved in the maintenance and manipulation of information in working memory (Cornette et al., 2001; D'Esposito et al., 2000) such that they could act as mediators of the interplay between episodic long-term and working memory processes (Lee et al., 2003; Ranganath et al., 2003). Successful encoding and retrieval of information in laboratory episodic memory tasks particularly depend on strategic "online" manipulation of relevant information. It is thus conceivable that laboratory episodic memory makes higher demands on working memory functions and relies more on lateral PFC regions than autobiographical recollections.

(2) Although the hippocampus is involved in laboratory episodic learning and memory, the degree to which an experimental task approaches the cognitive demands of autobiographical recollections (reference to one's autobiographical life-time context, re-experience of episodes, mental time travel, and self-referential cognition, emotional evaluation) modulates hippocampal and adjacent medial temporal involvement in episodic memory functions (see also Maguire and Frith, 2003b).

(3) The autonoetic conscious awareness which is uniquely associated with autobiographical episodic memory most likely emerges from fine-tuned interactions of circumscribed medial prefrontal, hippocampal, and retrosplenial brain areas. Therefore, it might be the whole cognitive set of autobiographical encoding and retrieval that allows for autonoetic consciousness. The cognitive set of autobiographical recollection is thus likely to differ qualitatively from that of experimental episodic memory. This assumption agrees with recent research on the brain substrates of diverse aspects of consciousness (Egan et al., 2003; Tononi, 2005; Vogt and Laureys, 2005).

Conclusion

The empirical data on laboratory and autobiographical episodic memory reviewed here indicate that the neuropsychological and neurofunctional differences between experimental and autobiographical forms of episodic memory call for an integrative view of the two memory types which considers both their overlapping and differential components. Currently, the laboratory and the autobiographical form of episodic memory may best be modeled as different subsystems of a large-scale neural circuit supporting basic episodic memory functions. To deal with the unresolved issues such as automatic episodic autobiographical memory encoding, the formation of autonoetic conscious awareness during autobiographical recollection, and the role of intentional (in the sense of experimentally induced) cognitive processing in laboratory episodic memory, further cognitive-behavioral and neurofunctional investigations are needed. The suggestions of this review may open the door for the elaboration of novel approaches to both laboratory and autobiographical episodic memory which are qualified for the assessment of such intricate questions.

Acknowledgements

MP is supported by the Hans Lungwitz Foundation, Berlin and the START program of the Rheinisch-Westfälische Hochschule (RWTH) Aachen.

References

Addis, D.R., Moscovitch, M., Crawley, A.P., McAndrews, M.P. (2004). Recollective qualities modulate hippocampal activation during autobiographical memory retrieval. *Hippocampus* 14, 752-762.

Aggleton, J.P., McMackin, D., Carpenter, K., Hornak, J., Kapur, N., Halpin, S., Wiles, C.M., Kamel, H., Brennan, P., Carton, S., Gaffan, D. (2000). Differential cognitive effects of colloid cysts in the third ventricle that spare or compromise the fornix. *Brain* 123, 800-815.

Aron, A.R., Robbins, T.W., Poldrack, R.A. (2004). Inhibition and the right inferior frontal cortex. *Trends Cogn Sci* 8, 170-177.

Backman, L., Small, B.J., Fratiglioni, L. (2001). Stability of the preclinical episodic memory deficit in Alzheimer's disease. *Brain* 124, 96-102.

Barr, W.B., Goldberg, E., Wasserstein, J., Novelly, R.A. (1990). Retrograde amnesia following unilateral temporal lobectomy. *Neuropsychologia* 28, 243-256.

Bolhuis, J.J., Stewart, C.A., Forrest, E.M. (1994). Retrograde amnesia and memory reactivation in rats with ibotenate lesions to the hippocampus or subiculum. *Q. J. Exp. Psychol. B* 47, 129-150.

Bowers, D., Verfaellie, M., Valenstein, E., Heilman, K.M. (1988). Impaired acquisition of temporal information in retrosplenial amnesia. *Brain Cogn* 8, 47-66.

Braak, H., Braak, E., Yilmazer, D., de Vos, R.A., Jansen, E.N., Bohl, J. (1996). Pattern of brain destruction in Parkinson's and Alzheimer's diseases. *J. Neural. Transm.* 103, 455-490.

Buckner, R.L. (2004). Memory and executive function in aging and AD: multiple factors that cause decline and reserve factors that compensate. *Neuron.* 44, 195-208.

Buckner, R.L., Raichle, M.E., Miezin, F.M., Petersen, S.E. (1996). Functional anatomic studies of memory for auditory words and visual pictures. *J. Neurosci.* 16, 6219-6235.

Buckner, R.L., Koutstaal, W., Schacter, D.L., Wagner, A.D., Rosen, B.R. (1998a). Functional-anatomic study of episodic retrieval using fMRI: I. Retrieval effort versus retrieval success. *Neuroimage* 7, 151-162.

Buckner, R.L., Koutstaal, W., Schacter, D.L., Dale, A.M., Rotte, M., Rosen, B.R. (1998b). Functional-anatomic study of episodic retrieval. II. Selective averaging of event-related fMRI trials to test the retrieval success hypothesis. *Neuroimage* 7, 163-175.

Burgess, N., Maguire, E.A, Spiers, H.J., O'Keefe, J. (2001). A temporoparietal and prefrontal for retrieving the spatial context of lifelike events. *Neuroimage* 14, 439-453.

Cabeza, R., St. Jacques, P. (2007). Functional neuroimaging of autobiographical memory. *Trends Cogn. Sci.*, epub ahead of print.

Cabeza, R., Prince, S.E., Daselaar, S.M., Greenberg, D.L., Budde, M., Dolcos, F., Labar, K.S., Rubin, D.C. (2004). Brain activity during episodic retrieval of autobiographical and laboratory events. *J. Cogn. Neurosci.* 16, 1583-1594.

Cansino, S., Maquet, P., Dolan, R.J., Rugg, M.D. (2002). Brain activity underlying encoding and retrieval of source memory. *Cereb. Cortex* 12, 1048-1056.

Cohen, N.J., Eichenbaum, H. (1993). *Memory, amnesia, and the hippocampal system.* Cambridge, MA: MIT Press.

Conway, M.A. (2001). Sensory-perceptual episodic memory and its context: autobiographical memory. *Philos Trans R Soc Lond B. Biol. Sci.* 356, 1375-1384.

Conway, M.A., Pleydell-Pearce C.W. (2000). The construction of autobiographical memories in the self-memory system. *Psychol. Rev.* 107, 261-288.

Cornette, L., Dupont, P., Salmon, E., Orban, G.A. (2001). The neural substrate of orientation working memory. *J. Cogn. Neurosci.* 13, 813-828.

Crovitz, H.F., Schiffman, H. (1974). Frequency of episodic memories as a function of age. *Bull. Psychon. Soc.* 5, 517-518.

Dalla Barba, G., Mantovan, M.C., Ferruzza, E., Denes, G. (1997). Remembering and knowing the past: a case study of isolated retrograde amnesia. *Cortex* 33, 143-154.

D'Esposito, M., Postle, B.R., Rypma, B. (2000). Prefrontal cortical contributions to working memory: evidence from event-related fMRI studies. *Brain Res.* 133, 3-11.

Egan, G., Silk, T., Zamarripa, F., Williams, J., Federico, P., Cunnington, R., Carabott, L., Blair-West, J., Shade, R., McKinley, M., Farrell, M., Lancaster, J., Jackson, G., Fox, P., Denton, D. (2003). Neural correlates of the emergence of consciousness of thirst. *Proc. Natl. Acad. Sci. USA* 100, 15241-15246.

Eustache, F., Desgranges, B., Giffard, B., de la Sayette, V., Baron, J.C. (2001). Entorhinal cortex disruption causes memory deficit in early Alzheimer's disease as shown by PET. *Neuroreport* 12, 683-685.

Fink, G.R., Markowitsch, H.J., Reinkemeier, M., Bruckbauer, T., Kessler, J., Heiss, W.D. (1996). Cerebral representation of one's own past: neural networks involved in autobiographical memory. *J Neurosci* 16, 4275-4282.

Fletcher, P.C., Shallice, T., Frith, C.D., Frackowiak, R.S., Dolan, R.J. (1998). The functional roles of prefrontal cortex in episodic memory. II. Retrieval. *Brain* 121, 1249-1256.

Fletcher, P.C., Stephenson, C.M., Carpenter, T.A., Donovan, T., Bullmore, E.T. (2003). Regional brain activations predicting subsequent memory success: an event-related fMRI study of the influence of encoding tasks. *Cortex* 39, 1009-1026.

Fujii, T., Suzuki, M., Okuda, J., Ohtake, H., Tanji, K. Yamaguchi, K., Itoh, M., Yamadori, A. (2004). Neural correlates of contex memory with real-world events. *Neuroimage* 21, 1596-1603.

Gaffan, D., Parker, A., Easton, A. (2001). Dense amnesia in the monkey after transection of fornix, amygdala, and anterior temporal stem. *Neuropsychologia* 39, 51-70.

Gainotti, G., Almonti, S., DiBetta, A.M., Silveri, M.C. (1998). Retrograde amnesia in a patient with retrosplenial tumour. *Neurocase* 4, 519-526.

Gallagher, H.L., Happe, F., Brunswick, N., Fletcher, P.C., Frith, U., Frith, C.D. (2000). Reading the mind in cartoons and stories: an fMRI study of "theory of mind" in verbal and nonverbal tasks. *Neuropsychologia* 38, 11-21.

Gallagher, I.I. (2000). Philosophical conceptions of the self: implications for cognitive science. *Trends Cogn. Sci.* 4, 14-21.

Gardiner, J.M., Java, R.I. (1993). Recognizing and remembering In: A.F. Collins, S.E. Gathercole, M.A. Conway, P.E. Morris (Eds.), *Theories of Memory* (pp. 163-188). Hove (UK): Erlbaum.

Geday J., Gjedde, A., Boldsen, A.S., Kupers, R. (2003). Emotional valence modulates activity in the posterior fusiform gyrus and inferior medial prefrontal cortex in social perception. *Neuroimage* 18, 675-684.

Gilboa, A. (2004). Autobiographical and episodic memory - one and the same? Evidence from prefrontal activation in neuroimaging studies. *Neuropsychologia* 42, 1336-1349.

Gilboa, A., Winocur, G., Grady, C.L., Hevenor, S.J., Moscovitch, M. (2004). Remembering our past: functional neuroanatomy of recollection of recent and very remote personal events. *Cereb. Cortex* 14, 1214-1225.

Gilboa, A., Ramirez, J., Köhler, S., Westmacott, R., Black, S.E., Moscovitch, M. (2005). Retrieval of autobiographical in Alzheimer's disease: relation to volumes of medial temporal lobe and other structures. *Hippocampus* 15, 535-550.

Habib, R., Nyberg, L., Tulving, E. (2003). Hemispheric asymmetries of memory: the HERA model revisited. *Trends Cogn Sci* 7, 241-245.

Heilman KM, Bowers D, Watson RT, Day A, Valenstein E, Hammond E, Duara R. (1990). Frontal hypermetabolism and thalamic hypometabolism in a patient with abnormal orienting and retrosplenial amnesia. *Neuropsychologia* 28, 161-169.

Henson, R.N., Rugg, M.D., Shallice, T., Josephs, O., Dolan, R.J. (1999). Recollection and familiarity in recognition memory: an event-related functional magnetic resonance imaging study. *J. Neurosci.* 19, 3962-3972.

Henson, R.N.A., Rugg, M., Shallice, T., Dolan, R.J. (2000). Confidence in recognition memory for words: dissociating right prefrontal roles in episodic retrieval. *J. Cogn. Neurosci.* 12, 913-923.

Hunkin, N.M., Mayes, A.R., Williams, S.C.R., Gregory, L.J., Nunn, J.A., Nicholas, A,K., Brammer, M.J., Bullmore, E.T. (2000). Does frontal lobe activation during retrieval reflect complexity of retrieved information? *Neuroreport* 11, 557-561.

Incisa della Rocchetta, A., Milner, B. (1993). Strategic search and retrieval inhibition: the role of the frontal lobes. *Neuropsychologia* 31, 503-524.

Insausti, R., Amaral, D.G., Cowan, W.M. (1987). The entorhinal cortex of the monkey II: Cortical afferents. *J. Comp. Neurol.* 264, 356-395.

Kapur, N., Ellison, D., Smith, M.P. McLellan, D.L., Burrows, E.H. (1992). Focal retrograde amnesia following bilateral temporal lobe pathology. A neuropsychological and magnetic resonance study. *Brain* 115, 73-85.

Kapur, N., Ellison, D., Parkin, A.J., Hunkin, N.M., Burrows, E., Sampson, S.A., Morrison, E.A. (1994). Bilateral temporal lobe pathology with sparing of medial temporal lobe structures: lesion profile and pattern of memory disorder. *Neuropsychologia* 32, 23-38.

Kapur, S., Craik, F.I., Jones, C., Brown, G.M., Houle, S., Tulving, E. (1995). Functional role of the prefrontal cortex in retrieval of memories: a PET study. *Neuroreport* 6, 1880-1884.

Kim, J.J., Fanselow, M.S. (1992). Modality-specific retrograde amnesia for fear. *Science* 256, 675-677.

Kircher, T.T.J., Brammer, M., Bullmore, E., Simmons, A., Bartels, M., David, A.S. (2002). The neural correlates of intentional and incidental self processing. *Neuropsychologia* 40, 683-692.

Knowlton, B.J., Squire, L.R. (1995). Remembering and knowing: two different expressions of declarative memory. *J. Exp. Psychol. Learn Mem. Cogn.* 21, 699-710.

Konishi, S., Wheeler, M.E., Donaldson, D.I., Buckner, R.L. (2000). Neural correlates of episodic retrieval success. *Neuroimage* 12, 276-286.

Lee, A.C.H., Robbins, T.W., Owen, A.M. (2003). Episodic memory meets working memory in the frontal lobe: functional neuroimaging studies of encoding and retrieval. *Crit. Rev. Neurobiol.* 14, 165-197.

Leveroni, C.L., Seidenberg, M., Mayer, A.R., Mead, L.A., Binder, J.R., Rao, S.M. (2002). Neural systems underlying the recognition of familiar and newly learned faces. *J. Neurosci.* 20, 878-886.

Maddock, R.J. (1999). The retrosplenial cortex and emotion: new insights from functional neuroimaging of the human brain. *Trends Neurosci.* 22, 310-316.

Maddock, R.J., Buonocore, M.H. (1997). Activation of left posterior cingulate gyrus by the auditory presentation of threat-related words: an fMRI study. *Psychiatry Res.* 75, 1-14.

Maguire, E.A. (2001). The retrosplenial contribution to human navigation: a review of lesion and neuroimaging findings. *Scand. J. Psychol.* 42, 225-228.

Maguire, E.A., Mummery, C.J. (1999). Differential modulation of a common memory retrieval network revealed by positron emission tomography. *Hippocampus* 9, 54-61.

Maguire, E.A., Frith, C.D. (2003a). Lateral asymmetry in the hippocampal responses to the remoteness of autobiographical memories. *J. Neurosci.* 23, 5302-5307.

Maguire, E.A., Frith, C.D. (2003b). Aging affects the engagement of the hippocampus during autobiographical memory retrieval. *Brain* 126, 1511-1523.

Maguire, E.A., Henson, R.N., Mummery, C.J., Frith, C.D. (2001a). Activity in the prefrontal cortex, not hippocampus, varies parametrically with increasing remoteness of autobiographical memories. *Neuroreport* 12, 441-444.

Maguire, E.A., Vargha-Khadem, F., Mishkin, M. (2001b). The effects of bilateral hippocampal damage on fMRI regional activations and interactions during memory retrieval. *Brain* 124, 1156-1170.

Maratos, E.J., Dolan, R.J., Morris, J.S., Henson, R.N., Rugg, M.D. (2001). Neural activity associated with episodic memory for emotional context. *Neuropsychologia* 39, 910-920.

Markowitsch, H.J. (1995). Which brain regions are critically involved in the retrieval of old episodic memories? *Brain Res. Brain Res. Rev.* 21, 117-127.

Markowitsch, H.J. (2003) The functional anatomy of learning and memory. In: P. Halligan, U. Kischka, G. Beaumont (Eds.), *Handbook of Clinical Neuropsychology* (pp. 724-740). Oxford (UK): Oxford University Press.

Markowitsch, H.J., Vanderkerkhove, M.M., Lanfermann, H., Russ, M.O. (2003). Engagement of lateral and medial prefontal areas in the ecphory of sad and happy autobiographical memories. *Cortex* 3, 643-665.

Mayes, A.R., Downes, J.J. (1997). What do theories of the functional deficit(s) underlying amnesia have to explain? *Memory* 5, 3-47.

Mayes, A.R., Montaldi, D. (2001). Exploring the neural bases of episodic and semantic memory: the role of structural and functional neuroimaging. *Neurosci. Biobehav. Rev.* 25, 555-573.

McDonald, R.J., White, N.M. (1993). A triple dissociation of memory systems: hippocampus, amygdala, and dorsal striatum. *Behav. Neurosci.* 107, 3-22.

Meilandt, W.J., Barea-Rodriguez, E., Harvey, S.A., Martinez, J.L. (2004). Role of hippocampal CA3 mu-opioid receptors in spatial learning and memory. *J. Neurosci.* 24, 2953-2062.

Mellet, E., Briscogne, S., Tzourio-Mazoyer, N., Ghaem, O., Petit, L., Zago, L., Etard, O., Berthoz, A., Mazoyer, B., Denis, M. (2000). Neural correlates of topographic mental exploration: the impact of route versus survey perspective learning. *Neuroimage* 12, 588-600.

Nadel, L., Moscovitch, M. (1997). Memory consolidation, retrograde amnesia, and the hippocampal complex. *Curr. Opin. Neurobiol.* 7, 217-227.

Niki, K., Luo, J. (2002). An fMRI study on the time-limited role of the medial temporal lobe in long-term topographical autobiographic memory. *J. Cogn. Neurosci.* 14, 500-507.

Nolde, S.F., Johnson, M.K., Raye, C.L. (1998a). Left prefrontal activation during episodic remembering: an event-related fMRI study. *Neuroreport* 9, 3509-3514.

Nolde, S.F., Johnson, M.K., Raye, C.L. (1998b). The role of prefrontal cortex during tests of episodic memory. *Trends Cogn. Sci.* 2, 399-406.

Nyberg, L., Tulving, E., Habib, R., Nilsson, L.G., Kapur, S., Houle, S., Cabeza, R., McIntosh, A.R. (1995). Functional brain maps of retrieval mode and recovery of episodic information. *Neuroreport* 7, 9-10.

Nyberg, L., Forkstam, C, Petersson, K.M., Cabeza, R., Ingvar, M. (2002). Brain imaging of human memory systems: between-systems similarities and within-systems differences. *Brain Res. Cogn. Brain Res.* 13, 281-192.

Otten, L.J., Henson, R.N., Rugg, M.D. (2001). Depth of processing effects on neural correlates of memory encoding: relationship between findings from across- and within-task comparisons. *Brain* 124, 399-412.

Piefke, M., Weiss, P., Zilles, K., Markowitsch, H.J., Fink, G.R. (2003). Differential Remoteness and emotional tone modulate the neural correlates of autobiographical memory. *Brain* 126, 650-668.

Piefke, M., Weiss, P., Markowitsch, H.J., Fink, G.R. (2005). Gender differences in the functional neuroanatomy of emotional episodic autobiographical memory. *Hum. Brain Mapp.* 24, 313-324.

Piefke, M., Fink, G.R. (2005). Recollections of one's own past: the effects of aging and gender on the neural mechanisms of episodic autobiographical memory. *Anat. Embryol.* 210, 497-512.

Ranganath, C., Johnson, M.K., D'Esposito, M. (2000). Left anterior prefrontal activation increases with demands to recall specific perceptual information. *J. Neurosci.* 20, 1-5.

Ranganath, C., Johnson, M.K., D'Esposito, M. (2003). Prefrontal activity associated with working memory and episodic long-term memory. *Neuropsychologia* 41, 378-389.

Remondes, M., Schuman, E.M. (2004). Role for a cortical input to hippocampal area CA1 in the consolidation of long-term memory. *Nature* 43, 699-703.

Rempel-Clower, N.L., Zola, S.M., Squire, L.R., Amaral, D.G. (1996). Three cases of enduring memory impairment after bilateral damage limited to the hippocampal formation. *J. Neurosci.* 16, 5233-5255.

Rugg, M.D., Fletcher, P.C., Frith, C.D., Frackowiak, R.S.J., Dolan, R.J. (1996). Differential activation of the prefrontal cortex in successful and unsuccessful memory retrieval. *Brain* 119, 2073-2083.

Ryan, L., Nadel, L., Keil, K., Putnam, K., Schnyer, D., Trouard, T., Moscovich, M. (2001). Hippocampal complex and retrieval of recent and very remote autobiographical memories: evidence from functional magnetic resonance imaging in neurologically intact people. *Hippocampus* 11, 707-714.

Schacter, D.L., Curran, T., Galluccio, L., Milberg, W.P., Bates, J.F. (1996a). False recognition and the right frontal lobe: a case study. *Neuropsychologia* 34, 793-808.

Schacter, D.L., Alpert, N.M., Savage, C.R., Rauch, S.L., Albert M.S. (1996b). Conscious recollection and the human hippocampal formation: evidence from positron emission tomography. *Proc. Natl. Acad. Sci. USA* 93, 321-325.

Scoville, W.B., Milner, B. (1957). Loss of recent memory after bilateral hippocampal lesions. *J. Neurol. Neurosurg. Psychiatry* 20, 11-20.

Shah, N.J., Marshall, J.C., Zafiris, O., Schwab, A., Zilles, K., Markowitsch, H.J., Fink, G.R. (2001). The neural correlates of person familiarity: A functional magnetic resonance imaging study with clinical implications. *Brain* 124, 804-815.

Shallice, T., Fletcher, P., Frith, C.D., Grasby, P., Frackowiak, R.S., Dolan, R.J. (1994). Brain regions associated with acquisition and retrieval of verbal episodic memory. *Nature* 368, 633-635.

Smith, A.P., Henson, R.N., Dolan, R.J., Rugg, M.D. (2004). FMRI correlates of the episodic retrieval of emotional contexts. *Neuroimage* 22, 868-878.

Squire, L.R. (1992). Memory and the hippocampus: a synthesis from findings with rats, monkeys, and humans. *Psychol. Rev.* 99, 195-231.

Squire, L.R. (1998). Memory systems. *CR Acad. Sci. III* 321, 153-156.

Squire, L.R., Knowlton, B.J. (2000). The medial temporal lobe, the hippocampus, and memory systems of the brain. In: M.S. Gazzaniga (Ed.), *The New Cognitive Neurosciences* (pp. 765-779). Cambridge, MA: MIT.

Squire, L.R., Zola-Morgan, S. (1991). The medial temporal lobe memory system. *Science* 253, 1380-1386.

Squire, L.R., Zola, S.M. (1996). Structure and function of declarative and nondeclarative memory systems. *Proc. Natl. Acad. Sci. USA* 93, 13515-13522.

Stuss, D.T., Alexander, M.P., Palumbo, C.L., Buckle, L., Sayer, L., Pogue, J. (1994). Organizational strategies of patients with unilateral or bilateral frontal lobe injury in word list learning tasks. *Neuropsychology* 8, 355-373.

Sugiura, M., Shah, N.J., Zilles, K., Fink, G.R. (2005). Cortical representations of personally-familiar objects and places: functional organization of the human posterior cingulate cortex. *J. Cogn. Neurosci.* 17, 183-198.

Tononi, G. (2005). Consciousness, information integration, and the brain. *Progr. Brain Res.* 150, 109-126.

Tulving, E., (1972). Episodic and semantic memory. In: E. Tulving, W. Donaldson (Eds.), *Organization of Memory* (pp. 381-403). New York: Academic Press.

Tulving, E. (1983). Elements of Episodic Memory. Oxford: Claredon Press.

Tulving, E. (1995). Organization of memory: Quo vadis? In: M.S. Gazzaniga (Ed.), *The Cognitive Neurosciences* (pp. 839-847). Cambridge, MA: MIT Press.

Tulving, E., Markowitsch, H.J. (1998). Episodic and declarative memory: Role of the hippocampus. *Hippocampus* 8, 198-204.

Tulving, E., Kapur, S., Craik, F.I.M., Moscovitch, M., Houle, S. (1994). Hemispheric encoding/retrieval asymmetry in episodic memory: Positron emission tomography findings. *Proc. Natl. Acad. Sci.* 91, 2016-2020.

Valenstein, E., Bowers, D., Verfaellie, M., Heilman, K M., Day, A., Watson, R.T. (1987). Retrosplenial amnesia. *Brain* 110, 1631-1646.

Vanderkerckhove, M.M., Markowitsch, H.J., Mertens, M., Woermann, F.G. (2005). Bi-hemispheric engagement in the retrieval of autobiographical episodes. *Behav. Neurol.* 16, 20-210.

Vargha-Khadem, F., Gadian, D.G., Watkins, K.E., Connelly, A., Van Paesschen, W., Mishkin, M. (1997). Differential effects of early hippocampal pathology on episodic and semantic memory. *Science* 277, 376-380.

Viard, A., Piolino, P., Desgranges, B., Chetelat, G., Lebreton, K., Landeau, B., Young, A., de la Sayette, V., Eustache, F. (2007). Hippocampal activation for autobiographical memories over the entire lifetime in healthy aged subjects. An fMRI study. *Cereb. Cortex*, epub ahead of print.

Vogeley, K., Bussfeld, P., Newen, A., Herrmann, S., Happe, F., Falkai, P., Maier, W., Shah, N.J., Fink, G.R., Zilles, K. (2001). Mind reading: neural mechanisms of theory of mind and self-perspective. *Neuroimage* 14, 170-181.

Vogt, B.A., Laureys, S. (2005). Posterior cingulate, precuneal, and retrosplenial cortices: cytology and components of the neural network correlates of consciousness. *Prog. Brain Res.* 150, 205-217.

Wager, T.D., Smith, E.E. (2003). Neuroimaging studies of working memory: a meta-analysis. *Cogn Affect Behav Neurosci* 3, 255-274.

Walker, A.E. (1957). Recent memory impairment in unilateral temporal lesions. *Arch. Neurol. Psychiatry* 78, 543-552.

Zola-Morgan, S., Squire, L.R., Amaral, D.G. (1986). Human amnesia and the medial temporal region: enduring memory impairment following a bilateral lesion to field CA1 of the hippocampus. *J. Neurosci.* 6, 2959-2967.

Zysset, S., Huber, O., Samson, A., Ferstl, E.C., von Cramon, D.Y. (2003). Functional specialization within the anterior medial prefrontal cortex: a functional magnetic resonance imaging study with human subjects. *Neurosci. Lett.* 335, 183-186.

In: Brain Mapping Research Developments
Editor: Lars N. Bakker, pp. 129-153
ISBN 978-1-60456-007-7

Chapter V

REAL-TIME FUNCTIONAL MAGNETIC RESONANCE IMAGING AND ITS APPLICATIONS

Shaolin Yang, Thomas J. Ross and Yihong Yang
Neuroimaging Research Branch, National Institute on Drug Abuse
5500 Nathan Shock Drive, Building C Room 383, Baltimore, MD, USA

ABSTRACT

Functional magnetic resonance imaging (fMRI) is a noninvasive imaging technique that is able to detect hemodynamic changes associated with neuronal activity in vivo. In the past decade, it has been used extensively for mapping functional neuroanatomy in basic neuroscience and clinical applications. A typical fMRI study includes acquisition of a time series of images (during which the subject is instructed to perform certain tasks) and offline processing and analysis of the image series. In real-time fMRI (rtfMRI), however, image processing and analysis start shortly after the beginning of the scan and then follow the image acquisition procedure as closely as possible. Real-time fMRI provides not only a useful tool for effective quality assurance of fMRI studies, but also opportunities for designing functional examinations with interactive controls and feedback.

In this chapter, we describe the basic concept and technical solution of rtfMRI, with a focus on a technique that we have recently developed and implemented on a Siemens 3T MRI scanner. We then demonstrate potential applications of rtfMRI techniques for neurofeedback and motion artifact reduction. In particular, we present a novel method of voluntary head-motion suppression using the feedback of the subject's own motion information in real time. This method was tested and the possible influence on the performance of tasks in fMRI study was assessed utilizing a commonly used working memory task. Our experiments showed that significant suppression of head motion was achieved consistently while the influence on the performance of task and the interference to brain activation could be minimized by careful design of the feedback system.

Keywords: functional magnetic resonance imaging (fMRI), real-time fMRI (rtfMRI), neurofeedback, head motion, BOLD.

INTRODUCTION

In the last decade, we have experienced a renaissance in neuroimaging with the emergence of functional Magnetic Resonance Imaging (fMRI). FMRI is a noninvasive imaging technique that is able to detect hemodynamic changes putatively associated with neuronal activity *in vivo*. The origins of this renaissance can be traced to a convergence of discoveries and technologies. Ogawa's discovery of the Blood Oxygen Level Dependant (BOLD) effect that documented changes in concentration of paramagnetic deoxyhemoglobin lead to changes in local magnetic field inhomogeneity and hence changes in the MRI signal [1,2]. The BOLD effect is consistent with an early discovery by Fox et al. [3] that reported a regional overperfusion in response to neuronal activation obtained from positron emission tomography. The availability of single-shot MRI imaging techniques such as echo planar imaging [4] and spiral imaging [5] made it possible to image the entire brain, at spatial resolution of the order of millimeters, in seconds. So we are now able to image in seconds changes in blood deoxyhemoglobin as a result of perfusion changes related to neuronal activation – BOLD fMRI.

FMRI based on the BOLD effect has become the cornerstone of neuroimaging research. In the past decade, it has been used extensively for mapping functional neuroanatomy in basic neuroscience and clinical applications. There are a number of steps to be performed between data acquisition and the final statistical map. These can include reconstruction of the thousands to tens of thousands of slices, motion correction, spatial normalization, spatial filtering, temporal filtering and modeling of the time-course data. Many of these steps are computationally intensive. However, Moore's law, the observation that number transistors – and hence computing power – doubles roughly every 18 months, has continued unabated [6] such that tasks like reconstruction that used to require expensive array processors are now done with desktop personal computers. Additionally, it has become relatively easy to combine PCs into a parallel processing cluster for greater performance [7]. By simplifying some of the processing steps, it is now possible to perform fMRI analysis in "real time."

What is meant by real-time fMRI (rtfMRI)? Clearly, despite computational improvements, the above steps take an appreciable amount of time. "Real-time" is typically defined as taking less time than other relevant time scales. For fMRI, the relevant time scale is the repetition time (TR), the time required to acquire one complete set of slices. Modern scanners reconstruct the data soon after each slice is acquired. The processing may be occurring on a slice by slice basis as well, although some steps such as 3D motion correction may require a full set of slices. If the processing is complete before the next TR is complete, thus leaving enough time for next TR's data to be processed itself during the TR after that, for our purposes we shall consider it done in real-time.

Given the extra hardware, software and setup requirements of rtfMRI, one might question the advantage of rtfMRI over traditional acquisition and processing. The largest gain is in a clinical setting. It is not uncommon for fMRI researchers to discard subject's data because of data quality, often related to motion.

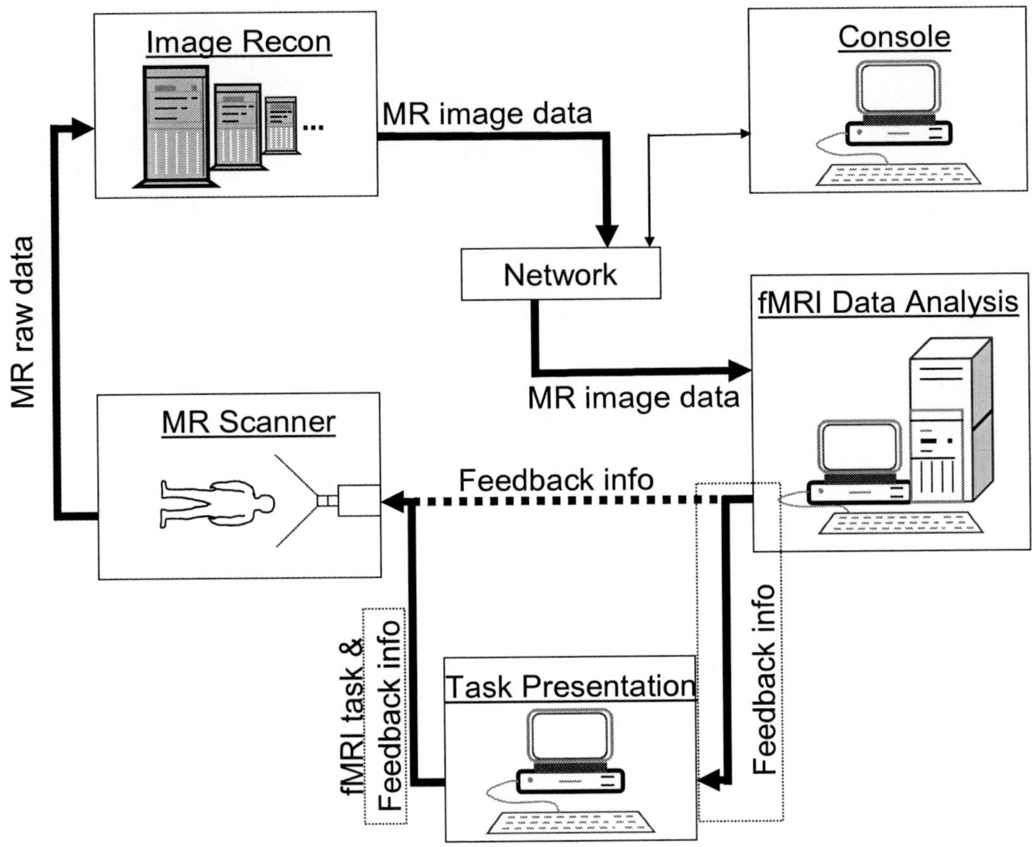

Figure 1. Schematic of a general real-time fMRI system, which is configured through close integration of the scanner, the online image reconstruction system, the task presentation system, the response monitoring system, and the online fMRI data analysis and/or real-time feedback system. The thick lines and arrows represent the data flow in real-time.

For a clinical scan of a patient, an immediate feedback of the quality, results and compliance of an fMRI scan is an enormous benefit. Real-time fMRI also opens intriguing biofeedback experiments for researchers, where subjects would receive information about the experiment, for example their brain's activation or their head position, in real-time. Finally, one can imagine creating dynamic experiment where the task itself changes as a result of a subject's neuronal activity.

In the remainder of this chapter, we will describe the basic concepts and technical solution of rtfMRI, with a focus on a technique that we have recently developed and implemented on a Siemens 3T MRI scanner. We will then elaborate on the potential applications of rtfMRI techniques mentioned above. In particular, we present a novel method of voluntary head-motion suppression using the feedback of the subject's own motion information in real time.

IMPLEMENTATION

Hardware Requirements and Data Flow

For conventional fMRI, the scanner and associated raw (or image) data storage facilities and task presentation system are the necessary parts of the hardware configuration. To perform fMRI in real-time, generally more stringent requirements must be met. The real-time fMRI hardware system is generally configured through close integration of the scanner, the online image reconstruction system, the task presentation system, the response monitoring system, and the online fMRI data analysis and/or real-time feedback system [8,9]. Additional hardware may be required for some specific real-time fMRI applications. Figure 1 shows a generic schematic of a real-time fMRI system with the parts in the boxes with dashed lines only for the implementation of feedback.

The real-time fMRI hardware determines the associated data flow during the fMRI experiments. The raw MR k-space (frequency space) data are acquired using the MR scanner and the raw data will immediately be transferred, via a fast connection such as an optical link, to a computer that is typically used exclusively for the image reconstruction due to the intensive computational load, especially for image reconstruction of whole-brain fMRI time series. Upon reconstruction, the image data are transferred slice by slice, or volume by volume, via internal network or local area network (LAN), to another computer which is running the real-time software. This software may be the public-domain AFNI [10], commercial software such as Turbo-Brain Voyager [11], or, most-commonly, custom-made software [8,12]. The real-time software is used for analyzing the fMRI image data, including various preprocessing steps, i.e., head motion detection and correction, detrending, and statistical analysis to get the activation maps. The intermediate analysis results, such as head motion parameters [12], activation maps [9,13] or activation intensity curves [13,14] can be simultaneously transferred to an independent feedback system for real-time presentation to the subject, or integrated into the task presentation system [12], making the fMRI experiments interactive by manipulating the ongoing paradigms according to the subject's responses. Additionally, the investigator and/or scanner operator can monitor the motion and activation of the subject [15], and stop the scan if the motion is excessive or if the activation has reached sufficient statistical power.

Image Reconstruction

In real-time fMRI experiments online image reconstruction follows immediately after the raw k-space data are sent out from the scanner. As one of the most computationally intensive tasks in real-time data processing, online image reconstruction requires powerful computer resources, often multiprocessor computers or even a cluster of PCs [15], to obtain sufficient processing speed. This is especially true for whole-brain studies. Besides hardware, image reconstruction algorithms strongly depend on the chosen fast imaging technique for fMRI data acquisition, such as single-shot echo-planar imaging (EPI) [8,12,13,14,16] or spiral imaging [17,18]. Spiral imaging acquires data along a spiral trajectory in k-space. The typical spiral image reconstruction algorithm first interpolates the raw spiral data onto an orthogonal, equidistant grid (so-called 'regridding') before a two-dimensional fast Fourier transformation [19]. In contrast, EPI acquires the raw data on a rectangular grid in k-space, therefore no regridding is necessary for EPI image reconstruction. Strategies to reduce the image reconstruction time commonly use parallel processing. Goddard et al. reported an fMRI system which includes the online image reconstruction using multiple parallel platforms [20]. Frank et al. distributed different volumes of data on different processors for image reconstruction and registration in parallel [18]. These arrangements substantially reduce the total image reconstruction time. For real-time fMRI studies, finishing all of the associated processing steps on one volume of data within the time window of one TR is necessary to achieve real-time imaging, which indirectly determines the upper limit of the time available for image reconstruction.

Motion Analysis and Correction

In fMRI data analysis, the signal intensity time series in each voxel are evaluated using various statistical methods. This is generally done under either the assumption that the subject's head remained motionless or that any residual motion can be accounted for in the statistical analysis with covariates. However, for most experiments, this is not the case [21, 22]. Subjects move substantially due to long scan times, unease over experimental procedures, orienting to experimental stimuli, swallowing, blood drawing or drug administration, or other experimental measures performed during data acquisition [12]. Although the absolute magnitudes of head movement in fMRI data are small, commonly within 1 mm, the influence of head motion cannot be ignored. The BOLD signal change generally is very small, i.e., usually 1-3% at 1.5 T magnetic field strength. If two adjacent voxels have 20% difference in their intensities (for example a gray matter voxel adjacent to a white matter voxel), a movement of 0.375 mm (10% of the voxel size of 3.75 mm, a typical image resolution in fMRI studies) will bring about 2% signal change, the same level as the BOLD signal change due to the neuronal activation [23]. If uncorrected, this motion-induced change to the voxel time series will lead to erroneous statistical inference. Depending upon the type of motion, false-positives/increased activation (for task-correlated motion) or false-negatives/decreased statistical significance (task-independent motion) volume will result, respectively. In other words, head motion will reduce the sensitivity and specificity of fMRI data analysis.

To combat this motion, image registration is normally used for motion detection and correction in fMRI data analysis [24,25]. Nearly all fMRI image registration techniques use the rigid body model, which assumes that the brain is rigid and does not deform due to head motion, breathing, and heart beat [26]. This is a reasonable assumption, although there does exist some brain motion and deformation, but only with a small amplitude in the cortex [24]. Non-rigid body models exist, but are far too computationally demanding for real-time applications.

The rigid body transformation in three-dimension (3D) space is described with six parameters, three translational parameters and three rotational parameters [24,25]. For image registration, a cost function is first defined as the measure of dissimilarity between the images, and then the transformation parameters are determined by minimizing the cost function. A least-squares criterion is widely used, where the cost function is defined as the square of the global difference between the reference image $I(\boldsymbol{r})$ and the source image $J(\boldsymbol{r})$ [24,27],

where $\mathbf{T}$ stands for the rigid body transformation, which, in theory, can be calculated using any technique for a multi-dimensional nonlinear least-squares problem [28]. However, these commonly used techniques are extremely time-consuming and thus inappropriate for real-time application. So special treatments targeted at reducing the computation time while maintaining sufficient motion estimation accuracy are needed for the associated implementation in real-time fMRI.

If the motion is small and the volumes are spatially smooth (by blurring if necessary), Eq. (1) can be linearized through expanding the source image as a first order Taylor series about the reference with respect to six rigid body transformation parameters [24,26,29]

where $m_1, \cdots, m_6$ are the rigid body transformation parameters. The linear equation, Eq. (2), can be solved iteratively with repeated "reslicing" of the volume in each intermediate step, providing the estimation of six rigid body transformation parameters when the iteration converges [24].

As stated before, for real-time applications the convergence of the iteration has to be rapid. Solving the linear equation, Eq. (2), is straightforward, so the key is how to more efficiently "reslice" or regrid the volume into new intermediate grid positions in each iterative step, which, to a great extent, determines the total calculation time and precision [30,31]. If only the computational speed is considered, simple linear interpolation of the volume to the new grid is the best. However, image blurring will result, which will degrade image quality and potentially impair the convergence. In contrary, sinc interpolation is the best for image quality [24,27], but is costly in terms of calculation time. Recently, a few new processing strategies have been proposed for this problem [23, 26, 30, 32].

As proposed by Eddy et al. [30], if regridding is performed in k-space, much lower computation load can be achieved while maintaining sufficient accuracy. This is due to the following reasons. First, a shift in image space (or i-space) is equivalent to simple phase multiplications in k-space according to the Fourier shift theorem. Second, rotation in i-space also corresponds to rotation in k-space; however, a rotation can be approximated by successive shearing operations. Shearing operations are realized through column/row-wise translations, which still can exploit the Fourier shift theorem in k-space to replace the translations with phase multiplications. As a result, "quite accurate approximation with only a moderate amount of computation" of rotation and shifting (translation) operations is achieved [30]. Cox et al. expanded Eddy's 2D shearing operation directly to 3D, which further speeded up the computation [23, 26]. The interested audience can refer to the references [23, 26, 30, 32] for the details. Using the above methods, an accurate real-time motion detection and correction can be achieved in an expedient fashion, leaving some time for real-time analysis of the fMRI data.

Statistical Analysis

The overriding issues in real-time fMRI statistical analysis parallel those of registration in many ways. Besides registration there are a number of steps in typical offline fMRI analysis such as distortion correction, spatial filtering, spatial normalization to a standard space and temporal filtering. These steps are a prelude to the statistical modeling, which is usually some variation of the general linear model (GLM) [29]. However, other more sophisticated, and computationally demanding, multivariate techniques are becoming more popular such as independent component analysis (ICA) [33] or partial least squares [34]. Unfortunately, many of these preprocessing steps and analysis methods are too time consuming to be practical for real-time fMRI. It is likely that this will always be the case – as computational resources increase, so will the complexity of the most sophisticated analysis as researchers are generally willing to expend that time. For real-time applications some steps must be omitted and some simplifications to the analysis or algorithm improvements must be made.

Some groups make a distinction between real-time and 'online' (sometime called 'in-time' or 'near real-time') analysis, the latter being finishing the analysis soon after the completion of the scan. Goddard et al. [20] used a variety of parallel computing platforms to complete a complicate processing stream including spiral reconstruction, motion correction, regridding and statistical analysis. This was done using the 'FIASCO' software package.

Offline analysis steps are typically designed to operate on an entire dataset at once (e.g., all of the slices in one image or all of the time points in a voxel). Thus as the number of time points increase so does the calculation time, eventually reaching a point where real-time processing becomes impossible. One solution is to operate only on the last N time points – the so-called 'sliding window' analysis used in software such as 'FIRE' [35,36]. This has the added advantage of being dynamic in the sense that the activation maps can change over the course of an experiment – a necessary condition for some real-time applications like neurofeedback, discussed below. Additionally, sliding-window analysis would be necessary for examining the dynamics of activation associated with changes in cognitive strategy and tasks that would take advantage of these changes and modify the stimuli based upon the activation. In contrast, one can imagine applications where real-time functional maps based upon the entire time course, the so-call cumulative approach, such as clinical scans where scanning to a criterion, such as a given region of the brain activating, is appropriate. With this approach the number of false-positives decreases with time, at the expense of losing the ability to see changes in activation with time.

Cox et al. [37] were the first group to perform real-time analysis using the entire time course, which is integrated into the AFNI analysis suite [10]. They modified the calculation of correlation coefficients to be calculated incrementally – that is each new image modifies the previously calculated correlation coefficient. They also include optional removal of nuisance terms such as a mean and linear trend. Cohen similarly reports an incremental correlation approach [8]. Others, such as Voyvodic et al. [38] calculate t-statistics in an incremental fashion. Their software package, FSCAN, then calculates a more complicated model including cardiac and respiratory effects at the end of scanning. The advantage of using correlation over a t-statistic is that the former allows for a reference vector whose shape varies with time. This is critical for so-called event-related experiments where the stimuli are brief compared to the hemodynamic response such that each event is expected to result in a hemodynamic response.

The above approaches are limited in that they produce a single statistical quantity. Whereas that may be sufficient for simple designs that may occur in clinical settings, in current fMRI research there are typically several conditions in each run, with the data processed using GLM. By using a least-squares algorithm designed for limited computation time and memory, Smyster et al. were able to achieve real-time analysis and display for high-resolution EPI (128x128), but a limited number of slices/brain volume [39]. The speed depended on both the number of voxels and the number of regressors. A notable feature of their approach is the incorporation of an input mask and an output mask. The former restricts data aggregation to intracerebral voxels – reducing memory and computational costs, and the later restricts where the regression parameters and statistics are computed, again reducing computational costs. The output mask can be changed during the experiment without any computational penalty. Using a cluster of PCs, Bagarinao et al. were able to perform a comprehensive processing pipeline including realignment, smoothing and a full GLM model in real-time [15]. Their cluster consisted of 16 nodes using off-the-shelf PC components. The GLM coefficients were computed using a recursive algorithm that permitted incremental calculations that they implemented [40]. Using this system, they were able to process a 30 slice 64x64 dataset in just over 1 second and a 20 slice 128x128 dataset in just over 2.5 seconds.

As mentioned earlier, one of the most promising multivariate analysis approaches is independent components analysis (ICA). ICA is a non-hypothesis driven approach which decomposes fMRI data into independent spatial maps, each associated with a component timecourse. Until recently, it has been used exclusively for offline analysis. However, Esposito et al. demonstrated a real-time analysis strategy using ICA [41]. They used a limited subset of time points in a sliding-window fashion, but cleverly averaged the sliding-window maps of the component of interest to create an accurate cumulative map. One of its complications is choosing the component(s) of interest. This group used a ROI approach where the experimenter chooses a brain region expected to be activated, and the program automatically chooses the component most active in that region. Unfortunately, their implementation precluded full-brain imaging as even a single slice (128x128) could take greater than one second to process.

APPLICATIONS

Due to its incomparable power in detecting brain functions noninvasively with high sensitivity and spatial specificity, the use of fMRI has increased dramatically in recent years [8, 38]. Real-time implementation of fMRI greatly enhances the utility of this technique in various aspects. We will discuss, in this section, applications of rtfMRI in quality assurance, interactive manipulation of tasks, biofeedback, and a detailed example of head-motion reduction using online feedback of subject's own head motion information.

Quality Assurance and Interactive Control

At the simplest level, routine real-time fMRI can be used to assure data quality by having the scan operator stop the scan if the online analysis indicates that the subject is performing poorly (i.e., excessive head motion, or misunderstanding the instructions, etc.) and reacquire the data before the subject leaves the scanner. The MRI environment – the confined space, constricting restraints and loud noises – can easily distract the subjects from the task at hand. Additionally, subjects simply don't have sufficient proprioception to detect the minute motions that critically affect the fMRI data, especially when the subject is occupied with the task.

Information from rtfMRI can be used to evaluate whether the paradigm is followed by the subject or if the research aim has been reached, during the scan or at least while the subject remains in the scanner bore [15, 18]. This ability to 'scan to criteria' could be a great benefit to clinical scans like pre-surgical mapping where one must collect sufficient data to define a certain functional region of the brain. Online analysis also makes it possible for investigator to manipulate the paradigm for subsequent scans according to the analysis results of the ongoing scan. With interactive real-time paradigm control and online fMRI analysis, fMRI experiments will become more flexible and the data reliability will be improved. The subjects will benefit from this technique as well, especially for patients with neurological and/or psychiatric disorder where monitoring is strongly needed in the scanner [18, 38].

Biofeedback and Self-Regulation

Biofeedback is a technique of monitoring one's own physiological parameters, such as heart rate, skin temperature, skin conductance, and specific frequency components of brainwaves, therefore gaining a certain level of voluntary manipulation or self-regulation of these biological measures by conscious mental control [9, 13]. Among the various applications of biofeedback, there is a more specific area that targets the self-regulation of a subject's own brain function with EEG (electroencephalogram) biofeedback, also know as "neurofeedback" [9]. Training and therapeutic intervention with EEG neurofeedback are commonly applied in clinical practice for improving brain functions such as "concentration, short term memory, speech, motor skills, sleep, energy level, and emotional balance." [42] The high temporal resolution (on the order of a millisecond) achieved by EEG neurofeedback makes it easy to measure rapid changes in electrical brain activity and give immediate feedback. However, the source localization capability of EEG is limited. Since EEG electrodes are put on the scalp, in theory EEG signals collected come from a large volume of the brain. Due to the spatial smearing and various potential interferences in the large brain volume, EEG neurofeedback is mainly limited to autonomic and global physiological parameters, and thus traditionally is used for improving relaxation, attention and other generic behaviors that involve global brain process not tied to specific brain regions [17,42].

While EEG neurofeedback is still widely implemented, a new, more powerful, spatially constrained neurofeedback technique, fMRI-based neurofeedback, has been developed recently, which exploits the greater spatial localization capability inherent in magnetic resonance imaging [9,42]. Because the information derived from fMRI is required to be fed back during ongoing scan, shortly after each trial, or at least before subjects leave the MR scanner, the advent of this new type of neurofeedback greatly depends on the fMRI data acquisition and processing techniques. These have improved considerably in recent years, including increased gradient power and higher magnetic field strength allowing for faster MR imaging with an adequate signal-to-noise ratio (SNR), and faster computers and data processing software providing the possibility of reconstructing images and performing statistical analysis in real-time [13]. In other words, real-time fMRI lays down the technical basis for fMRI-based neurofeedback.

One of the first feasibility studies for fMRI-based neurofeedback was reported by Yoo and Jolesz [9], where they developed an fMRI infrastructure with a neurofeedback capability. In that study, the subjects were presented with visual feedback of their own brain activation maps during a motor task. It was demonstrated that neurofeedback successfully guided the subjects to expand the activation in the motor and somatosensory cortex. The subjects adjusted their motor strategies with the help of feedback, although the feedback was delayed approximately 20 s after the completion of each movement trial, therefore not exactly in real time [9]. Another fMRI neurofeedback study used a self-induced sadness task with randomized presentation of sad or neutral faces in each trial, 10 trials per scan [36]. The level of the neuronal activation in the amygdala, a main brain region involved in the response to the negative mood, was fed back to the subjects in each trial to enhance the induction of sadness. Although the study, as pointed out by other researchers [13,17], didn't try to separate the effects due to the feedback from the effects due to the visual presentation of sad facial expressions, it did demonstrate the capability of online feedback of fMRI information to the subjects [36]. In another study, researchers [13] directly fed back the local BOLD signals of the targeted brain region to the subjects in a time series, similar with the use of brain waves in EEG biofeedback. They emphasized the importance of immediate feedback (less than 2-second delay following the data acquisition), considering that in EEG neurofeedback minimum delays facilitate self-regulation [13]. The sole subject in that study successfully increased and decreased his own local BOLD signals following the task instructions, and the achieved BOLD-response was reported to increase with the help of feedback training. The revealed training effect suggested the potential of voluntary control of the circumscribed brain region using fMRI-based neurofeedback [13]. A more recent report represented the first full study of training a group of subjects to control their brain activation in a local brain region using real-time fMRI neurofeedback [17]. The subjects performed an imagined manual action task and were asked to achieve a dynamically-updated activation level in the target brain region with the help of real-time feedback of their current activation in that brain region. The voluntary control of the brain activation was enhanced in the group of subjects receiving the fMRI neurofeedback compared with the control group without neurofeedback. The brain activation in the subjects receiving feedback reached the same level in the imagined manual action task as when the subjects performed actual manual action. These effects of voluntary control continued even after fMRI neurofeedback was removed. This study systematically proved the possibility of the mental control of activation over the circumscribed regions using real-time fMRI neurofeedback.

Motion Reduction

Subject head motion is a common problem in fMRI experiments [21, 22]. Although various physical restraints including a bite bar, supporting pillows or compression pads are routinely used at most facilities, the problem remains with a significant cost of lost data. The common methods for dealing with moderate head motion, "retrospective" motion correction using image registration in post-processing [23,29,32,43,44,45] and "prospective" motion correction during ongoing scanning [26,46,47,48,49,50], are successful to varying degrees with some remaining motion artifacts [25,51]. Preventing motion during data acquisition is still preferred [12].

Real-time monitoring of the subject head motion parameters using online image registration has proved to be a very useful quality assurance (QA) tool [23]. If the estimated movements are too large, the subjects may be re-scanned immediately. However, the method is not suitable for many studies, such as the studies involving learning and/or practice effects, or drug administration, where a repeated acquisition would confound the experimental manipulations [12]. It is observed in practice that verbal feedback from investigators between scan runs can help to reduce the amount of head motion significantly. Most subjects simply don't have a good proprioceptive feel for how still they need to remain, or how much movement they are making in the magnet [23]. However, the feedback in this way is very operator dependent.

In the last section of the chapter, we demonstrate a specific application of real-time fMRI – a voluntary head-motion suppression method by consistent feedback to subjects of their own head motion information in real time [12]. The method was tested in two sets of experiments, the original design [52], herein called as Design I, and an improved design [12], herein called as Design II. In Design I, subjects watched six head motion curves in a full screen while performing an auditory verbal N-BACK task. In Design II, the feedback of head motion information was simplified to a visual cue shown within a visual N-BACK task. A real-time fMRI analysis system was developed for the above purposes on standard MR imaging hardware.

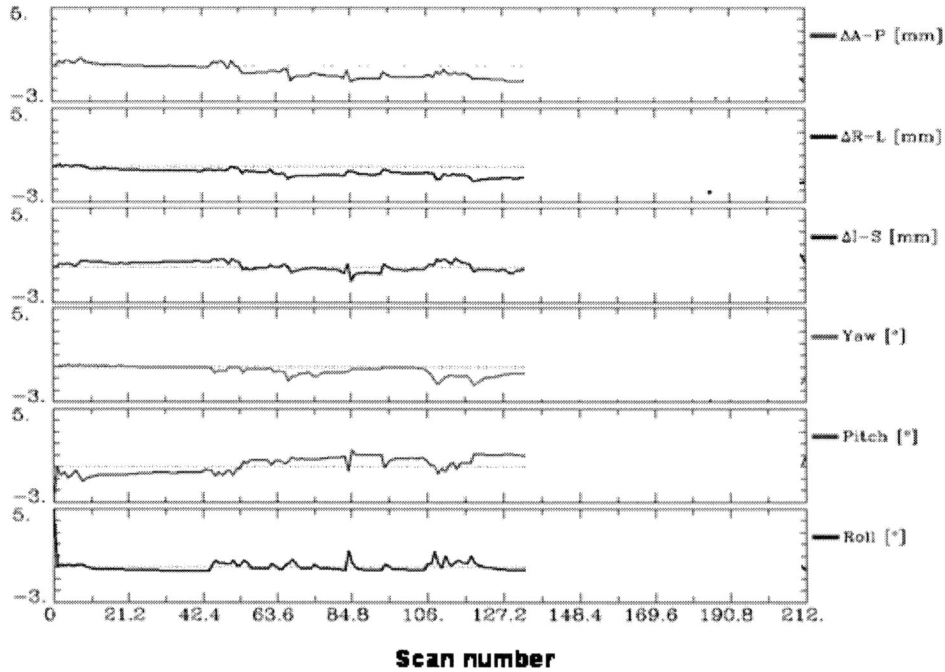

Figure 2. An example of six head motion curves shown in a whole screen, through which the subject could watch his (or her) own head motion status while he or she was performing an auditory N-BACK task. The six motion parameters, ΔA-P, ΔR-L, ΔI-S, Yaw, Pitch and Roll are the output of the AFNI real-time plug-in.

The real-time fMRI analysis system was developed on a Siemens 3T Allegra head-only scanner (Siemens, Erlangen, Germany). In Design I, the system hardware, involving the scanner HOST computer, the MRIR (MR Image Reconstruction) computer and the RT (real-time analysis) computer, are connected to each other in an internal network. The system software involves an ICE (Image Calculation Environment) program that we developed for real-time image reconstruction and image transfer and the AFNI package [10] for real-time motion correction and functional analysis.

The ICE program achieves the parallel processing of image reconstruction and image transfer with data acquisition. Upon reconstruction of one slice on the MRIR computer, the image is sent using TCP/IP sockets to the RT computer where AFNI waits for incoming data with its real-time plug-in. After each 3D volume is complete, online image registration is evoked, and the estimated motion parameters are displayed in a continually updating graph on the monitor of the server. The graph is also simultaneously displayed on the screen in the scanner bore that subjects can watch during the ongoing scan, as shown in Figure 2. The data transfer and motion parameter calculation are finished within about 100ms, much less than a TR. Due to parallel processing between the data acquisition and data processing, accurate real-time 3D registration and motion display are achieved. Online activation analysis can also be performed with this system, although it was not used in this study [52].

An auditory N-BACK paradigm was used in Design I. Auditory stimuli were presented in 30-s epochs to subjects via an air-conduction tube. Condition A is a rest period. During the epochs of 1-BACK (Condition B) and 2-BACK (Condition C), subjects listen to a series of 15 neutral words with an interstimulus interval of 2 s. Cycles of alternation between conditions were pseudorandomized within the 9 minute scan, e.g., ABCACBABCACBACBA. The N-BACK tasks were repeated in three scenarios with the subjects watching the their own real head motion curves (Real-Curve), watching the fake head motion curves (Fake-Curve, data from another subject) and without watching any curves (No-Curve). A head motion index is defined from the 6 motion parameters that AFNI outputs, ΔA-P, ΔR-L, ΔI-S, Yaw, Pitch and Roll (see Figure 2), i.e., $\sqrt{d_1^2 + d_2^2 + d_3^2 + r_1^2\theta_1^2 + r_2^2\theta_2^2 + r_3^2\theta_3^2}$, where d_i and θ_i stand for the three translational and the three rotational parameters, respectively, and r_i stands for the mean rotational semi-radii around the three directions. The head motion index, the performance accuracy and reaction time, and the activation map were evaluated. The experiments were performed on five healthy control subjects at our site and the subjects gave written informed consent for participation in this IRB-approved study. Thirty-seven sagittal slices were acquired using a 2D EPI-BOLD pulse sequences with TR=2500 ms, TE=27 ms, matrix size = 64×64, FOV = 220 mm, slice thickness/gap = 4/0 mm, flip angle = 80°, bandwidth = 3552 Hz/pixel, measurement # = 212.

Scan Number (TR)

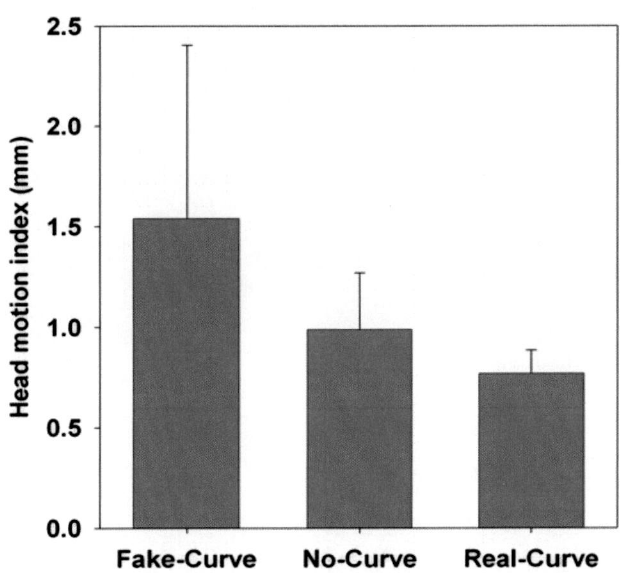

Figure 3. The mean head motion indexes for five subjects under the three scenarios, i.e., Fake-Curve, No-Curve, and Real-Curve, respectively. A reduction in head motion was seen as subjects watched their own head motion curves.

The mean head motion indexes under the three scenarios are shown in Figure 3. A reduction in head motion due to watching the real motion curves was seen, compared with the other two conditions, i.e., Fake_Curve and No_Curve. The performance accuracy was analyzed using two-way repeated-measures ANOVA where $F(2, 6) = 2.256$, $p = 0.186$ for the main effect of feedback. The same procedure was repeated for the reaction time where $F(2, 6) = 7.568$, $p = 0.023$. No significant differences were found in performance accuracy but there was a significant increase in reaction time. The group analyses of the functional MRI data were carried out offline using the 3dANOVA2 program of AFNI.

Figure 4 is the map of activation difference between No-Curve and Real-Curve with $p<0.001$ (*unadjusted*). Differences in brain activation are seen in the lateral frontal and posterior parietal regions that are closely related to the working memory task. The feedback of motion curves in this study significantly influences brain activation and reaction time of the N-BACK task, even though no effects on performance accuracy are observed. Thus it appears that the voluntary motion control may serve as a secondary cognitive task and alter the response to the primary cognitive task. Therefore, improvements of the motion suppression method are necessary to minimize the interference on the primary fMRI task. These results led to an improved design, i.e., Design II.

In Design II, the feedback of head motion information was simplified to a visual cue shown within a visual N-BACK task [12]. An additional computer, for integrating the head motion feedback information into the fMRI task and presenting both to subjects, i.e., the TASK computer, is added to the hardware components of the real-time fMRI system in Design II. The HOST, the MRIR and the RT computer were interconnected on an internal network via 100 Mbps Ethernet. The RT computer is connected to the TASK computer via RS-232 serial ports.

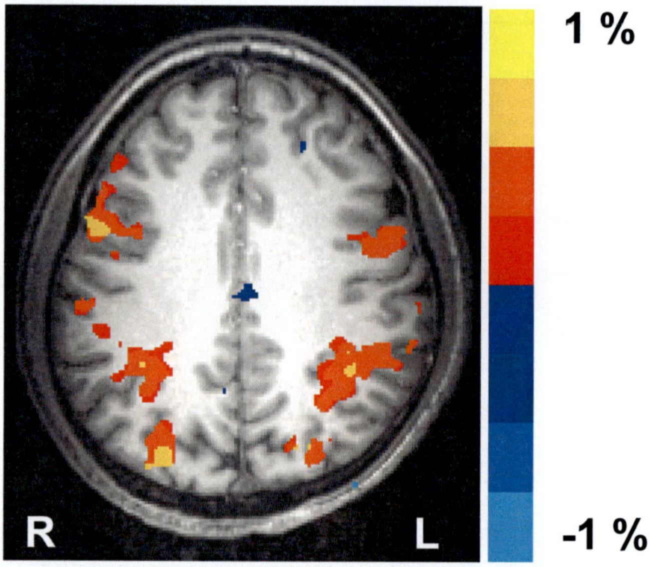

Figure 4. Map of activation difference between No-Curve and Real-Curve with $p < 0.001$ (*unadjusted*). Differences in brain activation are seen in the regions that are closely related to the working memory task, such as the lateral frontal and posterior parietal regions. The color bar in the right shows the BOLD signal difference as a percentage change from baseline.

The hardware components form a closed loop in which the MR raw data originate from the subject and the final head motion information estimated from the image data is fed back to the subject. The added software components of the real-time fMRI system in Design II include a separate program we developed on the RT computer for communications between a modified real-time plug-in in AFNI and the TASK computer, and a modified visual N-BACK task on the TASK computer written in E-Prime (Psychology Software Tools Inc., Pittsburgh, PA).

The motion parameters are displayed on the RT computer monitor in a continually updating graph similar to the one the subject saw in Design I – see Figure 2. This graph permits the investigator to observe subject head motion. Additionally, AFNI sends the data via UNIX sockets to the separate program mentioned above on the RT computer, which simply collects that motion data and sends it out through a serial port to the TASK computer, where the head motion information and fMRI task are integrated and presented, as described below.

Twelve healthy right-handed male volunteers (mean age 26.9 years) participated in this experiment after giving written informed consent to this IRB-approved study. The modified version of the visual N-BACK task consists of six 4'12" runs in a pseudo-randomized block design. Each run consists of one block each of 1, 2 and 3-BACK conditions (15 stimuli per block), separated by blocks of 0-BACK (control condition, 9 stimuli per block). The stimuli are letters, each presented for 500 ms with an inter-stimulus interval (ISI) of 2500 ms.

Our typical visual N-BACK task was modified to include the following new functions: reading the serial port for online head motion information, updating of motion feedback information, and synchronizing with the scanner. Motion information was conveyed to the subject via a group of arrows on the display (see Figure 5). During much of the ISI and instruction screens, the task polled the serial port for current motion information and updated the arrow group accordingly. To maintain accurate timing, resynchronization with the scanner was repeated each TR.

Each subject repeated the modified N-BACK tasks under two conditions in a counterbalanced design, once with feedback of the head motion information (MotFB) and once without feedback of the head motion information (No_MotFB). The two scenarios occurred in one session, one immediately after the other. The head motion information was displayed as a four-way arrow group changing color from green to red when a composite head motion index went beyond a specified threshold, which is detailed below. In the No_MotFB condition, the color of the arrow group remained the same (blue) at all times, irrespective of the subjects' motion. For the MotFB experiment, subjects were informed to observe any changes in the arrows, to try to stay still, especially if the arrows changed, but to not compensate for any motion. Critically, before each task, subjects were informed that the most important thing was to stay focused on the task and secondarily to be aware of arrow changes with their peripheral vision. They were further informed that the colors would change back to green just by them keeping still. No directional significance for the arrows was implied in the instructions and given that all four directions changed simultaneously (see Figure 5), it was impossible for subjects to infer a direction and try and compensate for the motion. For both conditions, subjects were told to stay as still as possible at all times.

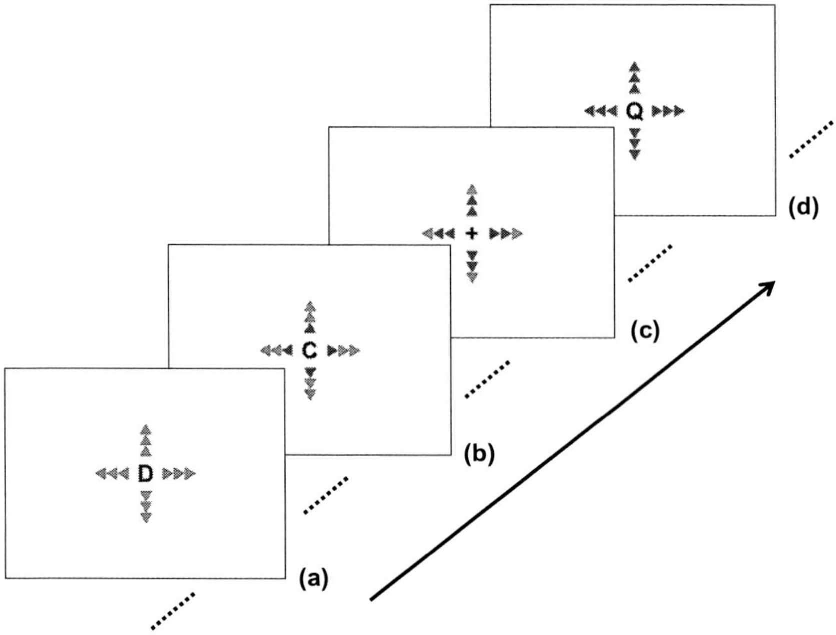

Figure 5. Example screens from the N-BACK task along with the four-way arrow group at different states based upon the value of the motion index, $M(t)$ in Eq. (3): (a) $M(t) < 0.2$ mm (b) 0.2 mm $< M(t) <$ 0.4 mm, (c) 0.4 mm $< M(t) <$ 0.6 mm, (d) $M(t) >$ 0.6 mm.

On a Siemens 3T Allegra head-only scanner, whole-brain scanning was performed using a 2D EPI pulse sequence with 39 sagittal slices, TR = 3000 ms, TE = 27 ms, matrix size = 64×64, FOV = 220 mm, slice thickness/gap = 4/0 mm, flip angle = 85°, bandwidth = 4112 Hz per pixel, number of measurements per run = 84. Additionally, 1 mm^3 resolution T1 weighted structural scans were obtained for spatial normalization using a MPRAGE pulse sequence.

The head motion feedback information was integrated into the fMRI task by presenting the arrow group along with the visual N-BACK task. The arrow group, along with the visual N-BACK stimuli, was back-projected onto a screen above the subject's head by a LCD projector, which the subjects viewed via a mirror. The letters and the fixation were displayed at the center of the screen. The four-way arrow group surrounded the screen center in the four perpendicular directions in the arrangement shown in Figure 5. The arrow group sections, the inner (I), middle (II) and outer (III), were related to three empirically derived thresholds based on the head motion index described below. When a subject's head motion index was below the 1st threshold, all three sections were green Figure 5a. When the head motion index went beyond the 1st threshold but below the 2nd threshold, Section I turned red Figure 5b. Sections II and III turned red analogously when the 2nd and 3rd threshold were exceeded, respectively Figure 5c-d.

The head motion index is defined as

$$M(t) = w\, M(t - \Delta t) + \Delta MOT\,, \tag{3}$$

where ΔMOT is written as

$$\Delta MOT = \sqrt{\begin{array}{l}[m_1(t) - m_1(t - \Delta t)]^2 + [m_2(t) - m_2(t - \Delta t)]^2 + [m_3(t) - m_3(t - \Delta t)]^2 \\ + r_\theta^2[m_4(t) - m_4(t - \Delta t)]^2 + r_\phi^2[m_5(t) - m_5(t - \Delta t)]^2 + r_\varphi^2[m_6(t) - m_6(t - \Delta t)]^2\end{array}}$$

and Δt = 1 TR. This is the total amount of head motion between two adjacent TRs, where $m_1(t)$, $m_2(t)$, and $m_3(t)$ are the three translational parameters, $m_4(t)$, $m_5(t)$, and $m_6(t)$ are the three rotational parameters, and r_θ, r_ϕ, and r_φ are the semi-radii around the three axes. Eq. (3) is a typical recurrent expression, which gives a weight, w, of 1 to the motion that just happened, ΔMOT, and a weight of less than 1 to the previous motion, $M(t-\Delta t)$. Based upon analysis of historic data, the three empirical thresholds were set as 0.2, 0.4, and 0.6 mm, respectively.

FMRI image analysis was performed using AFNI. Data were preprocessed with retrospective motion correction. Motion curves from this step were analyzed two ways to determine the effectiveness of head motion suppression. Figure 6 shows the mean number per session of greater than 0.2 mm head motion indices under the two scenarios. Mean head motion counts decreased significantly from a mean of 39.41 (No_MotFB) to a mean of 11.08 (MotFB) (Z=3.059, p=0.002), shown as the thick line and two big black dots. This head motion suppression was seen in every subject, shown as the thin lines and small black dots. A histogram of composite online head motion index, calculated from Eq. (3), along time in one run was evaluated for the MotFB and No_MotFB conditions. The histogram (shown in Figure 7) represents the number of motion excursions above 0.2 mm as a function of time, which is obtained by summing the number at each time point across 6 runs for each subject, then averaged across subjects. Examination of the histogram shows that task-related head motion was suppressed in the MotFB condition. Head motion data and behavioral data were analyzed with repeated-measures ANOVA and nonparametric Wilcoxon signed ranks tests using SPSS (SPSS Inc., Chicago, IL, USA).

No significant differences were found in the behavioral data between the MotFB and No_MotFB conditions. For accuracy, results of a 2 (feedback) X 4 (N-BACK task level) MANOVA were $F_{1,11} = 3.157$, $p = 0.10$ (n.s.) for a main effect of feedback and $F_{3,33} = 1.916$, $p = 0.146$ (n.s.) for the feedback X task interaction. Similar analysis for reaction time yielded $F_{1,11} = 2.497$, $p = 0.142$ (n.s.) for a main effect of feedback and $F_{3,33} = 2.046$, $p = 0.126$ (n.s.) for the feedback X task interaction. Results of voxel-wise analysis of brain activation indicated no significant difference between the MotFB and No_MotFB conditions. A more sensitive region of interest (ROI) analysis over 38 brain regions activated by the task found no regions with a significant feedback X task interaction and only 2 regions that had a significant main effect of feedback at $p < 0.05$, *uncorrected.* Interestingly, the two significant regions, posterior cingulate ($F_{1,11} = 5.281$, $p = 0.042$) and right superior temporal gyrus ($F_{1,11} = 5.5$, $p = 0.039$) were both regions that were *deactivated* by the N-BACK task. In both regions, there was less deactivation in the MotFB condition.

There is evidence that deactivation is more related to internal processing during rest than being task driven. The ROI map and average activation for 2 regions, including the posterior cingulate, are shown in Figure 8.

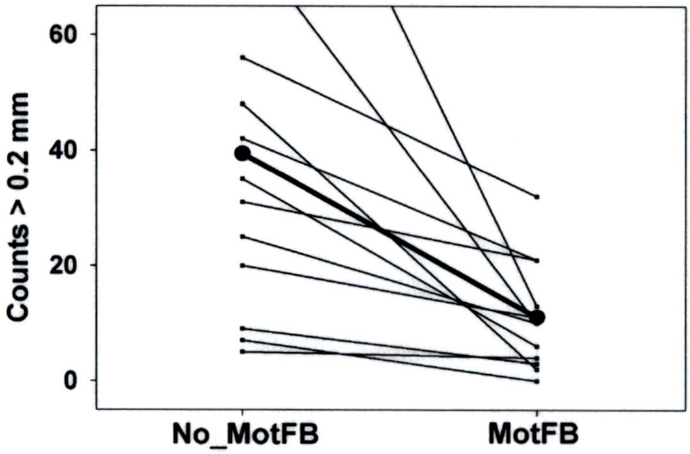

Figure 6. Mean times that the head motion index was larger than 0.2 mm with (MotFB) and without (No_MotFB) head motion feedback. The thick line and two big black dots represent the mean values for the twelve subjects, while the thin lines and small black dots are the data for each subject. Two large motion counts larger than 60 are cut off in the figure. Note that all subjects showed improvement.

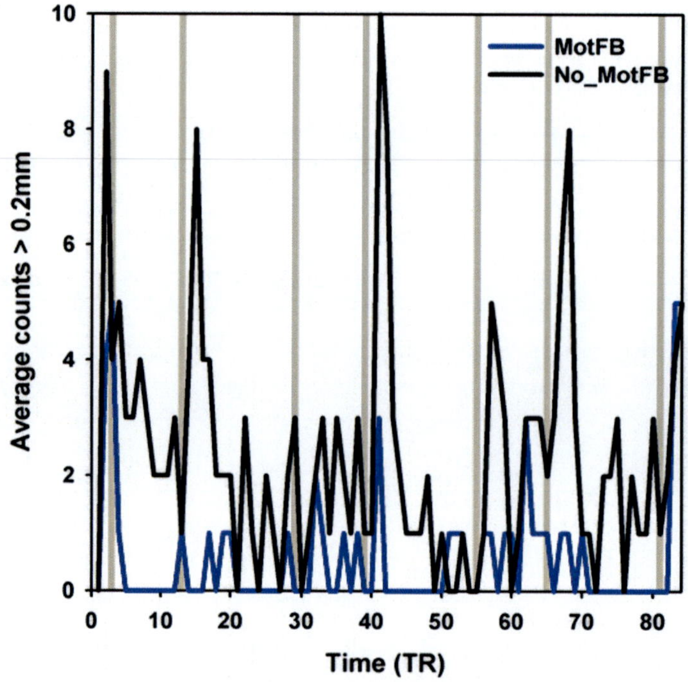

Figure 7. Histogram of counts of head motion index > 0.2 mm (from Eq. (3) with $w = 0$) along time in one run for MotFB (blue) and No_MotFB (black) conditions. Data were summed over 6 runs within subjects and then averaged across subjects. Shaded bars indicate times when instructions appeared and/or when task blocks ended. Examination of the histogram shows that task-related head motion was greatly suppressed in the MotFB condition.

In this section we demonstrated a new strategy, to address head motion confounds, that depends critically on the ability of rtfMRI to preprocess the data in real-time such that parameters of the processing can be feed back to the subject. Significant reduction in mean head motion was observed, along with a reduction of task-correlated motion. The influence on task performance and brain activation was minimal. The current design indicates that a concise, clear, simple, non-overwhelming feedback of head motion information is the key to implementing this idea. It is proposed that under certain experimental conditions and subject populations, voluntary head motion suppression may feasibly be employed without significant compromise of fMRI data. The real-time fMRI system has been developed on standard MR imaging hardware. Most of the hardware components of the real-time system are part of Siemens' standard equipment; the only additional hardware is a PC running LINUX. Other than the custom set of IDEA and ICE programs, the software components are also standard. Thus, it should be fairly straightforward to implement this procedure on other platforms.

Discussion and Conclusion

FMRI has been used extensively to study the functions of the human brain. A typical fMRI experiment usually acquires several hundred brain images. The intensive computational cost inherent in fMRI data analysis makes it more reasonable to perform the analysis offline. However, immediate analysis of fMRI data has unique advantages both for neuroscience studies and clinical applications, which are the underlying fuel for the development of real-time analysis of fMRI data.

As discussed in the previous sections, the advantages provided by rtfMRI include more effective QA monitoring on the task performance of the subject, more flexibility in allowing interactive paradigm manipulation, immediately locating brain regions with expected activation for subsequent scans, immediate feedback of the subject's brain activity to assist the subject in achieving a certain level of mental control of his own neuronal response, for either the recovery of lost brain function or basic research on internal cognitive mechanisms. Other applications that are not detailed in this chapter include pre-surgical planning, in which rtfMRI can be used immediately before surgery to define the functional brain regions that are targeted for surgery or, more commonly, to be avoided during the operation.

With the progress of computer hardware, MR scanner facilities and fMRI data processing algorithms, more subtle applications with rtfMRI are possible, such as the case given in the last section - voluntary head motion suppression with the help of immediate feedback of subject's own head motion information. The technique itself is complicated because the feedback information is not a part of the stimuli of the normal tasks that the subjects are performing during the scan. The interference from feedback to the normal task definitely exists; however, the degree of influence may vary depending on the feedback design. While Design II in the last section minimally influenced the task performance, further investigation on any subtle influence may be beneficial before this technique is applied more widely.

In contrast to conventional biofeedback of behavioral or physiological information, such as the subject's task performance accuracy, breathing or heart rate, etc., immediate feedback of the subject's own localized brain activation is only feasible with rtfMRI and several new fMRI research projects are thus possible. Mental control over localized brain activation with the help of feedback has been illustrated in a few rtfMRI reports in literature [17, 53, 54].

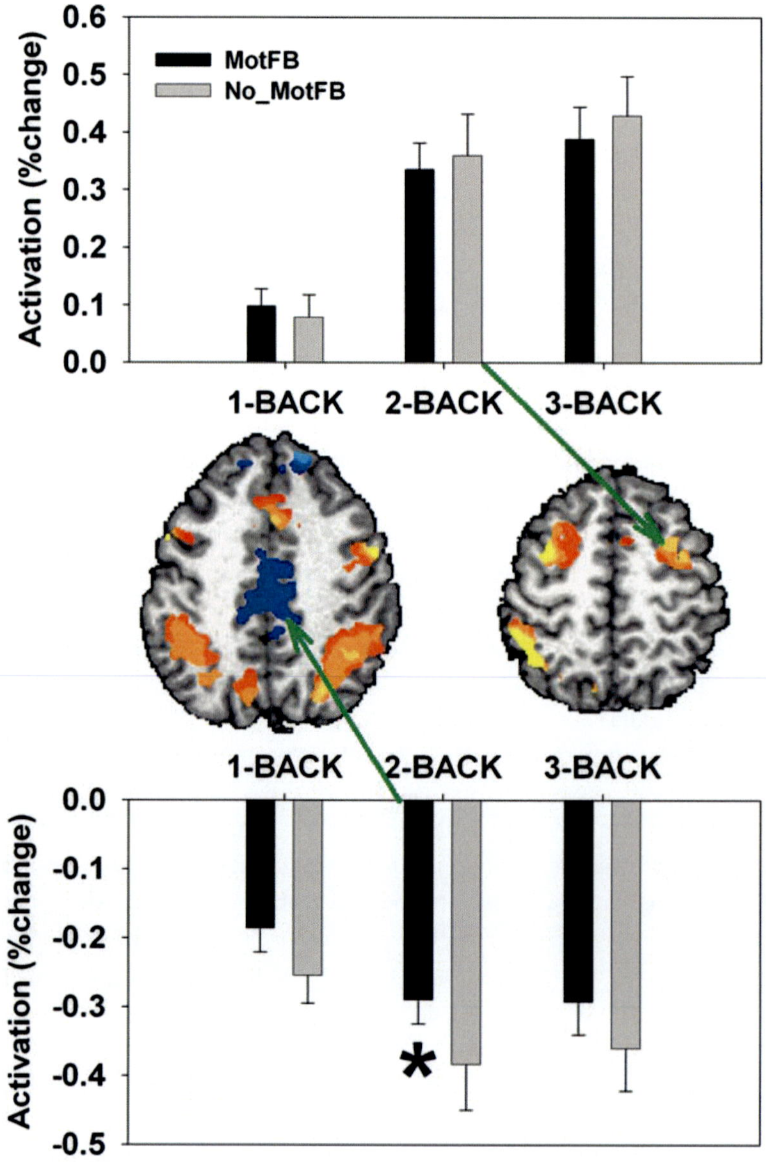

Figure 8. Regions used in a region of interest (ROI) analysis. The colors indicate the average magnitude of activation in the 3-BACK – 0-BACK contrast. The two graphs depict activation (% BOLD signal change) averaged over a given region for three task difficulties (all minus 0-BACK) with and without motion feedback (MotFB and No_MotFB, respectively). Of the regions shown, only the posterior cingulate had a significant main effect of feedback (deactivation decrease). One other region (right superior temporal gyrus) was significant for feedback; there were no significant interactions of feedback X task.

Until recently, the intention has been focused on feasibility studies, i.e., whether the localized brain activation can be manipulated with the feedback of brain activity (using the raw BOLD signals or activation levels) on one pre-specified brain region. The actual extent that mental control can achieve on different brain regions, such as the brain activation amplitude and spatial specificity, are unknown yet. Interesting questions like whether two regions can be simultaneously controlled with the help of feedback, or whether the subject can increase brain activation on one region and decrease those on the other region independently have yet to be addressed. How do the other brain regions behave when the brain activation on one target region is voluntarily manipulated with the help of feedback? The answer to the above questions will help reveal the internal working mechanisms of some brain functions and even the connectivity between different brain regions. The common procedure in neurofeedback studies using rtfMRI is to instruct the subject to achieve certain levels of brain activity; the subject needs to figure out what strategies to employ to achieve this goal. A statistical study on the various strategies that the subjects have employed after successful accomplishment of the experiments may help to reveal the relationship between the various brain activities and the different brain regions. Ultimately, this kind of study will be beneficial to the patients who are receiving recovery treatment with the help of rtfMRI neurofeedback. They can adopt the same strategies that have been reported successful in activating specific brain activation to gradually restore their lost brain function, or self-regulate the disturbed brain activation. There is already preliminary evidence that this approach may be helpful for the treatment of chronic pain [54].

With continuous progress of rtfMRI, we believe that the role of rtfMRI will gradually turn from a mainly complementary tool to fMRI at present into a more complete and comparably independent sub-area in the fMRI field, which may help us to understand how the brain works more clearly in basic research and at the same time improve the associated clinical applications and benefit patients.

REFERENCES

[1] Ogawa, S., Lee, T. M., Kay, A. R. and Tank, D. W. (1990) Brain magnetic resonance imaging with contrast dependent on blood oxygenation. *Proc. Natl. Acad. Sci. USA, 87*, 9868-9872.

[2] Ogawa, S. and Lee, T. M. (1990) Magnetic resonance imaging of blood vessels at high fields: in vivo and in vitro measurements and image simulation. *Magn. Reson.Med., 16*, 9-18.

[3] Fox, P. T. and Raichle, M. E. (1986) Focal physiological uncoupling of cerebral blood flow and oxidative metabolism during somatosensory stimulation in human subjects. *Proc. Natl. Acad. Sci. USA, 83*, 1140-1144.

[4] Mansfield, P. (1977) Multi-Planar Image-Formation Using NMR Spin Echoes. *Journal of Physics C-Solid State Physics, 10*, L55-L58.

[5] Ahn, C. B., Kim, J. H. and Cho, Z. H. (1986) High-Speed Spiral-Scan Echo Planar Nmr Imaging .1. *IEEE Transactions on Medical Imaging, 5*, 2-7.

[6] Lundstrom, M. (2003) Moore's law forever? *Science, 299*, 210-211.

[7] Becker, D., Ligon, W., Merkey, P. and Ross, R. (1999) Beowulf: Low-cost supercomputing using Linux. *IEEE Software, 16*, 79-79.

[8] Cohen, M. S. (2001) Real-time functional magnetic resonance imaging. *Methods, 25*, 201-220.

[9] Yoo, S. S. and Jolesz, F. A. (2002) Functional MRI for neurofeedback: feasibility study on a hand motor task. *Neuroreport, 13*, 1377-1381.

[10] Cox, R. W. (1996) AFNI: software for analysis and visualization of functional magnetic resonance neuroimages. *Comput. Biomed. Res., 29*, 162-173.

[11] Goebel, R. (2001) Cortex-based real-time fMRI. *NeuroImage, 13*, 129-129.

[12] Yang, S., Ross, T. J., Zhang, Y., Stein, E. A. and Yang, Y. (2005) Head-Motion Suppression Using Real-Time Feedback of Motion Information and its Effects on Task Performance in fMRI. *NeuroImage, 27*, 153-162.

[13] Weiskopf, N., Veit, R., Erb, M., Mathiak, K., Grodd, W., Goebel, R. and Birbaumer, N. (2003) Physiological self-regulation of regional brain activity using real-time functional magnetic resonance imaging (fMRI): methodology and exemplary data. *NeuroImage, 19*, 577-586.

[14] Weiskopf, N., Mathiak, K., Bock, S. W., Scharnowski, F., Veit, R., Grodd, W., Goebel, R. and Birbaumer, N. (2004) Principles of a brain-computer interface (BCI) based on real-time functional magnetic resonance imaging (fMRI). *IEEE Trans. Biomed. Eng, 51*, 966-970.

[15] Bagarinao, E., Matsuo, K. and Nakai, T. (2003) Real-time functional MRI using a PC cluster. *Concepts in Magnetic Resonance Part B-Magnetic Resonance Engineering, 19B*, 14-25.

[16] Mathiak, K. and Posse, S. (2001) Evaluation of motion and realignment for functional magnetic resonance imaging in real time. *Magn. Reson. Med., 45*, 167-171.

[17] deCharms, R. C., Christoff, K., Glover, G. H., Pauly, J. M., Whitfield, S. and Gabrieli, J. D. E. (2004) Learned regulation of spatially localized brain activation using real-time fMRI. *NeuroImage, 21*, 436-443.

[18] Frank, J. A., Ostuni, J. L., Yang, Y., Shiferaw, Y., Patel, A., Qin, J., Mattay, V. S., Lewis, B. K., Levin, R. L. and Duyn, J. H. (1999) Technical solution for an interactive functional MR imaging examination: application to a physiologic interview and the study of cerebral physiology. *Radiology, 210*, 260-268.

[19] Jackson, J. I., Meyer, C. H., Nishimura, D. G. and Macovski, A. (1991) Selection of A Convolution Function for Fourier Inversion Using Gridding. *IEEE Transactions on Medical Imaging, 10*, 473-478.

[20] Goddard, N. H., Hood, G., Cohen, J. D., Eddy, W. F., Genovese, C. R., Noll, D. C. and Nystrom, L. E. (1997) Online analysis of functional MRI datasets on parallel platforms. *Journal of Supercomputing, 11*, 295-318.

[21] Friston, K. J., Williams, S., Howard, R., Frackowiak, R. S. and Turner, R. (1996) Movement-related effects in fMRI time-series. *Magn. Reson. Med., 35*, 346-355.

[22] Hajnal, J. V., Myers, R., Oatridge, A., Schwieso, J. E., Young, I. R. and Bydder, G. M. (1994) Artifacts due to stimulus correlated motion in functional imaging of the brain. *Magn. Reson. Med., 31*, 283-291.

[23] Cox, R. W. and Jesmanowicz, A. (1999) Real-time 3D image registration for functional MRI. *Magn Reson.Med., 42*, 1014-1018.

[24] Cox, R. W. (1996) *Motion and funcitonal MRI: Informal notes for the Boston '96 workshop on functional MRI* Available from http://afni.nimh.nih.gov/old/afni/regnotes.ps

[25] Frackowiak, R. S., Friston, K. J., Firth, C. D., Dolan, R. J., Price, C. J., Zeki, S., Ashburner, J. and Penny, W. (2004) *Human brain function* (second edition). San Diego:Academic Press.

[26] Thesen, S., Heid, O., Mueller, E. and Schad, L. R. (2000) Prospective acquisition correction for head motion with image-based tracking for real-time fMRI. *Magn. Reson. Med., 44*, 457-465.

[27] Hajnal, J. V., Saeed, N., Soar, E. J., Oatridge, A., Young, I. R. and Bydder, G. M. (1995) A registration and interpolation procedure for subvoxel matching of serially acquired MR images. *J. Comput. Assist. Tomogr., 19*, 289-296.

[28] Press, W. H., Teukolsky, S. A., Vetterling, W. T. and Flannery, B. P. (2002) *Numerical recipes in C++: The art of scientific computing* (second edition). Cambridge:Cambridge University Press.

[29] Friston, K. J., Ashburner, J., Frith, C. D., Poline, J. B., Heather, J. D. and Frackowiak, R. S. J. (1995) Spatial registration and normalization of images. *Human Brain Mapping, 3*, 165-189.

[30] Eddy, W. F., Fitzgerald, M. and Noll, D. C. (1996) Improved image registration by using Fourier interpolation. *Magn. Reson. Med., 36*, 923-931.

[31] Thesen, S., Henselmans, N. and Schad, L. R. (2000) BOLD Magnetic resonance imaging in real time. *Electromedica, 68*, 45-52.

[32] Tong, R. and Cox, R. W. (1999) Rotation of NMR images using the 2D chirp-z transform. *Magn. Reson. Med., 41*, 253-256.

[33] McKeown, M. J., Makeig, S., Brown, G. G., Jung, T. P., Kindermann, S. S., Bell, A. J. and Sejnowski, T. J. (1998) Analysis of fMRI data by blind separation into independent spatial components. *Human Brain Mapping, 6*, 160-88.

[34] McIntosh, A. R., Bookstein, F. L., Haxby, J. V. and Grady, C. L. (1996) Spatial pattern analysis of functional brain images using partial least squares. *NeuroImage, 3*, 143-57.

[35] Gembris, D., Taylor, J. G., Schor, S., Frings, W., Suter, D. and Posse, S. (2000) Functional magnetic resonance imaging in real time (FIRE): sliding-window correlation analysis and reference-vector optimization. *Magn. Reson.Med., 43*, 259-268.

[36] Posse, S., Fitzgerald, D., Gao, K., Habel, U., Rosenberg, D., Moore, G. J. and Schneider, F. (2003) Real-time fMRI of temporolimbic regions detects amygdala activation during single-trial self-induced sadness. *NeuroImage, 18*, 760-768.

[37] Cox, R. W., Jesmanowicz, A. and Hyde, J. S. (1995) Real-time functional magnetic resonance imaging. *Magnetic Resonance in Medicine, 33*, 230-6.

[38] Voyvodic, J. T. (1999) Real-time fMRI paradigm control, physiology, and behavior combined with near real-time statistical analysis. *NeuroImage, 10*, 91-106.

[39] Smyser, C., Grabowski, T. J., Frank, R. J., Haller, J. W. and Bolinger, L. (2001) Real-time multiple linear regression for fMRI supported by time-aware acquisition and processing. *Magn. Reson.Med., 45*, 289-298.

[40] Bagarinao, E., Matsuo, K., Nakai, T. and Sato, S. (2003) Estimation of general linear model coefficients for real-time application. *NeuroImage, 19*, 422-429.

[41] Esposito, F., Seifritz, E., Formisano, E., Morrone, R., Scarabino, T., Tedeschi, G., Cirillo, S., Goebel, R. and Di Salle, F. (2003) Real-time independent component analysis of fMRI time-series. *NeuroImage, 20*, 2209-2224.

[42] Hall, L. and Johansson, P. (2003) Neurofeedback and metacognition *Proceedings of 11th Int. Conference on Artificial Intelligence in Education AIED 2003 Supplementary Proceedings: Metacognition and Self-regulation in Learning with Metacognitive Tools*, 541-556.

[43] Jiang, A. P., Kennedy, D. N., Baker, J. R., Weisskoff, R. M., Tootell, R. B. H., Woods, R. P., Benson, R. R., Kwong, K. K., Brady, T. J., Rosen, B. R. and Belliveau, J. W. (1995) Motion detection and correction in functional MR imaging. *Human Brain Mapping, 3*, 224-235.

[44] Maas, L. C., Frederick, B. D. and Renshaw, P. F. (1997) Decoupled automated rotational and translational registration for functional MRI time series data: the DART registration algorithm. *Magn. Reson. Med., 37*, 131-139.

[45] Woods, R. P., Cherry, S. R. and Mazziotta, J. C. (1992) Rapid automated algorithm for aligning and reslicing PET images. *J. Comput. Assist. Tomogr., 16*, 620-633.

[46] Lee, C. C., Jack, C. R., Jr., Grimm, R. C., Rossman, P. J., Felmlee, J. P., Ehman, R. L. and Riederer, S. J. (1996) Real-time adaptive motion correction in functional MRI. *Magn. Reson. Med., 36*, 436-444.

[47] Derbyshire, J. A., Wright, G. A., Henkelman, R. M. and Hinks, R. S. (1998) Dynamic scan-plane tracking using MR position monitoring. *J. Magn. Reson. Imaging, 8*, 924-932.

[48] Lee, C. C., Grimm, R. C., Manduca, A., Felmlee, J. P., Ehman, R. L., Riederer, S. J. and Jack, C. R., Jr. (1998) A prospective approach to correct for inter-image head rotation in fMRI. *Magn. Reson. Med., 39*, 234-243.

[49] Ward, H. A., Riederer, S. J., Grimm, R. C., Ehman, R. L., Felmlee, J. P. and Jack, C. R., Jr. (2000) Prospective multiaxial motion correction for fMRI. *Magnetic Resonance in Medicine, 43*, 459-69.

[50] Ward, H. A., Riederer, S. J. and Jack, C. R., Jr. (2002) Real-time autoshimming for echo planar timecourse imaging. *Magn. Reson. Med., 48*, 771-780.

[51] Muresan, L., Renken, R., Roerdink, J. B. and Duifhuis, H. (2002) Position-history and spin-history artifacts in fMRI time series, *Proceedings of SPIE 4683*, San Diego, CA, USA, 444-451.

[52] Yang, S., Ross, T. J., Zhang, Y., Feng, H., Stien, E. A. and Yang, Y. (2004) Head-motion suppression using real-time feedback of motion curves and its effects on performance of task in fMRI. *Proceedings of 12th scientific meeting of the International Society for Magnetic Resonance in Medicine (ISMRM),* Kyoto, Japan.

[53] Goebel, R., Sorger, B., Birbaumer, N. and Weiskopf, N. (2005) Learning to play BOLD Brain Pong: From individual neurofeedback training to brain-brain

interactions. *Proceedings of 11th annual meeting of the Organization for Human Brain Mapping,* Toronto, Canada.

[54] Maeda, F., Lutomski, L., MacLeod, S., Soneji, D., Mackey, S., Gabrieli, J. D. E., Glover, G. H., Pauly, J. M. and deCharms, R. C. (2005) Learned control over brain activation and pain in chronic pain patients achieved through repetitive training using real time fMRI (rtfMRI). *Proceedings of 11th annual meeting of the Organization for Human Brain Mapping,* Toronto, Canada.

In: Brain Mapping Research Developments
Editor: Lars N. Bakker, pp. 155-176

ISBN 978-1-60456-007-7

Chapter VI

Brain Functional Asymmetry Based on Brain BOLD Signal Dynamic Model

Huafu Chen and Dezhong Yao
School of Life Science and Technology, University of Electronic Science and Technology of China, 610054, China

Abstract

Blood oxygenation level-dependent (BOLD) contrast-based functional magnetic resonance imaging (fMRI) has been widely utilized to detect brain neural activities and great efforts are now stressed on the hemodynamic processes of different brain regions activated by a stimulus. The focus of this paper is the comparison of Gamma and Gaussian dynamic convolution models of the fMRI BOLD response. The convolutions are between the perfusion function of the neural response to a stimulus and a Gaussian or Gamma function. The parameters of the two models are estimated by a nonlinear least-squares optimal algorithm for the fMRI data of eight subjects collected in a visual stimulus experiment. The results show that the Gaussian model is better than the Gamma model in fitting the data. The model parameters are different in the left and right occipital regions, which indicate that the dynamic processes seem different in various cerebral functional regions. Further, the asymmetry of the left-right and upper-lower visual field is investigated by the differences of the Gaussian model parameters. The results from eight subjects show that reaction time is significant shorter and the response is significant stronger when the lower field is stimulated than that when the upper field is stimulated. For the left and right fields, the response is different. These results provide the fMRI BOLD response evidence of the asymmetry of spatial visual fields.

Keyword: fMRI, BOLD, asymmetry, Brain.

1. INTRODUCTION

A primary goal of functional MRI(fMRI) is to accurately characterize the underlying neural activities by the changes of the measured signals. The most common technique in fMRI is the gradient-echo imaging with blood oxygenation level dependent (BOLD) contrast to measure the hemodynamic changes accompanying neural activation (Kwonget al, 1992; Ogawa et al,1992; Bandettini et al,1993). Increase of neuronal activities lead to local increase of blood flow and blood volume. As a result, the increase of oxygen delivered to the activated region will cause changes in the local concentration of deoxyhemoglobin which magnetic resonance signal is sensitive to (Rasmus et al,2001). This BOLD effect is commonly utilized by researchers to detect position of activities in the brain, and great efforts are now putted on the hemodynamic processes of different brain regions activated by a stimulus, so that fMRI can be closely related with other functional brain imaging techniques such as the high temporal resolution EEG and MEG techniques (Yao, 2000).

In block design experiments the subject is instructed to perform a task that activates a certain region of the brain during a specific time interval(Chen et al, 2005b, 2006. The resultant hemodynamic response (HDR) of the cortex under investigation changes with the stimulus. Early fMRI experiments (Boynton et al, 1996; Rao et al,1996) suggested a linear relationship between the parameters in the stimulus and the resultant HDR, but later experiments (Miller et al, 2001; Buxton et al, 2001; Liu et al, 2000; Vazquez et al,1998; Aguirr et al,1998) showed an increasing amount of nonlinearity in the response. To analyze the nonlinear relationship, Miller et al proposed a fMRI dynamic model of convolution between the perfusion function of the neural response to a stimulus with a Gamma response function of the Cerebral Blood Flow (CBF) hemodynamics of neuron (Miller et al, 2001; Rasmus et al, 2001). Recently, we proposed an extended Gamma convolution model where a baseline is introduced into the original Gamma convolution model to represent the background activities (Chen 2004 b). In general, it is still a frontier problem to construct a better BOLD dynamic model to reveal the neural mechanism of cerebral activities and to investigate the dynamic pattern of various cerebral regions in brain function exploration and cognitive neuroscience (Logothetis et al, 2001; Rajapakse et al, 1998; Rosen et al, 1998).

In Miller's model (Miller et al, 2001; Chen 2004b), the Gamma function is originated from the characteristic of the CBF hemodynamic pulse response of neuron. Recently, according to the law of large number in probability, we proposed the Gaussian convolution model which was implemented using a Gaussian function replace the Gamma function to represent the neural cluster response to analysis the asymmetry of spatial visual fields(Chen et al, 2004a). In this paper, the effectiveness of the new model is evaluated by a comparison study between the extended Gamma model (Chen et al, 2004b) and the new Gaussian model.

As a preliminary application, the new model and the extended Gamma model are applied to a fMRI data of a visual stimulus where we concern the phenomena of hemispheric lateralization. Understanding the specific nature of how spatial abilities are lateralized in the brain is important for many reasons and is still a topic without common viewpoint (Vitouch et al, 1997; Wendt et al, 1994; Vogel et al, 2003). Many studies have shown that the human visual information process depends on the location of information in the visual field (VF)

(Naito,2000; Rubin 1996; Edwads, 1993; Okita, 1990; Yoshizaki, 1990; Casco,1988). The asymmetry of the neural process between the left and right visual fields (VFs) is considered to be the functional difference between the left and right hemispheres (Heilman,1980; Kinsbourne, 1970). In terms of stimulus or task properties, the left hemisphere primarily mediates verbal processing, while the right hemisphere mediates nonverbal processing. In terms of processing style, the left hemisphere is specialized in local (high spatial frequency) processing, while the right hemisphere is specialized in global (low spatial frequency) processing (Sergent, 1982). For asymmetry of the upper and lower VFs, some studies have shown that humans perform various visual tasks better when the stimulus is presented in the lower VF than in the upper VF (Previc, 1995; von Grunau, 1994; whishaw, 1994). Asymmetries in favor of the lower VF have been found for simple reaction time, global processing, and near stereoscopic vision. Asymmetries in favor of the upper VF have been found for local processing, far stereoscopic vision, visual search, and visual attention (Hagenbeek, 2002). Christman and Niebauer concluded that upper–lower VFs asymmetries are at least as strong and prevalent as left–right VFs asymmetries (Christman 1997, Niebauer 1998). In corroboration, findings for human studies done with behavior experimental evidence (He, 1996) and event-related brain potentials (OKita,1993) have shown that the magnitude of responses in the occipital lobe to the pattern onset presented in the lower VF are higher than in the upper VF. Furthermore, they suggested a systematic link between lower and left VFs processing and between upper and right VFs processing (Niebauer and Christman 1998; Christman and Niebauer 1997; Christman 1993). However, How and to what extent the asymmetry of the magnetic response is related to human perception or performance is unknown. LVF superiority has been reported in many attentional and perceptional tasks in previous reports (He, 1996; Previc, 1990), whereas there have been only a few reports of UVF superiority under a specific condition; e.g., crossed-phi apparent motion with low-frequency sine wave patch stimuli (Osaka,, 1993). Extensive psychophysical studies are needed to clarify the importance of the findings in this study (Naito, 2000). So, The asymmetry of the left–right and upper–lower VFs is still under investigation(Naito, 2000; Vogel, 2003).

The relation between left–right and upper–lower visual field (VF) asymmetries was examined for face matching, letter naming, and lexical decision with the VF quadrants experiment. Face matching resulted in a lower left and upper right VF advantage. Letter-naming resulted in a distinct upper–right VF advantage. For lexical decision, no upper/lower asymmetries were found. Words were processed faster in the right than in the left VF, while nonwords were processed equally fast in both VFs (Rogier, 2002; Christman,1997). A recent study on the difference of upper and lower VFs provided neuroscience evidence of visual evoked potential(VEP) recordings and functional magnetic resonance imaging (fMRI) data in study of the spatio-temporal patterns of cortical activity with VF quadrants experiment (Di Russo, 2001; 2003). In general, the brain asymmetries may be due to the physiologic differences between the processing of information in the visual fields and the anatomical influences on recordings. The distance and anatomical path from a specific scalp electrode to the activation points excited by upper, lower, left and right stimulus are different when VEPs and MEGs are used. On the other hand, fMRI directly image the activities on the actual anatomical positions the influence of anatomical asymmetry is limited (Toga, 2003).

However, the fMRI only shows us a spatial anatomic location, further quantitative study of the blood oxygenation level dependent (BOLD) dynamic response of spatial VFs with a mathematical model may provide us further information of the mechanism with various visual fields. For example, a similar study has been conducted on the discrimination of word and non-word with parametric changes in a Gaussian function BOLD model (Lundervold, 2002), and the result is that the response duration for word trials were generally wider/longer than for non-word trials. Moreover Henson concluded that word versus non-word elicited different magnitude and latency within several brain regions by implementing the general linear mode task (Henson, 2001).

In this paper, the parameters of the two fMRI models were estimated by a nonlinear least-square optimal algorithm and according to the parameter changes in the left and right cerebral visual region, the difference of the hemodynamic processes are discussed. Final, the different BOLD dynamic responses of the left and right, upper and lower VFs are investigated by the model parameters.

2. Brain BOLD Dynamic Model

2.1. The Perfusion Response

Many experiments indicate that there are neural adaptation between neural responses and stimulus, and it is the general tendency of the neural firing rate to decay from a high initial value to a lower steady-state value during a sustaining stimulus (Boynton et al, 1996; Miller et al, 2001; Rosen et al, 1998; Vogel et al, 2003). If the parameterization of the neural response to a block stimulus begins at t=0 and ends at t=T, then we have:

$$n(t) = \begin{cases} 1 + ae^{-t/t_n} & 0 \le t \le T \\ 0 & otherwise \end{cases} \tag{1}$$

where parameter t_n is a decay time constant, a is the amount that the initial response overshoots the steady-state response and $n(t)$ is assumed being the perfusion function of neural response(Chen et al, 2004ab).

2.2. Gaussian Response of a Neural Cluster

It has been shown that the regional response of collectively activated neural cluster to a stimulus is a normal distribution, and it is consistent to the law of large numbers in probability (Hwang et al, 1997; Kruggel et al, 2000), so the response of a neural cluster may be expressed by a Gaussian function:

$$g(t) = \frac{\theta_0}{\theta_1} \exp(-\frac{(t-\theta_2)^2}{2\theta_1^2}) \tag{2}$$

where θ_0 and θ_1 are two constants, θ_2 is the time interval from the presentation of a stimulus to the maximum neural response, namely it is a response delay parameter.

2.3. Gaussian Convolution Model

The BOLD signal of the cerebral activation is a collective response of an activated region and it can be explained as a mutual interaction process between the perfusion of the neural response to a stimulus and the Hemodynamic change due to the activation of a neural cluster. Therefore, the BOLD signal $x(t)$ of a cerebral activation can be expressed by convolution of this perfusion response of the neural response with a Gaussian function of the CBF hemodynamic response of a neural cluster(Chen et al 200ab):

Model I

$$x(t) = n(t) \otimes g(t) + (1 + \alpha \times t) \times \eta + e(t) \tag{3}$$

where $(1 + \alpha \times t) \times \eta$ is introduced to represent the background fMRI signal. The η is a constant, and the time dependence is assumed being a linear function $\alpha \times t \times \eta$ with a baseline shift factor α , $e(t)$ represents various additive noises. Figure 1 is the simulation result of model I without $e(t)$.

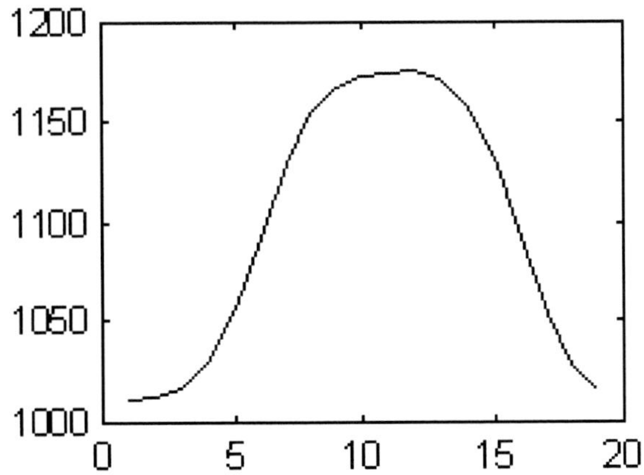

Figure 1. Gaussian convolution model. The parameters are η=1010, $\alpha = 0$, a=3.0, t_n=0.5,T=10, $\theta_0 = 20.10$, $\theta_1 = 1.5$, $\theta_2 = 8.83$. The horizontal axial is the temporal sampling point, the vertical axial is the response signal intensity.

2.4. Gamma Convolution Model

Miller et al proposed that BOLD response of neural activity $x(t)$ can be expressed as the convolution between the perfusion function of the neural response to a stimulus and a gamma function of the CBF hemodynamic response of neuron:

Model II

$$x(t) = n(t) \otimes h(t) \tag{4}$$

where the gamma function $h(t)$, shown below, denotes the CBF hemodynamic response of neuron.

$$h(t) = \frac{c}{\tau_h m!}\left(\frac{t - t_d}{\tau_h}\right)^m e^{-(t-t_d)/\tau_h} \tag{5}$$

where t_d shows the time delay, τ_h signifies the blurring effect, m is a response scale which will affect the shape of h(t), and c is an amplitude factor of the response which does not affect the shape of the function (Miller et al 2001). Figure 2 is the simulation result of the Gamma convolution model II.

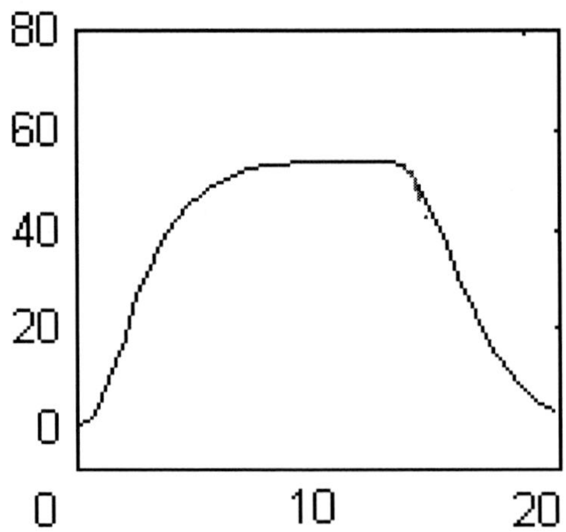

Figure 2. Gamma convolution model. The parameters are t_n=0.5, t_d=1.5,a=3.0, τ_h=1.5,c=54, m=3, the horizontal axial is the time points and the vertical axial is the response signal intensity.

Due to that a vivo fMRI signal actually exists in various background noises, the background fMRI signal should be taken into account in the model II, so we proposed an extended Gamma convolution model (Chen et al, 2005a, 2004ab):

Model III

$$x(t) = n(t) \otimes h(t) + (1 + \alpha \times t) \times \eta + e(t) \tag{6}$$

The response of the extended Gamma model III is similar to Figure 2 of the Gamma model II except a baseline, so the simulation result of model III is omitted. However, in the following text, the model III is actually utilized because it includes the original Model II as one of its special case.

3. Nonlinear Least-Squares Estimation

Gaussian convolution model I is composed of two nonlinear functions with parameters $a, t_n, \theta_0, \theta_1, \theta_2$, $\eta, e(t)$ and α. Gamma convolution model III is composed of another two nonlinear functions with parameters a, t_n, t_d, τ_h, m, $c, \eta, e(t)$ and α. These parameters are estimated with a nonlinear least-squares algorithm as follow.

1) Equations (3) and (6) are reformulated as

$$x(t) = f(t, \vec{\beta}) + e(t) \tag{7}$$

where $x(t)$ is the observed signal value at time t, $\vec{\beta}$ is an unknown parameter vector including all the above noted unknown parameters except the $e(t)$. f is the nonlinear function with respect to parameter t and $\vec{\beta}$.

2) Using a nonlinear least-squares estimator, the parameter $\vec{\beta}$ is estimated as following

$$\vec{\beta}^* = \arg\max\left[-\frac{1}{n}\left[x(t) - f(t, \vec{\beta})\right]^T \left[x(t) - f(t, \vec{\beta})\right]\right] \tag{8}$$

In our model, the detail cost function to be minimized is

$$\sum_{t=1}^{n} [x(t) - (1 + ae^{-t/t_n}) \otimes \varphi(t) - (1 + \alpha \times t) \times \eta]^2 \tag{9}$$

where $x(t)$ is the measured BOLD signal at time t, $t = 1, 2, \cdots, n$. $\varphi(t)$ is the Gaussian function (model I) or the Gamma function (model III).

4. VISUAL fMRI APPLICATION

4.1. In Vivo fMRI Experiment

For comparison of the Gamma model and Gaussian model in fMRI experiments in vivo, eight normal subjects were involved in a visual task with a Block paradigm. Experiment conducted at Beijing MRI center, Chinese Academy of Sciences, with SIEMENS 3 TESLA MAGNETOM TRIO. EPI: repetition time TR=1.0s, matrix size=64×64, voxel size=3.00×3.00×2mm.TE=30ms, flip angle 90°. The first 4 scans of each run were discarded to allow for magnetic saturation effects. Then 320 volume images comprised time-series were analyzed.

The stimuli consisted of circular black-and-white checkerboards (the checkerboards subtend 10' of arc), each stimulus with a 2° diameter visual angle and a spatial frequency of 3.2 cycles per degree. Stimuli pattern is block design, each stimulus were presented for 50 msec. These stimuli were presented randomly in the left and right VFs (stimulus onset asynchronies (SOAs) varying between 250 and 500 msec) in 16-sec blocks, where the stimuli were presented at a time. After the stimuli were presented to the left and right VFs, a blank block was followed. In this blank block, only the center fixation cross (0.8°) was displayed. Subjects were required to concentrate on the fixation cross and press a button upon detection of an infrequent brightness change of the fixation cross (Chen et al 2004a,).

4.2. fMRI Image Result

According to F-test statistical method (P value <0.05) and the prior response information, the data is analyzed with SPM principle (www.fil.ion.ucl.ac.uk/spm;). Shown in Figure3 is the result of the fMRI activations of eight subjects in Talairach brain corresponding to left and right VFs. The black points in Figure 3 represent the activated voxels in a brain slice, where regions of interest (ROIs) comprise those in the left and right occipital lobes of the primary visual cortex, respectively. Anatomical sites of the selected pixels are compiled in Table 1, which are the most active points in the primary visual cortex (human analogue of V1, area 17) of brain as shown in Figure 3.

Activation at these sites were positively correlated($r>0.6$) with the reference signal at a significance level of $p<0.005$ (Chen et al 2003).

Table 1. Average Talairach Coordinates of the most active points of the eight subjects in their primary visual cortexes (human analogue of V1, area 17). (values are in mm)

Stimulus Position \ Coordinates	X(mm)	Y(mm)	Z(mm)
A(left)	-16	-100	6
B(right)	10	-99	7

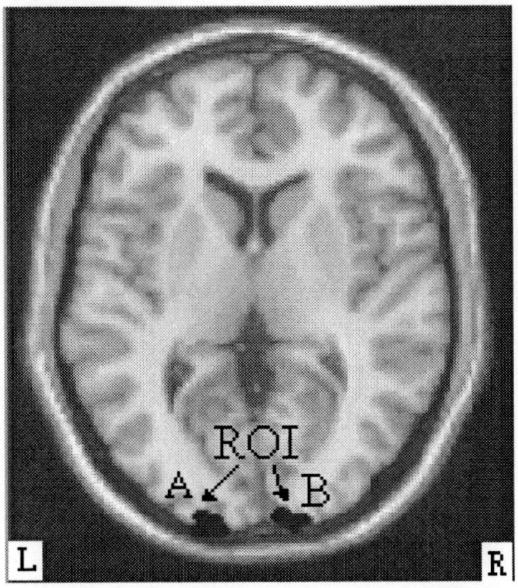

Figure 3. fMRI result.

4.3. Modelling Results of fMRI Signals

First, we choose two measured activated fMRI signals, marked them as A and B (Figure 3), from the selected ROIs in the left and the right primary visual cortexes, and minimize the cost function in Eq.(9) for the Gaussian model I and Gamma model III with optimal algorithm offered by MATLAB to get the model parameter estimations. Table 2 shows the result of a signal at voxel A , and Table 3 shows the result of a signal at voxel B in Figure 3.

Figure 4 and Figure 5 are the signal curves of the measured BOLD signals and the estimated BOLD signals of the model I and model III. Figure 4 is the result of the signal at voxel A in the left occipital lobe, where the solid lines in Figures 4(a) and 4(b) note the measured BOLD signal, the dotted solid lines note the signals estimated by the Gaussian model (Figure 4(a)) or and the Gamma model III (Figure 4(b)). Similarly, Figure 5 shows the results of the measured signal at voxel B and the related estimating signals.

Table 2. Model parameters of a BOLD signal in the left visual cortex (voxel A)

Parameter	η	t_n	a	α	θ_0 /c	θ_1 / τ_h	θ_2 / t_d	m	STD *
Gaussian Model I	1362	1.1	3.0	-0.012	θ_0 =45	θ_1=1.4	θ_2 =7.7		13.4
Gamma model III	1362	1.6	4.7	-0.012	c=100	τ_h =1.5	t_d =2.7	3	16.3

* STD= $std(x(t)-\overline{x}(t))$ i.e STD is the standard deviation of the difference between $x(t)$ and $\overline{x}(t)$. $x(t)$ is the measured signal and $\overline{x}(t)$ is the estimated signal.

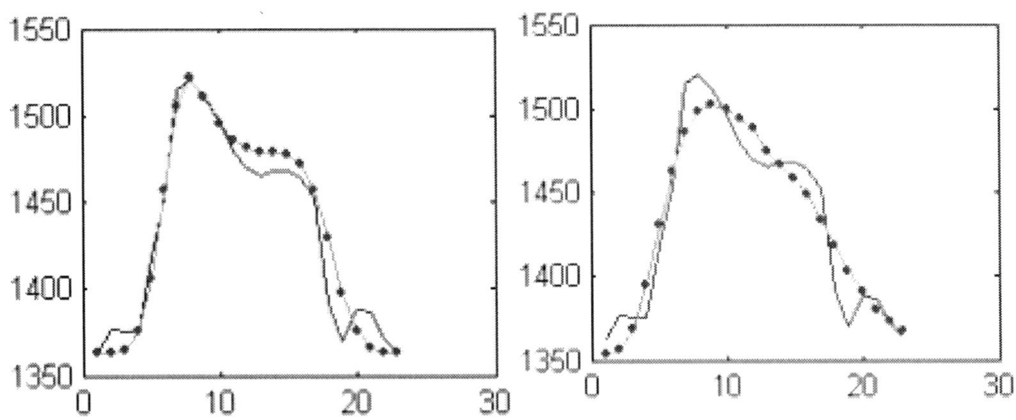

(a) Gaussian model I (b) Extended Gamma model III

Figure 4. BOLD signal in the left visual cortex (voxel A). The horizontal axis is the sample point, the vertical axis is the signal value.

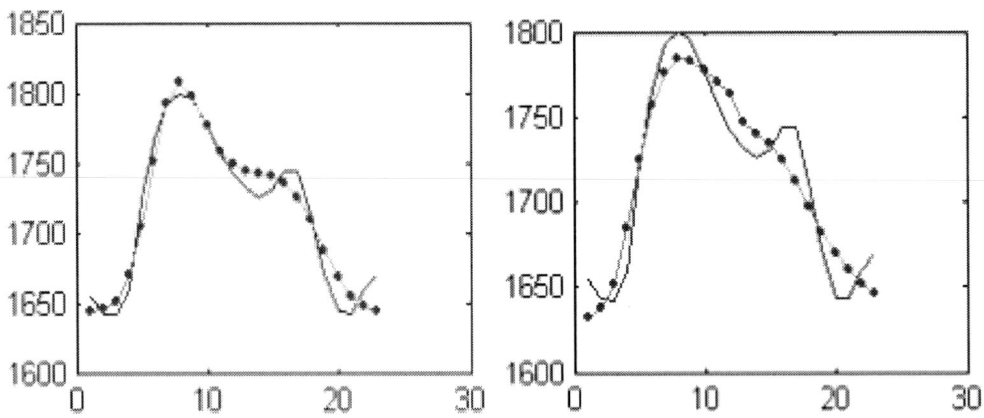

(a) Gaussian model I (b) Extended Gamma model III

Figure 5. BOLD signal in the right visual cortex (voxel B). The horizaontal axis is the sample point, and the vertical axis is the signal value.

Table 3. Model parameters of a BOLD signal in the right visual cortex (voxel B)

Parameter	η	t_n	a	α	θ_0 /c	θ_1/τ_h	θ_2/t_d	m	STD
Gaussian Model I	1642	0.46	35.	0.0051	θ_0 =40	θ_1= 1.8	θ_2= 1.8		13.2
Gamma model III	1642	1.0	9.4	0.0051	c=100	τ_h= 2.7	t_d =1.5	3	17.1

4.4. The Significance of Baseline and Baseline Shift

The baseline was corresponding to the fMRI structured noise and non-structured noise before the onset of the stimulation. As shown in Tables 2-3, the baselines of the two models are 1362 at voxel A and 1642 at voxel B of the two models, and such large baselines definitely mean the Gaussian model I (Figure4) and the extended Gamma model III (Figure 5) are more appropriate for simulating BOLD signals than the Gamma model II (Chen et al, 2004 ab). The shift factors of the two models are -0.012, i.e. the baseline shift is $-0.012 \times t \times 1362$, at voxel A and 0.0051, i.e. the baseline shift is $0.0051 \times t \times 1642$, at voxel B. The distinct differences of the baselines and their shift factors from the left voxel A to the right voxel B indicate different background activations of different brain regions.

4.5. Comparison of Gaussian Model I and Gamma Model III

The average standard deviation (STD) between $x(t)$ and $\overline{x}(t)$ of the two models are calculated over a totally eight subjects BOLD signals in ROIs (Figure3) in the left and right primary visual cortexes. The average STD of the Gaussian model is 13 with eight subjects. However, the average STD of the Gamma model III is 18. These results show the new Gaussian model not only of a better curve trend adapted to the measured BOLD signals (Figs. 4-5), but also of a smaller STD error (Tables 2-3). With SPSS (Statistics package for social science) software ANOVA method analysis for the eight subjects, it was found that the STD parameter of the Gauss model is significantly smaller than that of the gamma model ($F=5.31$, $p<0.05$). The reason is that the Gaussian model is based on the law of large numbers in probability, which considers BOLD signal as the collective response of neural cluster. Based on the available spatial resolution of fMRI, any measurable signal is actually due to a neuronal cluster, and the BOLD response is more likely a macroscopic response (Gaussian response), not a response of Gamma response.

4.6. A Preliminary Exploration of the Dynamic Difference of the Two Hemispheres

As shown in Tables 2-3, the parameters of the two models for the left visual cortex (voxel A) and right visual cortex (voxel B) are different. With SPSS software ANOVA method analysis for the eight subjects, the parameters of two models for the left visual cortex (voxel A) and right visual cortex (voxel B) are significant difference ($F=4.2$, $p<0.05$). The difference of the two models indicates that the nonlinear dynamic characteristics of BOLD signal evoked by the stimulus is different in the left and right occipital lobe region of the primary visual cortex in processing visual stimulus, which is in accordance with the main medical evidences (Chen et al, 2004 ab; Vitouch et al, 1997; Wendt et al, 1994; Voge et al, 2003). The more dominant analysis will be implemented in the future.

5. A Study on Asymmetry of Spatial Visual Field

5.1. Experiment Subject

Eight paid volunteer subjects participated in the fMRI study. All subjects are right-handed with normal or corrected- to-normal visual acuity.

5.2. Experiment Stimuli

The stimuli consisted of circular black-and-white checkerboards, each stimulus with a 2°diameter visual angle and a spatial frequency of 3.2 cycles per degree. These stimuli were presented for 50 msec. These stimuli were presented in the four quadrants of the left and right VFs at a fast rate (stimulus onset asynchronies (SOAs) varying between 250 and 500 msec) in 16-sec blocks, where the stimuli were presented in one quadrant at a time. The total of 480 stimuli were delivered. After the stimuli were presented to the four quadrants (four spatial location: left upper(A), right upper(B), left lower (C), right lower (D)) a blank block was followed. In this blank block, only the center fixation cross (0.8°) was displayed. Stimuli positions were centered along an arc that was equidistant (4°) from a central fixation cross and located at polar angles of 25° above and 45° below the horizontal meridian (Figure6). The purpose of the experimental paradigm is to activate the early visual areas corresponding to the four quadrants of VF, and this configuration was adopted from literature.(Di Russo et al, 2001).

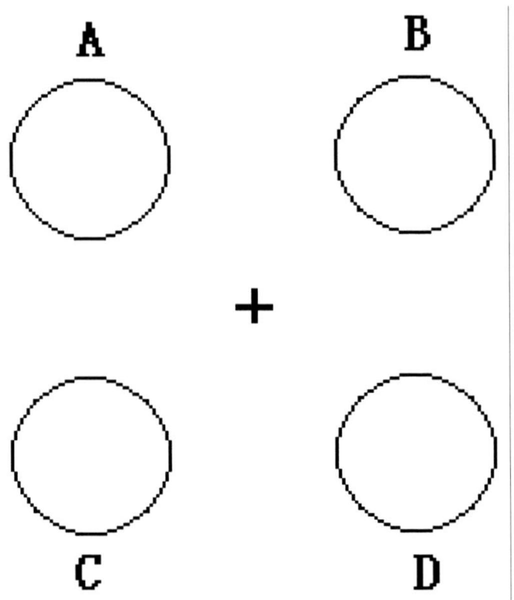

Figure 6. Experiment pattern.

5.3. Task

Subjects were required to concentrate on the fixation cross and press a button upon detection of an infrequent brightness change of the fixation cross. This target, event of brightness change of the fixation cross, lasted for 50 msec. The experiment is a block paradigm, during the period of stimulus, a circular checkerboard stimulus were presented in the four quadrants of the left and right VFs at a fast rate (SOAs varying between 250 and 500 msec). The target randomly occurred in both the stimulus block and blank block with a rare probability (5%).

5.4. Data Acquisition

The experiment was conducted at Beijing MRI center, Chinese Academy of Sciences, with SIEMENS 3 TESLA MAGNETOM TRIO. EPI: repetition time TR=1.0s, matrix size=64×64, voxel size=3.00×3.00×2mm.TE=30ms, flip angle 90°. The first 4 scans of each run were discarded to allow for magnetic saturation effects. Then 320 volume images comprised time-series were analyzed. Time-dependent echo-planar images were post-processed with AFNI software (Cox, 1996). After 3D motion correction, the raw time series data from each run were averaged within each individual. Group data were obtained by averaging the raw time series data over all subjects. A series of phase-shifted trapezoids representing the periodic alternation of conditions in the block design of the experiment (i.e., stimulus presentation at the four positions) was used as the reference waveform. Each trapezoid function was correlated on a pixel-by-pixel basis with the averaged (individual or group) signal strength time series by a least squares fit to generate a functional activation map(DiRusso,2001).

5.5. Results

Shown in Figures 7-10(a) are the results of the fMRI activations of eight subjects in Talairach brain corresponding to left upper (A), right upper (B) and left lower(C), right lower (D) VFs. Anatomical sites of selected pixels are compiled in Table 4, which are the most active points in the primary visual cortex (human analogue of V1, area 17) of brain as shown in Figures 7-10. The corresponding Gaussian convolution models of the four most active points were obtained according to the modeling method shown above. Figures 7-10 (b) are the resulted curves of one active point in Figures 2-5(a), respectively. The solid curve(blue curve) notes the measured BOLD signal and the dotted solid curve (green curve) denotes the signal of the estimated BOLD model. The model mainly parameters (t_n, θ_2,) and standard deviation STD (STD=$std(x(t)-\overline{x}(t))$ i.e STD is the standard deviation between $x(t)$ and $\overline{x}(t)$. $x(t)$ is the measured signal and $\overline{x}(t)$ is the estimated signal.) are shown the L-Lower in Table 5.

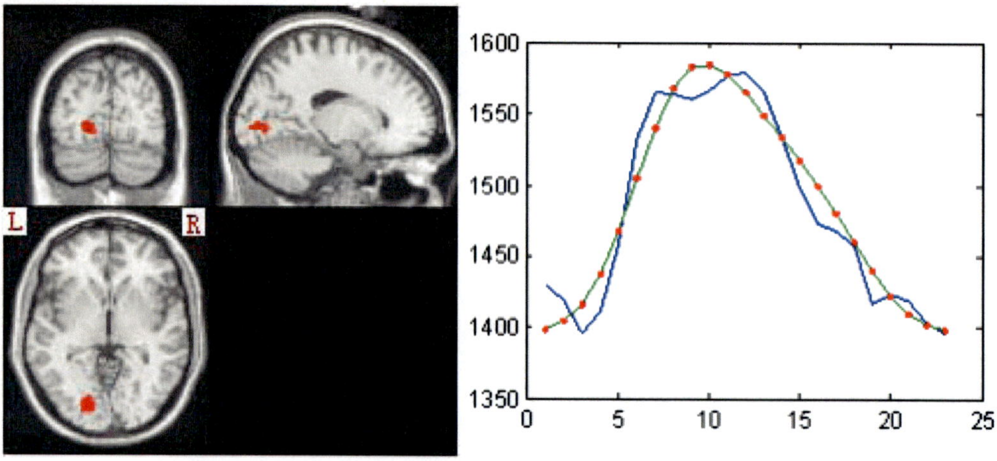

(a) (b)

Figure 7. The active points of the imaging result of the left upper VF (A in Figure 6) and its dynamic signal curves. (a) Talairach anatomic position of the active points of eight subjects; (b) BOLD signal curves of one pixel in (a), solid curve (blue curve) is the actual BOLD curve, the dotted solid curve (green curve) is the estimated BOLD with model mainly parameters (t_n, θ_2 ,) and standard deviation STD are the L-Lower in Table 5.

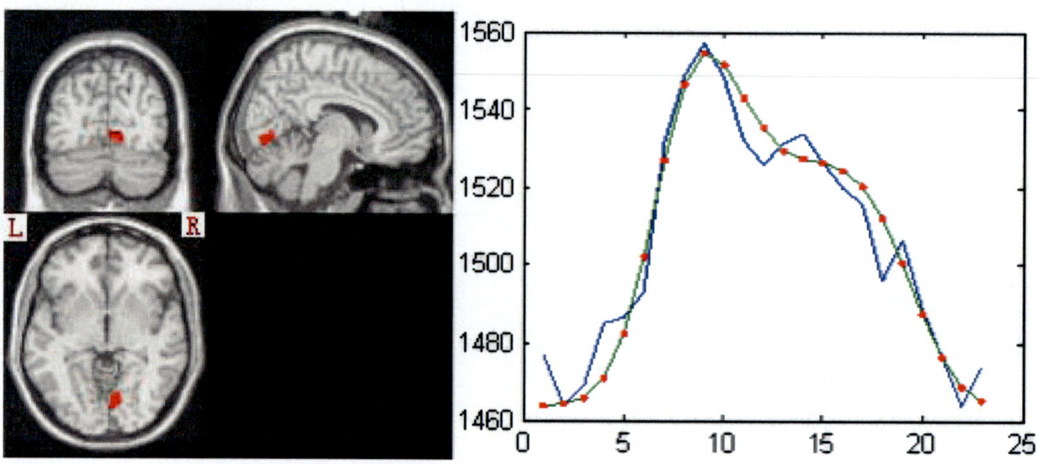

Figure 8. The active points of the imaging result of the right upper VF (B in Figure 6) and its dynamic signal curves. (a) Talairach anatomic position of the active points of eight subjects; (b) BOLD signal curves of one pixel in (a), solid curve (blue curve) is the actual BOLD curve, the dotted solid curve (green curve) is the estimated BOLD with model mainly parameters (t_n, θ_2) and STD are the R-Upper in Table5.

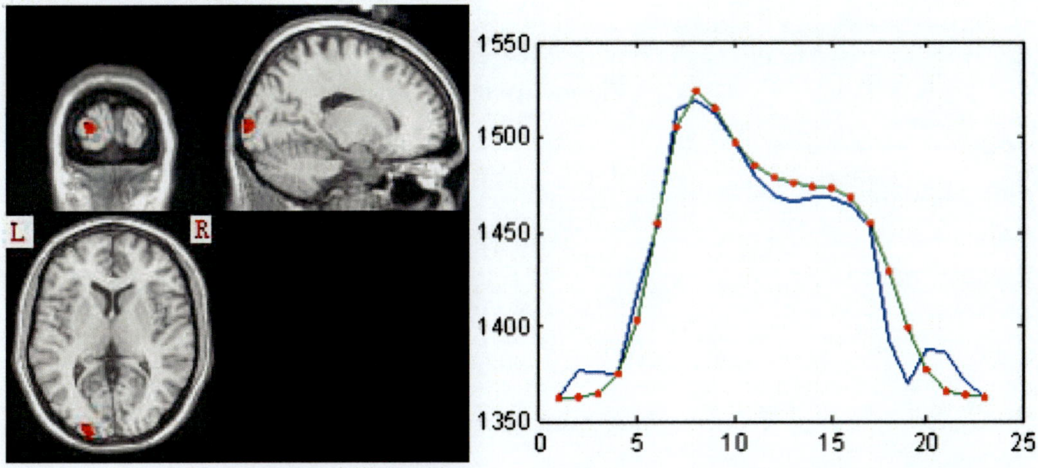

Figure 9. The active points of the imaging result of the left lower VF (C in Figure 6) and its dynamic signal curves. (a) Talairach anatomic position of the active points of eight subjects; (b) BOLD signal curves of one pixel in (a), solid curve (blue curve) is the actual BOLD curve, the dotted solid curve (green curve) is the estimated BOLD with model mainly parameters (t_n, θ_2) and STD are the L-Lower in Table 5.

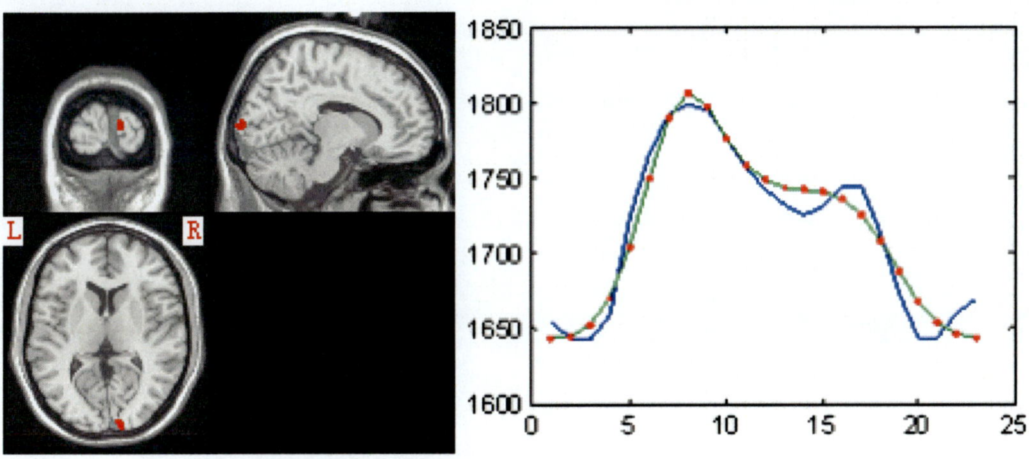

Figure 10. The active points of the imaging result of the right lower VF (D in Figure 6) and its dynamic signal curves. (a) Anatomic position of the active points of eight subjects; (b) BOLD signal curves of one pixel in (a), solid curve (blue curve) is the actual BOLD curve, the dotted solid curve (green curve) is the estimated BOLD with model mainly parameters (t_n, θ_2) and STD are the R-Lower in Table 5.

Activation at these sites were positively correlated(r>0.6) with the reference signal at a significance level of p<0.005(Chen et al, 2003)

Table 4. Average Talairach Coordinates of the most active points of the eight subjects was generated in the primary visual cortex (human analogue of V1, area 17) (Values are in mm)

Coordinates / StimulusPosition	X(mm)	Y(mm)	Z(mm)
A(upper left)	-16	-81	-1
B(upper right)	8	-74	-3
C(lower left)	-16	-100	6
D(lower right)	10	-99	7

Table 5. BOLD model parameters results

Parameter	L –Upper(A)	R-Upper(B)	L-lower (C)	R-Lower(D)	P
t_n	5.2	0.8	1.3	0.5	<0.05
θ_2	8.4	8.9	7.9	8.2	<0.05
STD	16.2±0.3	7.9±0.2	13.4±0.3	13.2±0.3	

where p <0.05 note the parameter t_n and θ_2 which is the significance level of difference between Left and Right fields, upper and lower fields. STD= $std(x(t) - \overline{x}(t))$ i.e STD is the standard deviation between $x(t)$ and $\overline{x}(t)$. $x(t)$ is the measured signal and $\overline{x}(t)$ is the estimated signal.

For comparing directly the four spatial fields, the activation point of Figure 7-10 are approximately set one transverse view in Figure 6, whose Talairach Coordinates is presented Table 15. The four spatial fields can easy be distinguished from the occipital area.

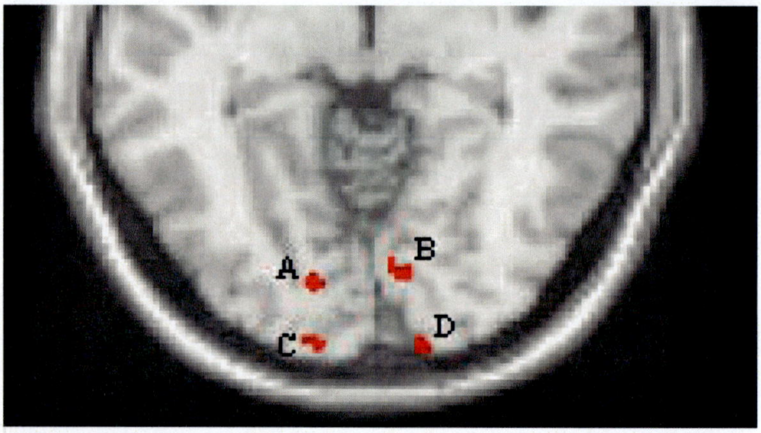

Figure 11. The active points of the spatial fields in transverse views.

Figure 11.is the mean parameters of the Gauss convolution BOLD model over eight subjects. Comparing the results in Figure 11, the parameters of the model for upper, lower and left, right VFs are different. And they provide the chance to discuss the asymmetry of the left–right and upper–lower visual field.

5.6. Asymmetries between the Lower VF and the Upper VF

With SPSS (Statistics package for social science) software ANOVA method analysis for the eight subjects, it was found that the delay parameter θ_2 of the lower VF is significantly smaller than that of the upper VF (F=4.3,p<0.05), Besides, the decay parameter t_n also shows an apparently different between upper and lower VFs (F=5.5,p<0.05).

Based on the model, Eq. (2), the reduction of the delay parameter t_n indicates a faster BOLD response; and according to Eq. (1), the reduction of the decay parameter θ_2 indicates a longer BOLD activation duration. Comparing the results in Figure 7, the decay parameter t_n reduces from 13.4 for the left upper VF (A) to 1.2 for the left lower VF (C), or from 13.9 in right upper VF (B) to 6.5 in right lower VF (D). The smaller decay parameter of the lower VFs than that of the upper VF suggests the neural activities are stronger in the lower field than that in the upper field. Meanwhile, the delay parameter θ_2 reduces from 18.6 at A to 8.9 at C and from 16.1 at B to 10.6 at D. The shorter delay parameter of the lower VF than that of the upper VF means the neural response to the lower VF is quicker. In conclusion, the same change trend of the two main parameters, the delay parameter and the decay parameter, tell us that the nonlinear dynamic characteristics of BOLD signal evoked by the visual stimuli are different in the upper and lower VFs. And both of these two evidences all suggest that the lower VF is dominant in processing visual stimulus. This result is in accordance with the earlier works that the perception of illusory contours (Rubin et al. 1996), achromatic motion processing (Edwards and Bad-cock, 1993) and chromatic motion processing (Bilodeau and Faubert, 1997) may be enhanced in the lower VF as opposed to the upper VF (He 1996; Natio, 2000).

5.7. Asymmetries between the Left VF and Right VF

According to Figure12, the delay parameter θ_2 of the left VF is an apparently different from the Right VF, while, with SPSS software ANOVA method analysis for the eight subjects, the difference is different (F=4.2, p<0.05). Meanwhile, the decay parameter t_n also shows an apparent difference between left and right VF, and the difference also is different (F=4.4, p <0.05).

Looking at the results in Figure12, the decay parameter t_n reduces from 13.4 for the left upper VF (A) to 13.9 in right upper VF (B), or from 1.2 for the left lower VF (C) up to 6.5 in right lower VF (D). The delay parameter θ_2 reduces from 18.6 at A to 16.1 at B and from 8.9 at C to 10.6 at D.

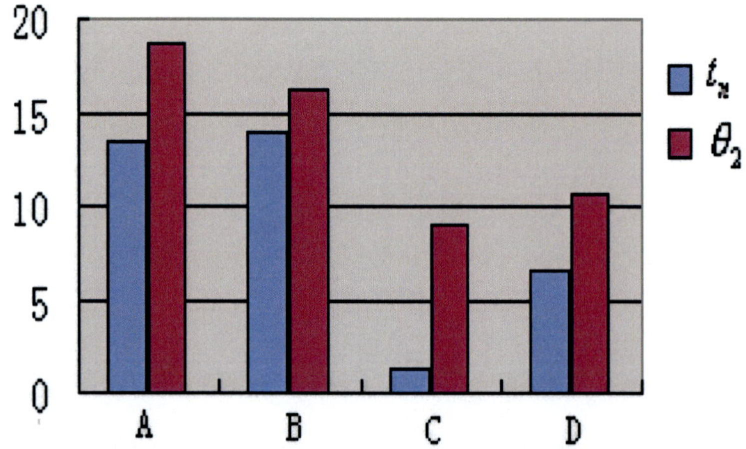

Figure 12. Mean parameters value of the Gauss convolution BOLD model over the eight subjects.

These results indicate that the dynamic responses are different between the left VF and the right VF. Both of these two evidences all suggest that it is asymmetry between the left VF and right VF for visual information process though the preponderant between left and right VFs is different. The result is also in accordance with the earlier works about the asymmetry of the neural process between the left and right VFs (Hagenbeek, 2002 ; Sergent, 1982; Heilman,1980; Kinsbourne, 1970).

CONCLUSION

In this paper, the comparison analysis was implemented between our Gaussian convolution model and the current Gamma model. The parameters were estimated for a vivo fMRI data evoked by a visual stimulation. The results show that the Gaussian model, which is based on the law of large numbers in probability thus may reflects the statistical characteristics of neural cluster activation, can simulate the BOLD response better than the Gamma model does. Both results of the two convolution models indicate that the nonlinear dynamic characteristics of BOLD signal evoked by the stimulus are different in the left and right occipital lobe region of the primary visual cortex in processing visual stimulus, and indicate that the dynamic processes seem different in various cerebral functional regions.

One the other hand, it was found that the model parameters for different visual spatial fields are different and the asymmetry of the left–right and upper–lower VF are analyzed. The results support that the lower VF is a dominant field than the upper VF in processing visual stimulus because it is of a stronger neural activities and shorter response delay. And the results show an apparent difference between the left VF and right VF for visual information process.

ACKNOWLEDGEMENT

This research was supported by the NSFC#30525030, 30570507, New Century Excellent Talents in University(NCET-05-0809) and key research project of science and technology of MOE(107097).

REFERENCES

Aguirre G. K., Zarahn E., and Esposito M.D(1998). The variability of human BOLD hemodynamic responses. *NeuroImage*. 8: 360-369.

Bandettini P.A., Jesmanowicz A., Wong E.C,.and Hyde J.S(1993). Processing Strategies for Time-Course Data Sets in Functional MRI of the Human Brain. *Magnetic Resonance in Medicine.* 30:161-173.

Bilodeau, L., and Faubert, J(1997).. Isoluminance and chromatic motion throughout the visual field. *Vision Research.*37: 2073– 2081.

Birn R M.; Saad, Z S.; Bandettini P A(2001). Spatial heterogeneity of the nonlinear dynamics in the fMRI BOLD response. *NeuroImage*. 14:817-826.

Boynton G.M.,. Engel S.A, Glover G.H. and Heeger D.J(1996). Linear systems analysis of functional magnetic resonance imaging in human V1. *J. of Neuroscience*. 16: 4207-4221.

Buxton, R.B., Liu, T.T.and Wong, E.C(2001). Nonlinearity of the Hemodynamic Response: Modeling the Neural and BOLD Contributions. *Proc. 9th ISMRM*: 1164.

Casco, C D. Spinelli(1998). Left-right visual field asymmetry in bistable motion perception, *Perception* .17: 721–727.

Chen, H., Yao, D., Becker, S., Zhuo, Y., Zeng, M. and Chen L(2002). A new method for fMRI data processing: Neighborhood independent component correlation algorithm and its preliminary application. *Science in China* (Series F). 45(5):373-382.

Chen H., Yao D., Zhuo Y, and Chen L(2003). Analysis of fMRI data by blind separation into independent temporal component. *Brain topography*. 15(4):223-232.

Chen H, Yao D, Liu Z(2004a). A Study on asymmetry of Spatial Visual field by Analysis of the fMRI BOLD Response. *Brain Topography*. 17(1):39-46.

Chen H, Yao D(2004b). An extended Gamma dynamic model of fMRI BOLD response. *Neurocomputing.* 61:395-400.

Chen H, Yao D, Liu Z(2005a). A comparison of Gamma and Gaussian dynamic convolution models of the fMRI BOLD response. *Magnetic Resonance Imaging*. 23: 83–88.

Chen H, Yao D, Chen W, Chen L(2005b). Delay Correlation Subspace Decomposition Algorithm and Its Application in fMRI. *IEEE Trans. Medical imaging*.24 （12） 1647-1650.

Chen H, Yuan H, Yao D, Chen L , Chen W(2006). An Integrated Neighborhood Correlation and Hierarchical Clustering approach of Functional MRI. IEEE Trans. *Biomedical Engineering.* 53(3):452-258.

Christman, S. D(1993). Local-global processing in the upper versus lower visual fields. *Bulletin of the Psychonomic Society*. 31: 275–278.

Christman, S. D., and Niebauer, C. L(1997). The relation between left–right and upper–lower visual field differences. In S. Christman (Ed.), *Cerebral asymmetries in sensory and perceptual processing*. Amsterdam: Elsevier.

Cohen, G(1982). Theoretical interpretation of lateral asymmetries. In J. G. Beaumont (Ed.), *Divided visual field studies of cerebral organisation*. London: Academic Press.

Cox RW (1996): AFNI: software for analysis and visualization of functional magnetic resonance neuroimages. *Comput. Biomed. Res*. 29:162–173.

Di Russo F, Martínez A and Hillyard S(2003).A Source Analysis of Event-related Cortical Activity during Visuo-spatial Attention. *Cerebral Cortex* May. 13:486 –499.

Di Russo F, Martínez A, Sereno M, Pitzalis S, and Hillyard SA(2001). Cortical Sources of the Early Components of the Visual Evoked Potential. *Human Brain Mapping*. 15:95–111.

Edwards, M., and Badcock, D. R. Asymmetries in the sensitivity to motion in depth: a centripetal bias. *Perception*,1993, 22: 1013–1023.

Friston K.J(2002). Bayesian estimation of dynamical systems: an application to fmri. *Neuroimage*. 16: 513-530.

Friston, K. J., Mechelli, A., Turner, R., Price, C. J(2002) .Nonlinear Responses in fMRI: The Balloon Model, Volterra Kernels, and Other Hemodynamics. *NeuroImage*. 12(4): 466-477.

Guillaume, M., Habib, B., Philippe, C., Me, P. I. and Jean, B. P(2003). Robust bayesian estimation of the hemodynamic response function in event- related BOLD fMRI using basic physiological information. *Human Brain Mapping*.19:1-17.

Hagenbeek, Rogier E.; Van Strien, Jan W(2002). Left–right and upper–lower visual field asymmetries for face matching, letter naming, and lexical decision. *Brain and Cognition*. 49(1): 34-44.

He S, Cavanagh P and Intriligator J(1996). Attentional resolution and the locus of visual a wareness. *Nature*., 1996, 383:334-337.

Heilman K.M., Van Den Abell T(1980). Right hemisphere dominance for attention: the mechanism underlying hemispheric asymmetries of inattention (neglect), *Neurology*. 30: 327–330.

Henson, R.N.A., Price, C.J., Rugg, M.D.,Turner R.and Friston, K. J.(2001): Detecting latency differences in event related BOLD responses: application to words versus nonwords and initial versus repeated face presentations. *NeuroImage*. 15: 83-97.

Hwang, K.S., Choi, Y.K.and Jung,J.S(1997). On superior limits for the increments of Gaussian processes. *Statistics and Probability Lette*.35(3): 289-296.

Kinsbourne M(1970). The cerebral basis of lateral asymmetries in attention, *Acta Psychol*. (Amsterdam).33: 193–201.

Kruggel, F., Zysset, S. and Von Cramon, F. D. Y(2000). Nonlinear regression of functional MRI data: an item recognition task study. *NeuroImage*. 12:173-183.

Kwong K. , Belliveau J. , Chesler D. et al(1992). Dynamic magnetic resonance imaging of human brain activity during primary sensory stimulation. *Proc. Natl. Acad. Sci. USA*. 89:5675–5679.

Liu, H. L. and Gao, J. H(2000). An investigation of the impulse functions for the nonlinear BOLD response in functional MRI. *Mag. Res. Med.* 18: 931-938.

Logothetis N.K., Pauls J., Augath M., Trinath T.,and Oeltermann A(2001). Neurophysiological investigation of the basis of the fMRI signal. *Nature.* 412: 150-157.

Lundervold A, Khateeb IH(2002). Numerical estimation of the BOLD response in event-related fMRI. *Poster at the 25th Annual Mid-Year Meeting of the International Neuropsychological Society*, 2002,July 24-27, Stockholm, Sweden.

Miller K. L., Luh, W. M., Liu, T. T, Martinez, A., Obata, T., Wong, E.C., Frank, L. R.and Buxton, R. B(2001). Nonlinear temporal dynamics of the cerebral blood flow response. *Human Brain Mapping*.13:1-12.

Naito T, Kaneoke Y,Osaka, N Kakigi R.: Asymmetry of the human visual field in magnetic response to apparet motion. *Brain Research*, 2000, 865:221-226.

Niebauer, C. L., and Christman, S. D(1998). Upper and lower visual field differences in categorical and coordinate judgments. *Psychonomic Bulletin and Review*. 5:147–151.

Ogawa S, Tank D. W., Menon R., Ellermann J.M., Kim S.G., Merkle H., and Ugurbil K(1992). Intrinsic signal changes accompanying sensory stimulation: Functional brain mapping with magnetic resonance imaging. *Proc. Natl. Acad Sci. USA*.89:.5951-5955.

Okita T, Konishi K, Morotomi T,Tanaka H(1990). Effects of selective attention to upper and lower visual-field pattern stimuli on event-related brain potentials, *Jpn. J. Physiol. Psychol. Psychophysiol*.8: 81–93.

Osaka N(1993). Apparent motion in the upper and lower peripheral visual field, *Perception.* 33: S80–S81.

Previc F H, Breitmeyer B.G., Weinstein L.F.(1995) Discriminability of random-dot stereograms in three-dimensional space, *Int. J. Neurosci*. 80:247–253.

Previc F H(1990). Functional specialization in the lower and upper visual fields in humans: its ecological origins and neurophysiological implications, *Behav. Brain Sci*. 13: 519–575.

Rajapakse J.C., Kruggel F., Maisog J.M. and Von Cramon D.Y(1998). Modelling hemodynamic response for analysis of functional MRI time-series. *Human Brain Mapping*. 6: 283-300.

Rao S.M., Bandettini P.A., Binder J.R., Bobholz J.A., Hammeke T.A., Stein v, and Hyde v(1996). Relationship between finger movement rate and functional magnetic resonance signal change in human primary motor cortex. *J. of Cerebral Blood Flow and Metabolis*. 16:1250-1254.

Rasmus M.B., Ziad S.S., and Peter A.N(2001).Spatial heterogeneity of the nonlinear dynamics in the fMRI BOLD response. *NeuroImage*.14: 817-826.

Rieke F., Warland D., van Steveninck R., and Bialek W(1997). *Spikes: exploring the neural code.* Cambridge, MA: MIT Press.

Rogier E. Hagenbeek and Jan W. Van Strien(2002). Left–Right and Upper–Lower Visual Field Asymmetries for Face Matching, Letter Naming, and Lexical Decision. *Brain and Cognition.* 49: 34–44.

Rosen B.R., Buckner R.L. and Dale A(1998). Event-related functional MRI: past, present, and future. *Proc. Natl. Acad. Sci. USA*.. 95:.773-780.

Rubin, N., Nakayama, K., and Shapley, R(1996). Enhanced perception of illusory contours in the lower versus upper visual hemifields. *Science*. 271: 651–653.

Se Fukusima, Sérgio S.; Faubert(2001). Jocelyn Perceived length in the central visual field: evidence for visual field asymmetries. *Vision Research*,.41: 2119–2126.

Sergent, J(1982).. The cerebral balance of power: Confrontation or cooperation? *Journal of Experimental Psychology: Human Perception and Performance*.8: 253–272.

Tanabe J, Miller D, Tregellas J, Freedman R, and Meyer FG(2002). Comparison of detrending methods for optimal fMRI preprocessing. *NeuroImage*. 15: 902–907.

Toga W and Thompson PM(2003), Mapping brain asymmetry, *Nature Reviews Neuroscience*. 4: 37 -48.

Underwood G, Whitfield A(1995). Right-hemisphere interactions in picture-word processing, *Brain Cogn*.4: 273–286.

Vazquez A.L., and Noll D.C(1988). Nonlinear aspects of the BOLD response in functional MRI. *Neuroimage*. 7:108-118.

Vitouch O., Bauer H., Gittler G., Leodolter M., and Leodolter U(1997). Cortical activity of good and poor spatial test performers during spatial and verbal processing studied with slow potential topography. *International Journal Psychophysiology*, 27:183 -199.

Vogel,J.J, Bowers,C. A Vogel, D.C(2003). Cerebral lateralization of spatial abilities: A meta-analysis. *Brain and Cognition*.52: 197-204.

von Grunau M, Dube S(1994) .Visual search asymmetry for viewing direction, *Percept. Psychophys*. 56:211–220.

Wendt P.E., and Risberg L(1994). Cortical activation during visual spatial processing: Relation between hemispheric asymmetry of blood flow and performance. *Brain and Cognition*. 24:87 -103.

Whishaw I.Q(1994). How do primates reach? *Behav. Brain Sci*. 1994,17: 173–174.

Yao D (2000). High-resolution EEG mappings: a spherical harmonic spectra theory and simulation results. *Clinical Neurophysiology*.111:81-92.

Yoshizaki K(1990). Shift toward left visual field advantage after short term learning experience, *Int. J. Neurosci*. 55:113–117.

In: Brain Mapping Research Developments
Editor: Lars N. Bakker, pp. 177-196
ISBN 978-1-60456-007-7

Chapter VII

MULTI-PARAMETRIC MAPPING OF GLIOMAS: DEMONSTRATION OF SEGMENTATION STRATEGIES

Kathryn M. McMillan and Ronald R. Price
Department of Radiology and Radiological Sciences
Vanderbilt Medical Center
Nashville, Tennessee, USA

INTRODUCTION

While MRI is well suited for examining post-treatment gliomas, there are often ambiguous results when attempting to interpret T1- and T2-weighted images, even with the use of an extravascular contrast agent. To provide additional clarity when distinguishing recurrent disease from radiation necrosis, edema, and normal tissue, a host of MRI parameters that probe physiology have been developed and continue to be optimized. These include specialized MR sequences that yield descriptive maps of tissue perfusion and diffusion [1-4]; chemical shift imaging that provides biochemical measures (choline, creatine, N-acetyl aspartate, lactate) [5]; and a blood oxygenation level dependent (BOLD)-based scan that provides hypoxia maps [6, 7].

The multi-parametric techniques now being used for recurrent Glioblastoma Multiforme (GBM) patients could be applied to many cancer management situations (e.g. diagnosis, surgical and radiation planning, monitoring therapy). When prescribing radiation therapy, for example, greater knowledge of the tumor environment would allow advances in radiation delivery systems (e.g. Intensity Modulated Radiotherapy) to deliver more focused, patient-specific treatment [8]. However, the imaging techniques yield a variety of maps that all require interpretation. The quantity of parameter maps and complexity of the dataset obtained from multi-parametric approaches emphasizes the need for further work to make these techniques more user-friendly in clinical settings.

Table 1. Processing Strategies, Specific Techniques and Relevant Software

Category	Technique	Software
Feature Extraction	Edge Detection	ImageJ
Composite Mapping	Percent Overlap Method	AFNI
Unsupervised clustering	ISODATA	Eigentool
Random Field Models	Hidden Markov	FSL
Artificial Neural Networks	INSECT	MINC

Segmentation, classification and composite mapping are critical needs for improved cancer management. Though a number of investigators are exploring the utility of multi-parametric imaging analyses [9-14], no consensus approach currently exists for presenting the results. The most useful composite map would clearly note the area of disease that most needed intervention. However, the tumor environment, especially post-treatment, is characterized by its heterogeneity in that some tumor areas are aggressive while others are necrotic. An efficient mapping system and prioritization of a range of tumor behaviors displayed by the imaging data is therefore of high interest.

A number of methods to automatically segment tissue have been introduced and a number of authors have covered pre-processing steps, general theory and the various available algorithms [15, 16]. Given a dataset that has been preprocessed and registered [17], we have applied five methods for processing the multi-parametric data. This chapter will cover techniques selected from the five broad categories listed in Table 1 by selecting freely available software packages. The algorithms were applied to the sample GBM dataset and discussed in terms of theory and the resulting maps.

Multi-Parametric Imaging in a Recurrent GBM Patient

Before demonstrating processing techniques, it is important to understand the underlying dataset used throughout this chapter. This section describes the acquisition parameters, offers some relevant details regarding the patient's history and provides background and references for the individual imaging techniques.

Figure 1 shows six MRI maps for a single patient who provided informed consent to an IRB approved clinical protocol. This patient is a male, age 51, and presented with right field visual loss. He completed external beam radiotherapy thirteen months after a craniotomy was performed. MR scanning was performed on a clinical 1.5T GE Signa Horizon magnet (GE Medical Systems, Milwaukee, Wisconsin). The diagnosis of recurrence was based on clinical information and the MR scan illustrated in figure 1. The recurrence occurred 16 months after completion of radiotherapy. This patient declined further treatment at that time.

T1-weighted images show nodular enhancement suggestive of recurrence around the resection bed and underlay the maps in figure 1A-D. The large area of elevated choline (figure 1A) extends past the medial edge of the abnormal enhancement, suggesting malignant processes in that region. The peak of the NAA color map is located outside the enhancing region in figure 1B, denoting the lack of normal neuronal tissue near the resection bed [18]. NAA levels are depleted in destructive, degenerative, or infiltrative tumor processes [19, 20]. The region of high lactate in figure 1C encompasses much of the posterior section of the recurrence.

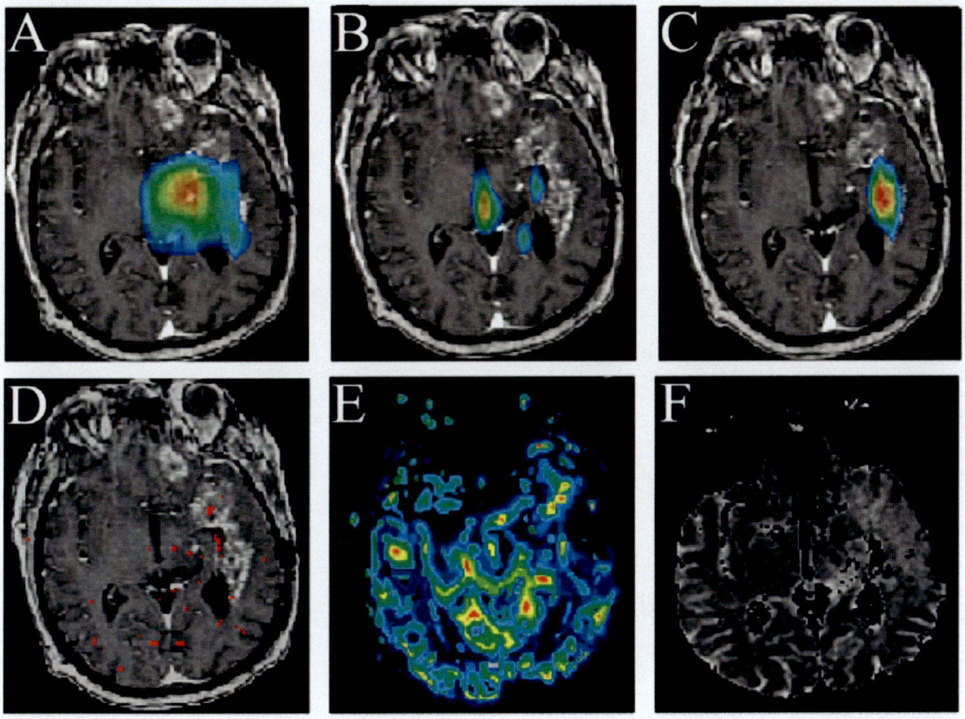

Figure 1. Scan where recurrence was diagnosed. (A) Choline (B) NAA and (C) lactate maps, (D) significant changes in T2* between air and carbogen breathing that represent hypoxia, (E) regional cerebral blood volume (rCBV), and (F) apparent diffusion coefficient (ADC) each have the potential to map the tumor environment but require additional processing for increased clinical utility.

Two multi-echo scans were acquired while breathing, respectively, air and carbogen (95%O_2, 5%CO_2) to obtain maps of hypoxic regions. Voxels with significantly different values of T2* ($p<0.02$) are displayed as red voxels in figure 1D. It has been found that hypoxic regions will preferentially experience increases in the oxygen tension during hyperoxygenation caused by carbogen breathing [7, 21]. Conversely, changes in response to hyperoxygenation in well-oxygenated and necrotic regions would be expected to be relatively small [22, 23].The maps appear moderately noisy, but do highlight regions of enhancement toward the anterior and medial portions of recurrent disease.

Regional cerebral blood volume (rCBV) values, illustrated in figure 1E, appear high in the anterior and medial edges of the enhancing region, suggesting neovascularity in those hyperintense spots. Many quickly growing tumors outgrow their blood supply and form new vasculature in an attempt to deliver nutrients and oxygen necessary for future growth. These vascular networks also offer an avenue for growth into new regions [24]. While rCBV maps are nonspecific to angiogenesis, high blood volume measures away from normal vasculature could indicate areas of growing tumor. As permeability measurements are increasingly applied to cancer protocols, an additional map of interest will be added to many multi-parametric datasets such as these [25].

Table 2. Multi-Parametric Acquisition Details

Scan	**Acquisition Details (TR, TE, Flip, Slice thickness/gap, FOV, matrix)**	**Parameter Map**	**Ideally characterizes**
Spin Echo Diffusion (b = 0, 1000 s/mm^2)	5s, 86ms, 90°, 5/0mm, 22cm, 128x128	Apparent diffusion coefficient (ADC)	Cellularity
2 Multi-echo EPI (air breathing, 10 minute equilibration, then carbogen breathing)	2s, 35-80ms (10 steps of 5ms), 90°, 5/1mm, 24cm, 128x128	Student's t-test map of changes in T2* between air and carbogen (95% O_2, 5% CO_2) breathing	Hypoxia
Gradient Echo Perfusion (gadodiamide injection)	2s, 60ms, 60°, 7/2mm, 22cm, 128x128	Relative cerebral blood volume (rCBV)	Angiogenesis
Post-contrast SPGR	21ms, 6ms, 20°, 1.5/0mm, 24cm, 256x256	T1-weighted image	Anatomy
Post-contrast T2-FLAIR	8s, 120ms, 90°, 5/1mm, 22cm, 256x256	Fluid attenuated T2-weighted image	Anatomy
Chemical Shift Imaging	1s, 144ms, 90°, 15mm (single slice), 24cm, 18x18	Metabolite ratios (Cho:NAA, Lac:Cre)	Metabolite values associated with cancer processes, normal brain tissue and anaerobic metabolism

Increased cellularity can restrict diffusion by decreasing the availability of extracellular space. Voxels with decreased intensity in figure 1F show reduced apparent diffusion coefficient (ADC) and are located in small regions to the right of the posterior section of the resection bed. While tumor cellularity is thought to be a major factor when determining the ADC values of brain tumors, it is not the only variable [26]. Post-treatment changes in ADC, for example, could relate to cell density changes resulting from necrosis or apoptosis. In addition, changes in ADC over time could show reorganization of the tumor environment [27].

Figure 2 shows an attempt at using various MR parameters in a radiation treatment plan. While the individual maps are condensed to the abnormal regions they contain via tracing by a radiologist, it is not clear from this map as to which areas should be treated, the actual tumor extent, or exactly where boost fields should be directed. A more compelling map would make future work in this area more attractive to clinical staff unfamiliar with the imaging techniques. Automating the process would reduce the labor required from Radiology and could increase reproducibility. To that end, several methodologies that attempt to identify likely recurrent regions, define tumor extent and describe the heterogeneous environment contained in high grade tumors were applied to this patient dataset.

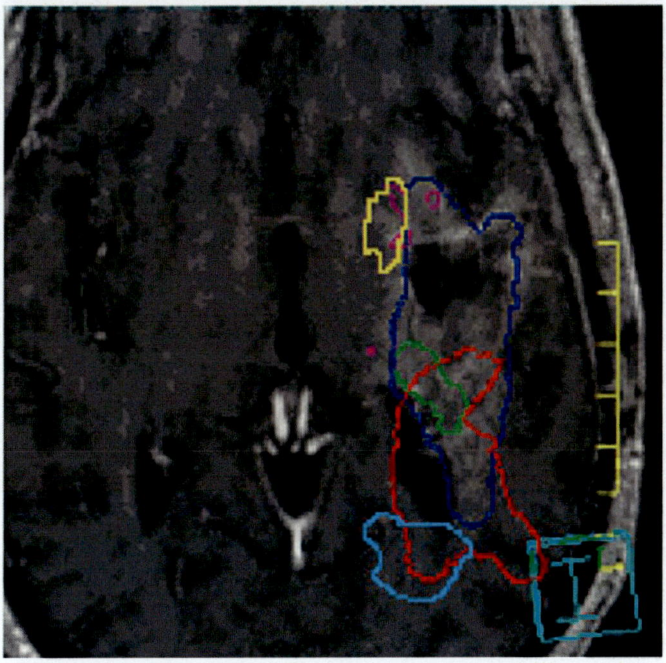

Figure 2. Clinical target volumes (CTVs) used in radiation treatment planning as traced by a neuroradiologist. A 2 cm margin around the gross tumor volume (GTV) is typically used to define the radiation target. Physiologic parameters indicate regions of interest outside the GTV region as well as areas that may benefit from boost fields, but the ideal treatment plan resulting from this map remains unclear.

GTV= dark blue CTV_{rCBV}= green $CTV_{Hypoxia}$= pink

$CTV_{Cho:NAA}$ = red $CTV_{Lac:Cre}$ = yellow CTV_{ADC} = light blue

Feature Extraction: Edge Detection

While expert tracing by a radiologist is advantageous, it is also somewhat subjective and very time consuming. When seeking to automate the process of highlighting voxels of interest, an automatic method should be relatively fast and highly reproducible. There are several methods of extracting features from the individual parameter maps (e.g. thresholding based on pixel intensity or texture; region growing techniques), but we have selected an edge detection algorithm for use in our dataset [15].

To detect edges, discontinuities in the intensity distribution are highlighted. That process should define several regions within the image through the use of gradient based operators in various forms [28]. Among the operators that may be applied within edge detecting schemes are the Canny [29] , Marr-Hildreth [30], and Sobel filters [31].

ImageJ (http://rsb.info.nih.gov/ij/) was used to perform the edge detection analyses on the individual parameter maps. This software utilizes a Sobel operator to convolve a single image (e.g. T1) with two 3x3 kernals – one in the horizontal and one in the vertical direction, providing an estimate of the gradient in both directions. If G_x is the horizontal gradient of the image intensity, it would be represented such that

$$G_x = \begin{bmatrix} -1 & 0 & 1 \\ -2 & 0 & 2 \\ -1 & 0 & 1 \end{bmatrix} * T1$$

Likewise, G_y for the T1-weighted image could be expressed such that

$$G_y = \begin{bmatrix} 1 & 2 & 1 \\ 0 & 0 & 0 \\ -1 & -2 & -1 \end{bmatrix} * T1$$

The gradient magnitude is therefore given by

$$G = \sqrt{G_x{}^2 + G_y{}^2}$$

Once the first derivative is calculated for each pixel, a threshold can be applied and the suprathreshold voxels can be traced to form edges of the image. This method of extracting relevant features tends to be restricted for use in distinguishing relatively simple structures with sharp boundaries. Automated analysis, however, is an important step, solving problems of subjectivity and the need for extensive user-interaction. The edge detection approach was able to locate some relevant tumor characteristics for the maps presented [32].

When considering T1, T2 and ADC maps (Figure 3A-3C), and their edge detected results ($3A_e$-$3C_e$) the edges of the ventricles are clearly defined and good separation of the brain from surrounding skull is achieved. Large, continuous regions lend themselves well to edge detection and the tumor region appears to be outlined on the T1 image (Figure $3A_e$). Edge detection approaches may fail in the presence of excessive noise, partial volume effects, motion artifacts, and non-optimal window/level settings [15]. RCBV and hypoxia maps are quite noisy and it appears as though there are excessive edges detected in $3D_e$.

Hypoxia results ($3E_e$) fail to give a meaningful segmentation in our case. The original t-test map does not offer distinct features or edges, likely due to small differences in intensity and smooth boundaries between hypoxic, well-oxygenated, and necrotic tissue types.

Improvements in edge detection have been made to incorporate multi-resolution applications [28] and simultaneous consideration of region and boundary information [33]. The edge detection algorithms demonstrated here, as with many feature extraction methods, are applied to the images on an individual basis and provide no mechanism by which important features from several maps can be combined.

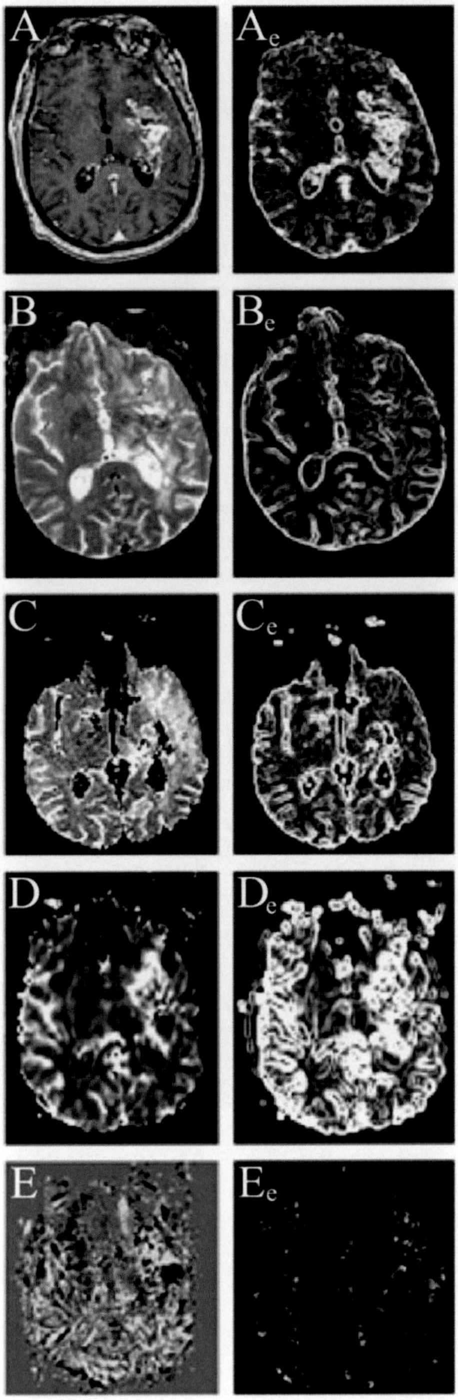

Figure 3. A single slice of the images acquired with a whole brain field of view are shown in the left column. (A) Post-contrast T1-weighted SPGR, (B) Post-contrast T2 FLAIR, (C) Apparent diffusion coefficient (ADC) (D) Regional cerebral blood volume (rCBV), (E) Hypoxia. The edge detection algorithm was applied in ImageJ to create the images in the right column: (A_e) Edge detected T1, (B_e) Edge detected T2, (C_e) Edge detected ADC, (D_e) Edge detected rCBV, (E_e) Edge detected Hypoxia.

Composite Mapping: Percent Overlap Method

Once features are extracted from the parameter maps in some meaningful way, there is then the question of how to combine the relevant tumor characteristics. The percent overlap method (POM) employs a global threshold to extract important regions from each physiologic map, evaluates the likelihood a given technique can characterize the tumor environment via a comparison with the contralateral hemisphere, then combines relevant parameters into a single map [34, 35].

The entire contralateral (non-tumor) hemisphere is used to establish appropriate global thresholds for each parameter by selecting the same percentile value (i.e. 95th percentile in the sample dataset shown here). Binary maps are then formed by thresholding each parameter map to contain only the extreme values (high Choline:NAA, Lactate:Creatine, high rCBV, low ADC, and highly significant T2* differences for hypoxia) such that suprathreshold voxels are equal to one, and all others are zero. Each thresholded parameter map contains a certain number of voxels, called $Voxels_x$, where x is the individual parameter (e.g. ADC, rCBV, hypoxia).

A single composite map containing all seven parameters can be formed where the signal intensity indicated the parameters that overlapped in each voxel. Unique values are first assigned to each of the seven thresholded parameter maps (e.g. rCBV = 1, hypoxia = 2, Cho:NAA = 4, Lac:Cre = 8, ADC = 16, Cho:Cre = 32) and sums are calculated voxel by voxel.

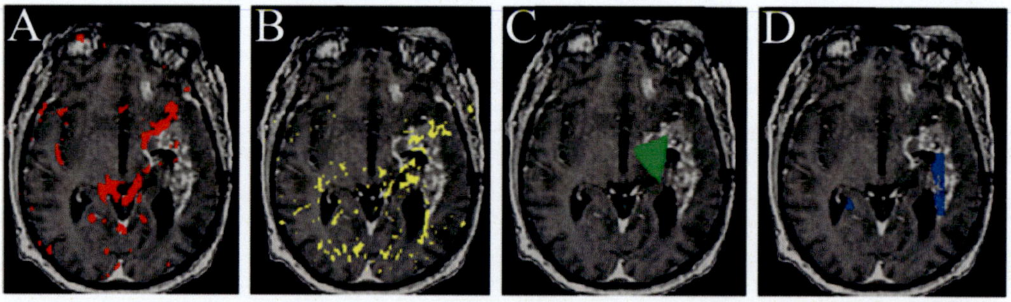

Figure 4. Global thresholds are applied to the various parameter maps such that a binary image is created for each. The suprathreshold voxels from each image are then assigned different values. (A) red voxels from rCBV = 1, (B) yellow voxels in hypoxia = 2, (C) green voxels in Cho:NAA = 4, (D) blue voxels of Lac:Cre = 8, then summed to form a composite map that should characterize the tumor environment.

A unique value then exists for every possible combination of techniques The assignment of unique values allows for the determination of which parameters overlap from color coding based upon which pure parameter maps contribute to the sum in each voxel. Voxels with a value of 10 indicate an overlap of Lac:Cre and hypoxia (displayed in the POM map – Figure 5 - as yellow), while green voxels have a value of 13, from an overlap of Cho:NAA, Lac:Cre and rCBV.

Voxels for each value are counted to calculate the percent overlap for each technique x, using

$$\%Overlap = \frac{Voxels_x - Voxels_{onlyx}}{Voxels_x}$$

where $Voxels_x$ was defined previously as the total number of voxels in a thresholded parameter map, and $Voxels_{onlyx}$ counts the voxels for technique x that do not show overlap with any other technique. Therefore, the numerator gives the number of voxels that overlap with any other technique and the denominator counts every voxel in the thresholded map regardless of overlap. Calculations of overlap percentage are performed for each hemisphere separately for each parameter. A parameter is considered successful at tumor characterization if the disease hemisphere shows increased percent overlap compared to the contralateral hemisphere.

The POM method makes use of the 3dcalc function in AFNI (http://afni.nimh.nih.gov/afni/) [36] once thresholds are determined. For this particular map, we used a command line such that:

3dcalc -prefix POMfinal -a rsrCBV+acpc. -b rsHypoxia+acpc. -c rsChoNAA+acpc. -d rsLacCre+acpc. -expr '1*step(a-$rCBV_{threshold}$)+2*step(b-$Hypoxia_{threshold}$)+4*step(c-$Cho:NAA_{threshold}$)+8*step(d-$Lac:Cre_{threshold}$)'

Note that all input parameters have been resampled and aligned. Once a POM map is formed, it should be loaded as an overlay on a T1- or T2-weighted underlay in AFNI. When defining the overlay, all voxels are positive and the number of colors should be changed to 15.

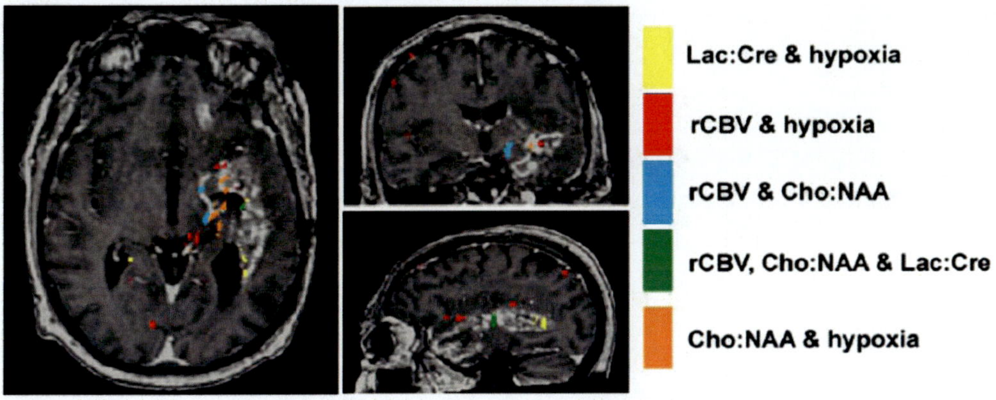

Figure 5. Lac:Cre (73% overlap), Cho:NAA (80% overlap), rCBV (13% overlap) and hypoxia (26%) were chosen as the most relevant parameters. Insight into the environment is offered, but extent is not clearly defined due to the lack continuous clusters.

Holding the mouse over the highest level will indicate the greatest integer calculated for a given map (i.e. Not every patient will display overlap in all four input parameters. The number of colors should be set to the highest integer calculated for each patient to appropriately display the map.) Clicking on the colors corresponding to pure parameters (e.g.

1, 2, 4 and 8) allows the user to assign no color to those values so that only overlapping voxels are displayed.

While an unlimited number of input techniques are feasible in when implementing POM, the color-coding for the final map becomes confusing when including more than four input parameters and the possible combinations thereof.

Hypoxic areas must resort to anaerobic metabolism, which makes lactate and hypoxia overlap reasonable as seen near the medial aspect of the posterior rim of enhancement. Hypoxic areas can be found in regions displaying elevated rCBV, possibly because tumor neovasculature is relatively dysfunctional, and the regions it serves may receive inadequate amounts of oxygenated blood [37]. Additionally, hypoxia promotes angiogenesis. Hypoxia-inducible factor 1 (HIF-1) is upregulated by hypoxic environments. Numerous genes, including glucose transporters, glycolysis enzymes and vascular endothelial growth factor (VEGF) are then activated to aid the adaptation of malignant cells to the hostile environment [38]. VEGF is the most important of the growth factors as it promotes angiogenesis, acts as a potent permeability factor [24], and is specifically required for survival of immature vasculature [39]. While the lack of histologic confirmation makes this explanation of tumor behavior conjecture, POM maps offer the ability to map behavior in individual voxels.

The concern with the overlap technique is that the subjectivity introduced by thresholding maps would result in missing areas since the complementary nature of the parameters is neglected in order to focus on redundant information. Falsely positive areas are avoided due to the nature of the overlap calculations, but finding an adequate amount of abnormal tissue is of interest. Users can alter the initial threshold or could implement code that utilized edge detection or contouring algorithms to extract features from the original parameter maps. The overall POM approach would be flexible to the incorporation of those changes as made appropriate by the specific goals and details associated with a given dataset. Additionally, the labeling of the classes is done automatically from the color-coded legend, aiding interpretation of these maps.

Additional work is clearly indicated in the initial feature extraction step, whether by choosing a threshold based on quantitative techniques or employing an edge detection or region growing algorithm instead of a global threshold. The method is, however, very simple to implement and provides an easily obtained map of some relevant features in the tumor environment.

Clustering: ISODATA

Clustering strategies offer some distinct advantages and are available as several algorithms. All approaches are designed to identify areas with high densities [15]. The unsupervised techniques limit user input to the selection of several initial parameters, then work automatically to separate the image set into tissue classes based on size, shape, contrast or connectivity [32]. Since tumor characteristics are time-dependent, an unsupervised approach is well-suited [40].

ISODATA, an iteratively self-organizing variation of the k-means algorithm, was validated against histology when considering multi-parametric datasets in stroke patients [41, 42]. While cancer processes are different than those seen in ischemic injury, the multi-parametric nature of imaging datasets in both disease states make a transition from stroke processes to cancer applications logical. ISODATA was chosen over other clustering methods since it does not require the knowledge of the number of clusters a priori. Rather, the initial guess at a number of clusters is iteratively altered until the algorithm finds an optimal solution. Since parameters vary from patient to patient in both identity and quantity an unsupervised algorithm is particularly important for our multi-parametric approach.

A space describing tumor characteristics can be created in n-dimensions by selecting relevant MR parameter maps, and placing each on a separate axis. Different tissue types can be differentiated by signal intensity, allowing visualization on MR images. These signal intensities provide the basis for classification of tissue type within clustering algorithms. The means to identify tissues is provided by the signature vector, S, defined for each pixel in our dataset as:

$$S = \left[S_{T1}, S_{T2}, S_{CBV}, S_{\Delta T2*}, S_{Cho\,:\,NAA}\right]^T$$

T notes that the matrix is transposed and input parameters are selected to contain post-contrast T1-SPGR, post-contrast T2-FLAIR, rCBV, hypoxia and Cho:NAA. After initialization with a user-defined number of cluster centers, intra-Euclidean distances to the cluster center are calculated pixel by pixel. Pixels with large distances will be placed in other clusters. Distances between cluster centers are also determined. Cluster centers located closely together will be merged. The distance calculations are continued and further merging and splitting stops at convergence, or when the maximum number of iterations is reached. The result from this analysis is a single theme map, where different clusters are shown by different colors [41, 43].

Eigentool image processing software (http://www.radiologyresearch.org/eigentoolhelp/) was used to perform the ISODATA analysis. As described in Shen *et al.*, the lumping parameter was chosen by defining a region of interest in the dominant tissue type for a given slice. The standard deviation parameter was then selected based upon another tissue type within that slice [42].

While cluster order schemes have been successfully implemented [44], there is some difficulty associated with interpreting the maps obtained. The colors that code the map could appear in different orders for different slices, though our results appear relatively constant. It is also not clear as to whether the yellow or olive green clusters note tumor behavior of interest. When comparing the ISODATA algorithm with POM maps in other patient datasets, we were able to note the appearance of similar regions from each strategy [34]. For the patient presented here, it is unclear as to whether the tumor behavior and lack of continuous regions contributes to the failure to isolate a large region that obviously requires treatment. There is also a question of how the metabolite maps contribute to the overall map. The brick red regions most clearly seen in Figure $6B_I$ and $6D_I$ require additional work with histologically confirmed images to better understand the method and how it might be optimized.

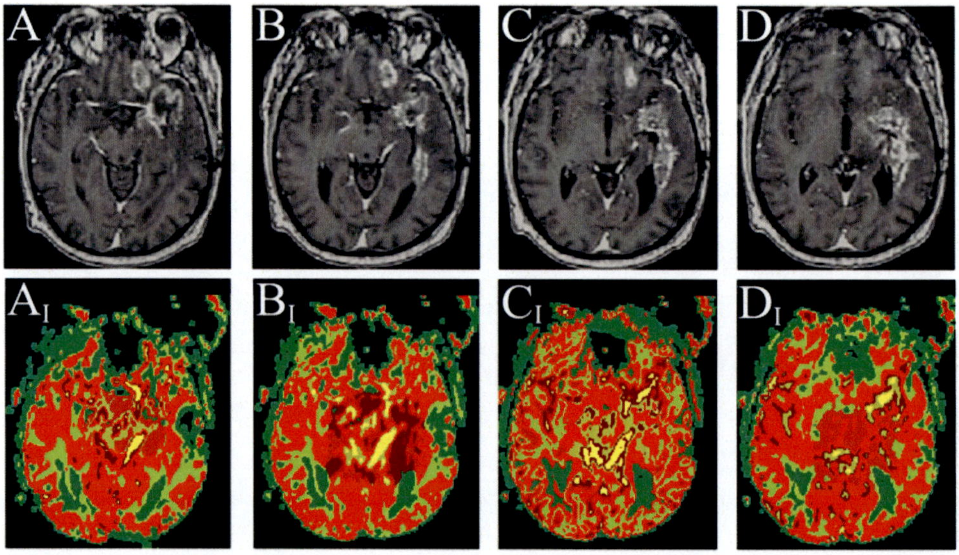

Figure 6. Four slices separated by 3 mm are shown in the post-contrast T1-weighted series of images (A-D). The corresponding slices created from an ISODATA clustering approach with input parameters including T1, T2, rCBV, Hypoxia and Cho:NAA are shown below (A_I-D_I).

Shen *et al.* implemented a Mahalanobis rather than Euclidean distance to deal with coordinate axis scaling, correct for correlation between different features, and allow for curved decision boundaries. [42]. Yovel and Assaf presented beautiful results for clustering regions within the thalamus using a technique they call virtual-dot-com imaging that applies *k*-means clustering within a multi-step algorithm [45].

Fuzzy c-means is a generalization of the k-means approach [16]. When fuzzy methods are applied, labels are descriptive of how well a pixel fits in a given cluster. This allows for better classification in the realistic view that pixels contain a mixture of tissue types. The idea that a voxel can fit partly in, for example, recurrent disease, and partly in a class representing edema could be powerful. In addition, noise and blur during acquisition and indistinct borders between tissues are handled elegantly in such algorithms [32]. Particle Swarm Optimization (PSO) algorithms have also been shown to perform very well in multi-parametric datasets [40].

Random Field Models: Hidden Markov

Many non-parametric methods require a large training set to label pixels based on the intensity distribution of the image. Conversely, parametric approaches like the finite mixture model [46] are based upon an assumed underlying distribution [47]. Modeling using random fields considers the interactions between neighboring pixels. Since most pixels tend to belong in the same class as those located close to them, the assumption is that a classifiable structure is unlikely to contain a single pixel. Despite being computationally intensive, they can be used to model segmentation classes, intensity inhomogeneities and texture properties [16].

Markov random fields (MRF) can systematically include constraints about known characteristics of the image as well as implementing reasonable algorithms to approximate optimal solutions [48]. The image segmentation problem can be viewed as a series of regions, each described by some modeled property. Estimating the parameters that characterize the model can be solved with the Estimation Maximization algorithm. Additional work has also been done to implement an Energy Minimization scheme [48].

The details of the model are explained elegantly by Zhang, *et al.* as they pertain to the processing performed using FSL's (http://www.fmrib.ox.ac.uk/fsl/) segmentation tool [47]. FMRIB Automated Segmentation Tool (FAST) can be performed on a single image set (e.g. T1, T2 or proton density) or using multi-spectral data.

Consider two random fields in a neighborhood system. X is the true classification of each pixel with state space denoted by L. Y is some observed characteristic of the pixel that depends on the true classification and has a state space denoted by D. A configuration of X and Y can be given, respectively, by:

$$X = \{x = (x_1, \cdots, x_N) \mid x_i \in L, i \in S\}$$
$$Y = \{y = (y_1, \cdots, y_N) \mid y_i \in D, i \in S\}$$

Since $X_i = l$ (realization of the random field by way of configuration), Y_i has the conditional probability such that

$$p(y_i \mid l) = f(y_i; \theta_l), \forall l \in L$$

θ_l is a set of parameters. A value from the set L is taken to assign a class label to each pixel that has an image intensity value y_i from the set D. The problem of assigning a proper x to each pixel based on y is solved by application of the HMRF.

$$\hat{x} = \arg\max_{x \in X}\{P(y \mid x)P(x)\}$$

The prior probability of x can be given by way of the Finite Mixture Model.

$$P(x) = \frac{1}{Z}^{-U(x)}$$

Given the class label $x = l$, one can assume the intensity, y_i, follows a Gaussian distribution.

$$p(y_i \mid x_i) = g(y_i; \theta_l) = \frac{1}{\sqrt{2\pi\sigma_l^2}}^{-\frac{(y_i - \mu_l)^2}{2\sigma_l^2}}$$

The joint likelihood probability can be expressed as

$$P(y \mid x) = \frac{1}{Z'}^{-U(y|x)}$$

where the likelihood energy is: $U(y \mid x) = \sum_{i \in S}\left[\frac{(y_i - \mu_{x_i})^2}{2\sigma_{xi}^2} + \log(\sigma_{x_i})\right]$

with a constant normalization: $Z' = (2\pi)^{\frac{N}{2}}$.

Therefore, $$\log P(x \mid y) \propto -U(x \mid y)$$ $$U(x \mid y) = U(y \mid x) + U(x) + c$$

U(x|y) is the posterior energy. Minimizing this function is achieved through iteratively solving $\hat{x} = \arg\min_{x \in X}\{U(y \mid x) + U(x)\}$ by using y (the signal intensities of the image) with their assigned labels $x^k_{S-\{i\}}$ by updating $x_i^{(k)}$ to $x_i^{(k+1)}$ and minimizing the conditional posterior probability, $U(x_i \mid y, x_{S-\{i\}})$. Model fitting in FSL is achieved through the use of the Expectation Maximization (EM) algorithm.

Results were obtained in three dimensions when the input parameter consisted of only a post-contrast T1-weighted image (Figure $7A_1$ (axial), $7B_1$ (coronal), $7C_1$ (sagittal)). Setting the number of clusters to 5, we obtained a white tumor region and some surrounding pale gray voxels. Since up to five input channels are allowed, a combination of T1 and T2-weighted maps was segmented. The tumor region (figure $7A_2$ (axial), $7B_2$ (coronal), $7C_2$ (sagittal)) is shown in pale gray, again in all three dimensions for a whole brain map.

We were able to segment an input dataset composed of T1, T2 and rCBV maps (figure $7A_3$ (axial), $7B_3$ (coronal), $7C_3$ (sagittal)), though the interpretation of that final map is less obvious. The algorithm failed to produce results when we attempted to include other physiologic parameters (e.g. ADC, Hypoxia, Choline:NAA). EM optimization schemes have failed on datasets with a large number of input parameters due to problems with numerical precision [40]. Ali, *et al.* were able to successfully include diffusion-weighted data when segmenting the mouse brain [49] so the future inclusion of differently-weighted maps is feasible.

A multi-spectral algorithm that operates in three dimensions is obviously of great utility. However, excessive noise in a region can cause non-ideal fragmentation of image regions, creating a result map that fails to truly map the tumor environment. Additionally, image quality issues due to technical or biological properties can cause imprecise segmentation [48]. Computation times tend to be long for image sets of this size. Despite these problems, FSL seems to be a valuable option for mapping the recurrent tumor environment.

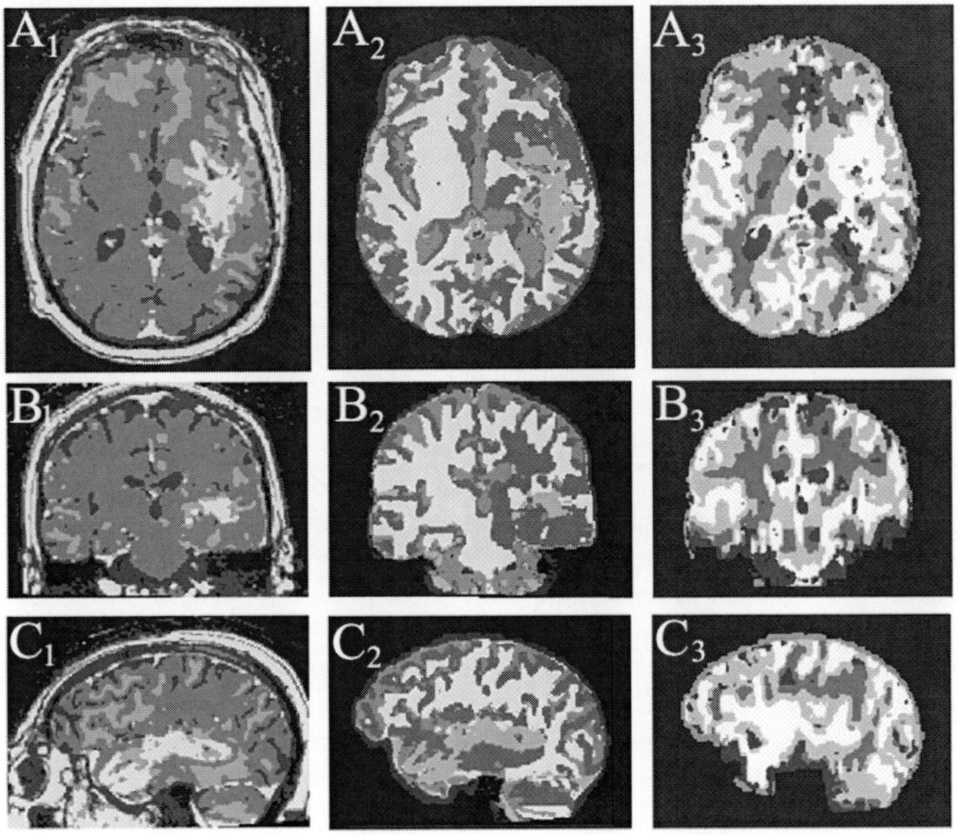

Figure 7. FAST (FMRIB's automated segmentation tool in 3D) was applied to the sample dataset using FSL software. T1 alone (A_1 (axial), B_1 (coronal), C_1 (sagittal)). T1- and T2-weighted images are combined (A_2 (axial), B_2 (coronal), C_2 (sagittal)), and the mixture of T1, T2 and rCBV are shown in A_3 (axial), B_3 (coronal), C_3 (sagittal), in a multi-channel segmentation using FSL.

Artificial Neural Networks: INSECT

The Brain Imaging Software Toolbox from the Montreal Neurological Institute (http://www.bic.mni.mcgill.ca/software/) was used to apply a model-based analysis to our patient data. The INSECT (Intensity Normalized Stereotactic Environment for the Classification of Tissue) algorithm employs a number of pre-processing steps in addition to an artificial neural network for the classification into four tissue classes – Grey Matter, White Matter, cerebrospinal fluid and background [50].

Preprocessing steps include intensity normalization, noise reduction and non-uniformity correction to account for low frequency variations in spatial intensity. The images are then registered to stereotactic space and resampled to match the training dataset. Voxels that do not correspond to brain tissue are masked and the subject maps are normalized to the training set [51].

To form the training set, a tissue probability map is formed in stereotactic space from a group of images acquired in healthy volunteers. Every voxel is therefore assigned a probability of containing a given tissue type (e.g. GM, WM). Based upon these probabilities, an initial classification of the input data is achieved [52]. Using an iterative loop based upon the previous classification, the algorithm identifies voxels with incorrect labels and removes them. This provides a set of labels that is optimized for the dataset in question. Various options are available within the algorithm (Figure 8). For our puposes, a standard error-backpropagation artificial neural network classified the final volume.

The number of input nodes for our dataset was five: T1, T2, rCBV, hypoxia and Cho:NAA maps were used. The output nodes are set to be the four tissue types: GM, WM, CSF and background. There is full connection between layers [50]. Figure 9 displays three axial slices from the whole-brain map created using the MNI tools. While impressive segmentation was obtained in the non-tumor hemisphere for the T2 map shown in figure 8, our results with the multi-parametric data are unlikely to find utility in treatment planning.

While elegant, this methodology is not likely to be ideal for treatment planning purposes. Once a brain is realigned and warped to fit in standard stereotactic space, there could be error associated with the exact tumor location in relation to fiducial markers. While impressive results were obtained in a large multiple sclerosis clinical trial [51], when considerable tissue is abnormal (i.e. tumor, edema, treatment effects) the algorithm fails to include additional classifications for such tissue. Cocosco *et al.* note that the healthy tissue should correctly be classified for such a dataset, given that the lesion burden is relatively small [52].

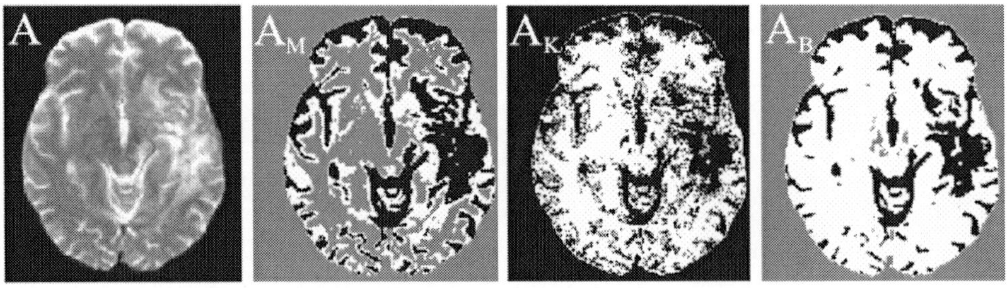

Figure 8. MNI software options. Left to Right: Original T2-weighted FLAIR (A), Minimum Distance classified (A_M), K-Nearest-Neighbor classified (A_K), and Bayesian classification (A_B).

While we certainly cannot rule out future work in this area, the present neural networks – with their registration and limited classes – seem a non-ideal choice for clinical implementation.

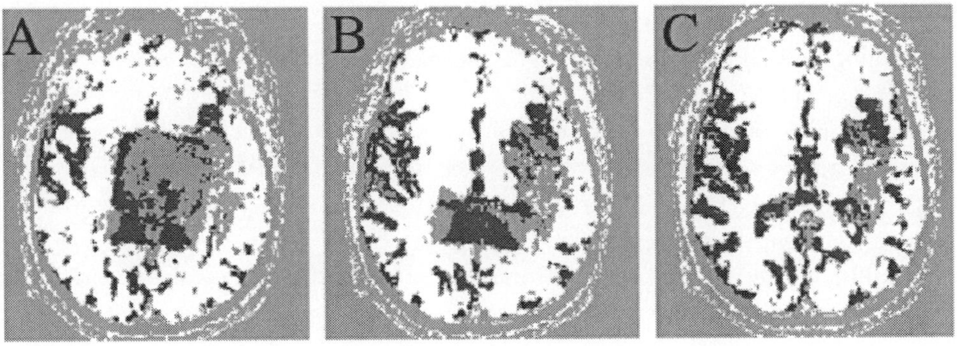

Figure 9. Multi-spectral classification using the neural network approach employed by MNI. Input parameters were T1, T2-FLAIR, rCBV, hypoxia and Cho:NAA maps.

CONCLUSION

There are a number of valuable strategies to map the tumor environment when given an imaging dataset, only a small number of which have been discussed here. The complexity of GBMs, especially post-treatment, may benefit from each of these techniques in some way. We have demonstrated several applicable methods with associated software available online for users who are attempting to process multi-parametric datasets with the goal of understanding brain cancer. While no method appears to be vastly superior to the others, a careful consideration of how the resulting map will be used can lead users to select a reasonable methodology.

REFERENCES

[1] Law, M., et al., High-grade gliomas and solitary metastases: differentiation by using perfusion and proton spectroscopic MR imaging. *Radiology,* 2002. 222(3): p. 715-721.

[2] Roberts, T., et al., Fiber Density Index correlates with reduced fractional anisotropy in white matter of patients with glioblastoma. *American Journal of Neuroradiology*, 2005. 26: p. 2183-2186.

[3] Tofts, P., et al., Estimating kinetic parameters from dynamic contrast-enhanced T1-weighted MRI of a diffusible tracer: standardized quantities and symbols. *Journal of Magnetic Resonance Imaging,* 1999. 10: p. 223-232.

[4] Tzika, A., et al., Neuroimaging in pediatric brain tumors: Gd-DTPA-enhanced, hemodynamic, and diffusion MR imaging compared with MR spectroscopic imaging. *American Journal of Neuroradiology*, 2002. 23(2): p. 322-333.

[5] Nelson, S., Magnetic resonance spectroscopic imaging: Evaluating response to therapy for gliomas. *IEEE*, 2004. 23: p. 30-39.

[6] Dunn, J., et al., Oxygenation of intracranial tumors with carbogen, an MR "BOLD" imaging and EPR oximetry study. *Journal of Magnetic Resonance Imaging*, 2002. 16(5): p. 511-521.

[7] Robinson, S., et al., Magnetic resonance imaging techniques for monitoring changes in tumor oxygenation and blood flow. *Sem. Rad. Onc.*, 1998. 8(3): p. 197-207.

[8] Chang, J., et al., Image-fusion of MR spectroscopic images for treatment planning of gliomas. *Medical Physics*, 2006. 33: p. 32-40.

[9] Castillo, M., et al., Apparent diffusion coefficients in the evaluation of high-grade cerebral gliomas. *American Journal of Neuroradiology*, 2001. 22: p. 60-64.

[10] Gupta, R., et al., Inverse correlation between choline magnetic resonance spectroscopy signal intensity and the apparent diffusion coefficient in human glioma. *Magnetic Resonance in Medicine,* 1999. 41: p. 2-7.

[11] Yang, D., et al., Cerebral gliomas: prospective comparison of multivoxel 2D chemical-shift imaging proton MR spectroscopy, echoplanar perfusion and diffusion-weighted MRI. *Neuroradiology*, 2002. 44: p. 656-666.

[12] Henry, R., et al., Comparison of relative cerebral blood volume and proton spectroscopy in patients with treated gliomas. *American Journal of Neuroradiology*, 2000. 21: p. 357-366.

[13] Batra, A., R.P. Tripathi, and A.K. Singh, Perfusion magnetic resonance imaging and magnetic resonance spectroscopy of cerebral gliomas showing imperceptible contrast enhancement on conventional magnetic resonance imaging. *Australasian Radiology*, 2004. 48: p. 324-332.

[14] Astrakas, L., et al., The clinical perspective of large scale projects: A case study of multiparametric MR imaging of pediatric brain tumors. *Oncology Reports*, 2006. 15: p. 1065-1069.

[15] Clarke, L., et al., MRI segmentation: methods and applications. *Magnetic Resonance Imaging,* 1995. 13(3): p. 343-368.

[16] Pham, D., C. Xu, and J. Prince, A survey of current methods in medical image segmentation. *Annual Review of Biomedical Engineering*, 1998. s: p. 1-27.

[17] Flusser, J. and B. Zitova, Image registration methods: a survey. *Image and Vision Computing,* 2003. 21(11): p. 977-1000.

[18] McKnight, T.R., et al., An automated technique for the quantitative assessment of 3D-MRSI data from patients with glioma. *J. Magn. Reson. Imaging*, 2001. 13(2): p. 167-77.

[19] Yamagata, N., B. Miller, and D. McBride, In vivo proton spectroscopy of intracranial infections and neoplasms. *J. Neuroimaging*, 1994. 4: p. 23-28.

[20] Shih, M., et al., Brain lesions with elevated lactic acid peaks on magnetic resonance spectroscopy. *Curr. Probl. Diagn. Radiol.*, 2004. 33: p. 85-95.

[21] Rijpkema, M., et al., Effects of breathing a hyperoxic hypercapnic gas mixture on blood oxygenation and vascularity of head-and-neck tumors as measured by magnetic resonance imaging. *International Journal of Radiation Oncology, Biology and Physics*, 2002. 53: p. 1185-1191.

[22] Robinson, S., et al., Tumor vascular architecture and function evaluated by non-invasive susceptibility MRI methods and immunohistochemistry. *Journal of Magnetic Resonance Imaging*, 2003. 17: p. 445-454.

[23] Taylor, N., et al., BOLD MRI of human tumor oxygenation during carbogen breathing. *Journal of Magnetic Resonance Imaging*, 2001. 14: p. 156-163.

[24] Gillies, R., et al., Applications of magnetic resonance in model systems: tumor biology and physiology. *Neoplasia*, 2000. 2: p. 139-151.

[25] Law, M., et al., Comparison of cerebral blood volume and vascular permeability from dyanamic susceptibility contrast-enhanced perfusion MR imaging with glioma grade. *American Journal of Neuroradiology*, 2004. 25: p. 746-755.

[26] Kono, K., et al., The role of diffusion-weighted imaging in patients with brain tumors. *American Journal of Neuroradiology*, 2001. 22: p. 1081-1088.

[27] Moffat, B., et al., Functional diffusion map: a noninvasive MRI biomarker for early stratification of clinical brain tumor response. *PNAS*, 2005. 102: p. 5524-5529.

[28] Tang, H., et al., MRI brain image segmentation by multi-resolution edge detection and region selection. *Computerized Medical Imaging and Graphics*, 2000. 24: p. 349-357.

[29] Canny, J., A computational approach to edge detection. *IEEE Trans Pattern Analysis and Machine Intelligence,* 1986. 8: p. 679-714.

[30] Bomans, M., et al., 3-D segmentation of MR images of the head for 3-D display. *IEEE Transactions on Medical Imaging,* 1990. 9(2): p. 177-183.

[31] Gibbs, P., et al., Tumour volume determination from MR images by morphological segmentation. *Phys. Med. Biol.*, 1996. 41: p. 2437-2446.

[32] Pan, J. and M. Li, Segmentation of MR Osteosarcoma Images. Proceedings of the Fifth International *Conference on Computational Intelligence and Multimedia Applications*, 2003. 5: p. 379.

[33] Xie, K., et al., Semi-automated brain tumor and edema segmentation using MRI. *European Journal of Radiology*, 2005. 56: p. 12-19.

[34] McMillan, K., et al., An Objective Method for Combining Multi-parametric MRI Datasets to Characterize of Malignant Tumors. *Medical Physics*, 2007. 35(3): p. 1053-1061.

[35] McMillan, K., et al., Physiologic Characterization of Glioblastoma Multiforme Using MRI-based Hypoxia Mapping, Chemical Shift Imaging, Perfusion and Diffusion Maps. *Journal of Clinical Neuroscience*, 2006. 13: p. 811-817.

[36] Cox, R., AFNI: Software for analysis and visualization of functional magnetic resonance neuroimages. *Computers and Biomedical Research*, 1996. 29: p. 162-173.

[37] Collingridge, D., et al., Polarographic measurements of oxygen tension in human glioma and surrounding peritumoural brain tissue. *Radiother Oncol.*, 1999. 53: p. 127-131.

[38] Kostourou, V., et al., Overexpression of Dimethylarginine Dimthylaminohydrolase enhances tumor hypoxia: an insight into the relationship of hypoxia and angiogenesis in vivo. *Neuroplasia*, 2004. 6: p. 401-411.

[39] Benjamin, L.E., et al., Selective ablation of immature blood vessels in established human tumors follows vascular endothelial growth factor withdrawal. *J. Clin. Invest*, 1999. 103: p. 159-165.

[40] Omran, M. and A. Engelbrecht, Particle swarm optimization method for image clustering. *International Journal of Pattern Recognition and Image Analysis*, 2005. 19: p. 297-321.

[41] Mitsias, P., et al., Multiparametric MRI ISODATA ischemic lesion analysis. *Stroke,* 2002. 33(12): p. 2839-2844.

[42] Shen, Q., et al., Dynamic tracking of acute ischemic tissue fates using improved unsupervised ISODATA analysis of high-resolution quantitative perfusion and diffusion data. *Journal of Cerebral Blood Flow and Metabolism*, 2004. 24: p. 887-897.

[43] Jacobs, M., et al., A model for multiparametric MRI tissue characterization in experimental cerebral ischemia with histologic validation in rat.. *Stroke*, 2001. 32(4): p. 943-957.

[44] Soltanian-Zadeh, H., et al., MRI tissue characterization of experimental cerebral ischemia in rat. *Journal of Magnetic Resonance Imaging*, 2003. 17: p. 398-409.

[45] Yovel, Y. and Y. Assaf, Virtual definition of neuronal tissue by cluster analysis of multi-parametric imaging (virtual-dot-com imaging). *NeuroImage*, 2007. 35: p. 58-69.

[46] Liang, Z., R. Jaszczak, and R. Coleman, Parameter estimation of finite mixtures using the EM algorithm and information criteria with application to medical image processing. *IEEE Trans Nuclear Science*, 1992. 39(4): p. 1126-1133.

[47] Zhang, Y., S. Smith, and M. Brady, Segmentation of brain MR images through a hidden Markov randomfield model and the expectation-maximization algorithm. *IEEE Trans Medical Imaging,* 2001. 20: p. 45-57.

[48] Marroquin, J., E. Santana, and S. Botello, Hidden markov measure field models for image segmentation. *IEEE Trans Pattern Analysis and Machine Intelligence*, 2003. 25: p. 1380-1387.

[49] Ali, A.A., et al., Automated segmentation of neuroanatomical structures in multispectral MR microscopy of the mouse brain. *Neuroimage*, 2005. 27(2): p. 425-35.

[50] Collins, D., et al., ANIMAL+INSECT: Improved cortical structure segmentation. *Lecture Notes in Computer Science*, 1999. 1613: p. 210-223.

[51] Zijdenbos, A., R. Forghani, and A. Evans, Automatic "pipeline" analysis of 3-D MRI data for clinical trials: application to multiple sclerosis. *IEEE Trans Medical Imaging*, 2002. 21: p. 1280-1291.

[52] Cocosco, C., A. Zijdenbos, and A. Evans, A fully automatic and robust brain MRI tissue classification method. *Medical Image Analysis*, 2003. 7: p. 513-527.

In: Brain Mapping Research Developments
Editor: Lars N. Bakker, pp. 197-209

ISBN 978-1-60456-007-7

Chapter VIII

THE EMOTIONAL S1-S2 PARADIGM FOR EXPLORING BRAIN MECHANISMS UNDERLYING AFFECTIVE MODULATION OF EXPECTANCY

Francisco Mercado[a*], Jose Antonio Hinojosa[b], Cecilia Peñacoba[a] and Luis Carretié[c]

[a] Facultad de Ciencias de la Salud, Universidad Rey Juan Carlos, Madrid, Spain.
[b] Instituto Pluridisciplinar, Universidad Complutense de Madrid, Spain.
[c] Facultad de Psicología, Universidad Autónoma de Madrid, Spain.

ABSTRACT

From the past decade to date, research on the interactive brain mechanisms between attention and emotion studied through event-related potentials (ERPs) has increasingly grown. This brain signal reflects fast and swift cognitive processing due to its excellent temporal resolution and it has become a suitable tool in order to study several issues concerning cognitive processing. In this chapter we present a detailed description of an 'emotional variant' of the S1 (cue)-S2 (target) task that has been typically used to explore vigilance-related attention. The application of the emotional S1-S2 paradigm elicits an affective modulation effect on a brainwave that has been related to expectancy, the early Contingent Negative Variation (eCNV). In this chapter we will present several issues concerning different methodological aspects to take into account when applying this paradigm and some details related to the procedures of quantification and analysis of the ERP data. Finally, some findings obtained through the use of the emotional S1-S2 protocol are summarized and some of its different application possibilities (e.g., clinical samples) are proposed.

* Corresponding author: Departamento de Psicología, Facultad de Ciencias de la Salud, Universidad Rey Juan Carlos, Avda. Atenas s/n, 28922 Alcorcón, Madrid, SPAIN. Phone: +34 91 488 8943. Fax: +34 91 488 8954. E-mail: francisco.mercado@urjc.es

Keywords: emotional S1-S2 paradigm; Attention; Emotion; Event-related potentials, eCNV.

INTRODUCTION

Selective attention constitutes a necessary cognitive process to effectively cope with our dynamic and changing world. Through this mechanism, relevant aspects such as affective information are prioritized in awareness not only to improve stimulus perception but also to prepare people for its forthcoming processing. The S1-S2 paradigm has shown to be a useful tool in order to cast light on the selective attentional aspects related to vigilance or expectancy processes towards next upcoming events. In its conventional form, this paradigm comprises of the presentation of a signal stimulus (S1) that indicates the target (S2) appearance in each trial (Walter et al., 1964; McCallum, 1988). Usually, the subject is instructed to respond to S2 as fast as possible.

Because attention involves short and fast subprocesses, some of them occurring during the first 500 milliseconds after the stimulus onset (Mangun and Hylliard, 1995), the use of event-related potentials (ERPs) methodology constitutes a helpful strategy that allows us, due to its privileged temporal resolution, to obtain data of the successive stages of these attentional subprocesses. The main ERP wave evoked by applying the S1-S2 protocol is the Contingent Negative Variation (CNV) (e.g., McCallum, 1988; Weinberg, 1972). This negative component that appears just after S1 (cue stimuli) reaching its end before S2 offset, is comprised of two adjacent but dissociable waves, the 'early' CNV (eCNV) and the 'late' CNV (lCNV). Whereas the lCNV seems to reflect preparation for motor activity (e.g., Van Voxtel and Brunia, 1994), the eCNV is directly linked to vigilance-related attention to forthcoming stimuli (Rohrbaugh and Gaillard, 1983; Basile et al., 1994). Vigilance-related attention refers to a general alert state that is necessary when a situation requires a sustained level of attention, such as that related to prioritize the processing of forthcoming relevant information (Posner and Petersen, 1990).

Neurocognitive scientists have developed several modifications of the S1-S2 experimental protocol to study particular cognitive processes. Thus, it has shown to be useful to study long-term memory encoding (Leynes et al., 1998), visuospatial orienting attention (Talsma et al., 2005), temporal attention (Miniussi et al., 1999; Correa et al., 2006) or developmental differences in the saccadic CNV (Klein et al., 2005), among other processes. However, the use of the S1-S2 paradigm for studying the interaction between vigilance-related attention and emotion is rather scarce in relation to brain activity, even though from past decade there has been an increased interest to explore these issues. This lack of data is surprising since the need to be prepared for situations that involve the processing of upcoming affective events are frequent in every day's life. Some ERP studies have shown that the eCNV is sensitive to cues signalling the appearance of emotional targets (Yee and Miller, 1987; Regan and Howard, 1995) as well as socially relevant information, such as faces (Mantsakanian and Tarkka, 2002). Also, CNV amplitude has been related to expectancy when high-anxious subjects performed a S1-S2 stressful task (McCallum and Walter, 1968; Proulx et al., 1984). Recent data have shown larger lCNV amplitudes related to the expectancy of aversive consequences following S1 stimulus in panic disorder patients

(Amrhein et al., 2005). Despite the interesting data provided by these experiments, however, most of these studies did not differentiate between early and late CNV subcomponents. Moreover, these studies did not manipulate the emotional meaning conveyed by S1 and S2.

In order to overcome these limitations, we propose in this chapter the emotional S1-S2 task, an experimental paradigm that consists of an 'emotional variant' of the S1-S2 task and an analytical procedure that allows for the differentiation of the early and late subcomponents of the CNV. As we will explain later in detail, in this paradigm, target stimuli are explicitly emotional while cue stimuli (which are neutral) signal in an implicit way the emotional category of the following target. Participants are asked to detect cue-target correspondences. The affective value of targets is manipulated according to two dimensions: valence (positive-negative) and arousal (arousing-relaxing) (for additional information see Russell, 1979; Lang et al., 1997). The combination of these two dimensions may yield to four emotional categories: arousing-positive, arousing-negative, neutral and relaxing stimuli. Some other combinations of the valence and arousal dimensions, such as relaxing-negative stimuli are virtually impossible (Lang et al., 1997).

The steps for the implementation of this paradigm in ERP research will be described in detail in the following section. Also, possible variants of some aspects of the emotional S1-S2 paradigm will be outlined.

Description and Application of the Emotional S1-S2 Paradigm

As indicated in the introduction section, the experimental design that will be described here is an emotional variant of the S1-S2 paradigm. This emotional S1-S2 paradigm comprises the sequential presentation of two stimuli, the S1 or *cue* stimulus and the S2 or *target* stimulus. This emotional S1-S2 task has two specific features. First, the target or S2 stimulus has emotional (or emotionally neutral) content. Second, the cue or S1 stimulus should be devoid of emotional content emotional but created in a way that lead the participants to conceive implicit expectancies concerning the emotional content of the forthcoming target stimulus. The reason for S1 stimuli to be non-emotional is that neural activity between S1 and S2 should reflect expectancy related differences, but not emotional reactions to S1. Although auditory stimuli (tones) have been used as cue stimuli (Carretié et al., 2004a), most of the studies employing this paradigm have used visual stimuli as both cue and target stimuli (e.g. Carretié et al. 2001; Amrheim et al., 2005). Whatever the case, it is important to equate the physical features of the stimuli (such as contrast, complexity or brightness in the case of the visual modality) so they differ only in their emotional content.

Target stimuli belong to different emotional categories that differ in valence, arousal, or both dimensions: negative stimuli (A-, negative valence and high levels of arousal), positive stimuli (A+, positive valence and high levels of arousal), relaxing stimuli (R, positive valence and low levels of arousal) and neutral stimuli (N, neutral in both valence and arousal). As mentioned before, cue stimuli are stimuli devoid of emotional content that have to be associated with target stimuli. It is important to notice that each cue stimulus has to be matched to a particular category of target stimuli. Several types of stimuli can be used as cues, such as schematic drawings, geometric figures or even tones. Each trial begins with the presentation of the cue followed by the presentation of the target after a variable time interval, both centred in the screen. A brief beep could be presented 1500 or 2000 milliseconds after the target that allows participants to provide a motor response that does not interfere with the recording of cognitive processing responses. For instance, eye-blinking and other eye movements usually constitute an important artefact when the experimenter carries out the correction and analysis of the ERP data (Picton et al., 2000). Although the use of algorithms for the correction of eye movements is a frequent practice in signal analysis, when EOG activity is intense the efficacy of these methods decreases. Since participants can not remain without blinking for long periods of time, it could be also helpful to tell them to blink at the same time they provide with a response (after the beep presentation, for instance). It should be noticed that this paradigm also allows investigating attentional processes related to input-processing (i.e., those appearing after post-target stimulation). Motor electrophysiological artefacts produced by the participants' responses during the experimental task could distort the amplitude and latency of some attentional ERP components (e.g., Picton et al., 1995). In this sense, the experimental design is free of this caveat since participants are asked to postpone their motor responses until the beep presentation. However, this way of proceeding has some limitations. In this regard, this task configuration does not allow collecting behavioural data about reaction times linked to target presentation.

The duration of the stimuli, the time interval between the presentation of the cue and the target stimulus and the inter-trial interval varies across studies. Thus, the duration of the cue and target stimuli usually ranges between 200 and 500 ms and the inter-trial interval usually ranges between 2500 and 4000 ms (e.g., Armheim et al., 2005; Mantsakanian and Tarkka, 2002). More relevant is the interval between the cue and the target stimulus, that usually ranges between 1500 and 4000 ms (Rockstroh et al., 1989; Rosahl and Knight, 1995). The temporal point at which target is cued to appear could modulate brain expectancy-related responses. Different time intervals between cue and target stimuli (short: around 500 or 600 ms; long: around 1500 ms) might be used to override this issue (Correa et al., 2006). Moreover, some studies have shown that several brain areas involved in cognitive expectations are differently activated as a consequence of this manipulation (e.g. Coull et al., 2000). Results of some studies suggest that, although the CNV is typically observed at long and fixed cue-target time intervals, a negative deflection with temporal and topographic characteristics resembling those of the eCNV could be attenuated or even eliminated at short cue-target time intervals, whereas its amplitude increases at long cue-target intervals (Talsma et al., 2005). Indeed, as some authors have pointed out, the time interval between the presentation of the cue and the target stimuli could influence the reliable dissociation on the two subcomponents of the CNV (Kropp et al., 2000; Brunia and van Boxtel, 2001). Figure 1 provides with a schematic description of the paradigm.

With respect to the experimental task, participants should be informed that they are going to see or hear a stimuli (S1) followed by a second stimuli (S2). The correspondence between each cue and each particular target stimulus has to be explicitly explained to participants and trained. In this sense subjects should have the opportunity to perceive all cue types and to associate them with each target type before the recording session.

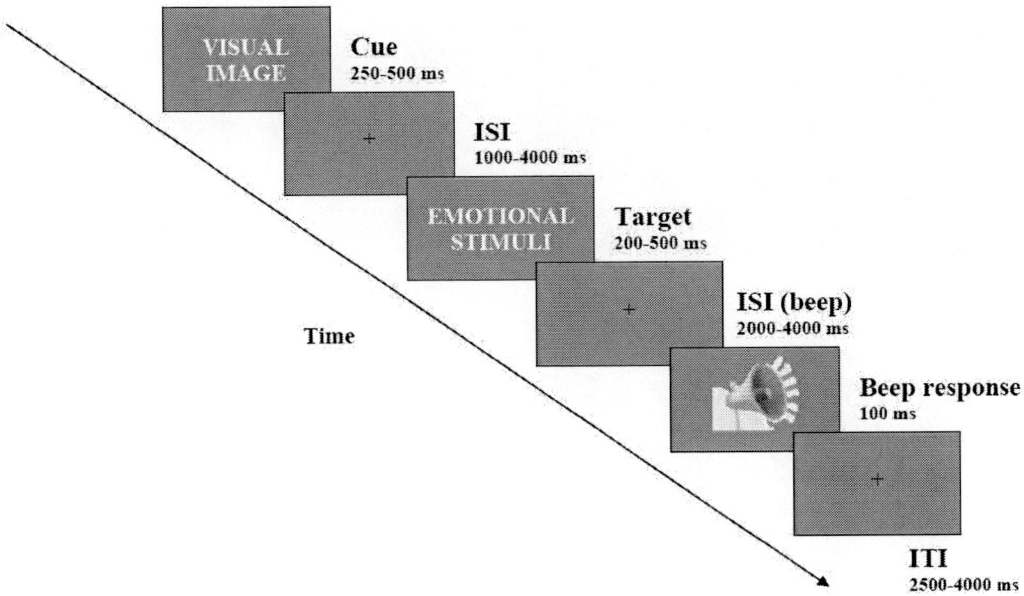

Figure 1. Schematic representation of the emotional variant of the S1-S2 paradigm described in the main text. ITI= Inter-trial interval; ISI= Inter-stimulus interval.

It is important to use an indirect task that keeps hidden the explicit objective of experiment (i.e., that it deals with emotional processing), since non-indirect procedures may lead participants to consider that some stimuli are more important than others (i.e., emotional, salient stimuli, more important than non-emotional ones for an experiment that deals with emotional reactions). This 'relevance-for-task effect' has often been described in previous research (e.g., Duncan Jonhson and Donchin, 1977). It showed that stimuli considered by subjects to be highly relevant for the task elicit higher amplitudes in certain endogenous components compared to less relevant stimuli. Indeed, the ERPs elicited by emotional stimuli in direct tasks are different from those elicited in indirect tasks (e.g., Carretié et al., 1997). Therefore, presenting the participants with a matching cue-target task ensures to distract their attention from the emotional meaning of stimuli so the allocation of the same amount of attentional resources towards every stimulus is guaranteed.

A good example of such a type of task is provided in Carretié et al. (2001). In this study the cue stimuli consisted of a pair of schematic drawings (one above the other) that implicitly provided information about the emotional content of target stimuli (pictures). Both drawings in the cue stimuli signalled targets belonging to the same emotional category (for instance a cue stimulus represented the schematic drawing of a wolf jaw and an insect, corresponding to targets of the negative category). Examples of stimuli are provided in Figure 2. Target pictures corresponded always to one of the two schematic drawings of the cue stimuli. Participants had to press a button whenever the target corresponded to the drawing that appeared in the top of the cue stimuli or a different button when the target corresponded to the bottom drawing.

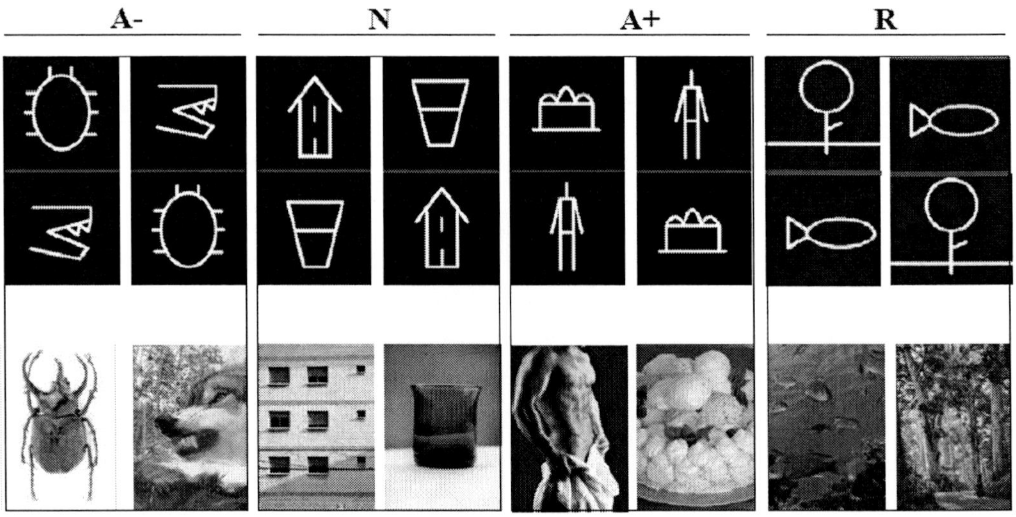

Figure 2. Examples of cue and target stimuli used in the task by Carretié et al. (2001). In the top of the Figure, starting from the left to the right schematic drawings of negative (A-), neutral (N), positive (A+) and relaxing (R) stimuli. In the bottom the pictures of the corresponding target stimuli are shown.

Another relevant aspect has to do with the choice of emotional stimulation which constitutes also a critical issue. A non-rigorous method for controlling stimuli might cause unexpected and unreliable results. For example, positive and negative stimuli should differ in valence but not in arousal. This would prevent from reaching an unequivocal conclusion about which of the two dimensions is explaining the results. In order to avoid these concerns, a careful selection of the emotional stimuli should be made. In this sense, the use of a validated database of emotional images, such as the IAPS (Lang, 2001) could be useful. However, this method is not free of some caveats. One has to do with the application of a standardized database on people of different cultural status (e.g., Latin and Anglo-Saxon populations), since these cultural differences could influence the emotional processing of the stimuli. Therefore, it is of the greatest importance to collect the particular assessment of the participants for every emotional target stimuli used in the study in order to confirm that the valence and arousal of the stimuli are those supposed a priori to be (e.g., Carretié et al., 1997). For this purpose a bidimensional scaling test (for instance with a five-point scale) can be supplied to participants after the recording session.

Issues Related to Electrophysiological Data Analysis

Concerning the statistical analysis of the ERP data, the use of some procedures might lead to a more reliable interpretation of the results. The waveform recorded at a site on the head over a period of several hundreds of milliseconds represents a complex superposition of different overlapping components. Although the visual inspection of grand-averaged ERPs has been the method more frequently used to detect components, its exclusive use should be taken with caution since this method may lead to several types of misinterpretation especially when high-density montages are employed (e.g, Chapman and McCrary, 1995; Dien et al., 2005; Donchin and Heffley, 1978). In order to override these shortcomings, temporal principal component analysis (tPCA) has been repeatedly recommended as the most reliable reduction, detection and quantification method for multivariate ERP data (e.g., Dien et al., 1998). Its main advantage is that it represents each ERP component with its 'clean' shape by extracting and quantifying them free of the influences of adjacent of subjacent components. Indeed, the application of tPCA avoids the subjectivity of selecting time windows for component analyses. In brief, the tPCA computes the covariance between all ERP time points, which tends to be high between those time points involved in the same component, and low between those belonging to different components. The solution is therefore a set of independent factors made up of highly covarying time points, which ideally correspond to ERP components. Temporal factor scores, the tPCA-derived parameter in which extracted temporal factors may be quantified, are equivalent to amplitude.

In the attention-research field, the usefulness of the PCA for disentangling spatiotemporally overlapping ERP components has been demonstrated recently in several studies (Beauducel et al., 2000; Debener et al., 2005; Dien et al., 2003). In this sense, despite of the fact that some studies have found that inter-stimulus intervals as long as 2-3 seconds are a necessary condition for a reliable dissociation of the two components of the CNV (Kropp et al., 2000), the use of the PCA allows for separation of the eCNV and the lCNV even with time-intervals shorter than 2 seconds (Carretié et al., 2001).

It is important to keep in mind some recommendations when the PCA is employed to analyze ERPs. For instance, the use of a covariance matrix has been strongly recommended with respect to correlation matrix-based analysis (Kaiser and Tenke, 2003; Dien et al., 2005). Also, the scree test is considered an optimal procedure to determine the number of factors that are retained or selected (Dien, 1998). Special caution should be taken in relation to the rotation method chosen since there is still not a total agreement. In this regard, whereas Kaiser and Tenke claim for the use of orthogonal rotations such as Varimax, Dien and co-workers have shown the advantages of oblique rotations such as Promax since this method considers brain components or factors as entities that are physiologically associated (see Dien et al., 2005; Kaiser et al., 2003, for a detailed discussion of caveats concerning the PCA analyses on ERP data). Our own experience also supports the advisability of oblique procedures such as Promax.

Additionally, the potential superposition of different ERP components can also complicate efforts when trying to apply source localization algorithms. Thus, PCA could be a suitable tool in order to increase the reliability for determining cortical sources (Richards, 2004). In particular, the introduction of factor scores instead of voltages in source localization procedures might be helpful in those ERP components altered or hidden in grand averages but detected by PCA. In fact, the results of a recent study strongly suggest that applying a source localization algorithm (LORETA, Pascual-Marqui et al., 1994) on factor scores is a more precise procedure than the application of this algorithm on voltage amplitude values (the traditional way) (see Carretié et al., 2004b for additional information).

DISCUSSION

As a consequence of the application of this emotional S1-S2 paradigm, several ERP experiments have provided with interesting data about the spatial and temporal characterization of the attentional processing linked to emotional events. Relatively recent experiments indicated that the eCNV elicited in this task seems to be reflecting interactive mechanisms between emotional and attentional processes, since its amplitude is modulated by the affective value conveyed by forthcoming stimulation (reduced eCNV amplitudes to negatively cued events; see Carretié et al., 2001). Furthermore, this processing could be enhanced in high anxious individuals because their vigilance-related attention resources tend to be captured by stimuli that represent threat (Carretié et al., 2004a). In a further study, Amrheim and coworkers (2005) have showed that the lCNV could also be reflecting a biased processing in panic patients while they are expecting aversive consequences following the disorder-relevant stimuli.

Also, the neural generators of the 'emotional expectancy' elicited by this paradigm have been analyzed. Evidence for neural sources of the eCNV seems to point to the anterior cingulate cortex (ACC) as the brain region generating it (Carretié et al., 2001). This brain area has been proposed to be implicated in anticipatory processes of affective events (e.g., Ploghaus et al., 1999). Regarding the lCNV, some findings suggest that the dorsolateral prefrontal cortex (DLPFC) might be critical for its generation. This structure has been suggested to be involved in motor preparatory processes (Rosahl and Knight, 1995). Taking together, ERP data obtained from the application of the emotional S1-S2 paradigm show that it seems to be a promising scientific methodology for studying some aspects of the influence of emotional stimulation on the attentional brain response. The spatiotemporal characterization of these processes might be helpful in order to develop current models of the psychobiological mechanisms involved in the interaction between emotion and attention (e.g., Bar, 2003; Vuilleumier, 2002; Vuilleumier, 2005).

Finally, a few words should be devoted to the use of different types of stimuli when applying this paradigm. Although affective pictorial stimulation has largely demonstrated to be an appropriate tool when trying to elicit intense attentional reactions to emotional stimuli as compared to other types of stimulus (Bradley et al., 1998), the use of such other types of emotional stimuli should not be disregarded. The results from recent experiments show that words (see Kissler et al., 2006 for a review) or even odours (Anderson et al., 2003) are able to evoke significant emotional responses. It would be thus interesting to complement and extend the results obtained with the application of this paradigm by using stimuli belonging to different sensorial modalities.

FINAL REMARKS

Although the emotional S1-S2 paradigm has probed to bee a valuable tool in order to address issues concerning the interaction between attention and emotion processes, it also suffers from some limitations. The most important one has to do with the involvement of cognitive processes apart from attention and emotion. In order to accomplished the task requirements it is necessary to take into account processes related to working memory (see Olton et al., 1979; Kartik and Amishi, 2007). Moreover, some authors have suggested that selective attention is closely linked to working memory processes (Awh et al., 2006). This situation may lead to some confusion when interpreting the contribution of the different cognitive processes involved in the task. This limitation might be mitigated by a careful experimental design.

Despite of its potential application possibilities for exploring emotional- attention interactions, the cue-target paradigm has been scarcely used to date and further research is needed in order to investigate in more detail the issues discussed here. The paradigm has been usually tested in healthy populations, although many aspects remain still unexplored. For instance, the application of the emotional S1-S2 paradigm could extend previous findings about the emotional habituation response (Carretié et al., 2003) or the attentional regulation in elder people (Bennet et al., 2004). Also, the fact that some clinical populations show an enhanced hipervigilance towards the threatening value of different events (e.g., fear or pain-related stimuli) such as fibromyalgic (e.g., Montoya et al., 2006), or anxious patients (Mogg and Bradley, 1998), makes this protocol a promising tool in order to explore the time course of expectancy-related attentional responses to emotional stimuli in these patients. Additionally, an emotional-spatial variant can be also used to study attentional deficits in hemineglect patients (Vuilleumier and Schwartz, 2001). Finally, it would be interesting to explore the paradigm through its implementation in alternative techniques with high temporal resolution, such as the magnetoencephalography (Onoda et al., 2006).

ACKNOWLEDGEMENTS

This work was supported by grants SEJ2005-08461-C02-02/PSIC and SEJ2004-08171/PSIC from the Ministerio de Ciencia y Tecnología of Spain.

REFERENCES

Amrheim, C., Pauli, P., Dengler, W., Wiedemann, G., 2005. Covariation bias and its physiological correlates in panic disorder patients. *J. Anx. Disord.* 19, 177-191.

Anderson, A.K., Christoff, K., Stappen, I., Panitz, D., Ghahremani, D.G., Glover, G., Gabrieli, J.D.E., Sobel, N., 2003. Dissociated neural representations of intensity and valence in human olfaction. *Nat. Neurosci.* 6, 196-202.

Awh, E., Vogel, E.K., Oh, S.H., 2006. Interaction between attention and working memory. *Neurosci.* 139, 201-208.

Basile, L.F.H., Rogers, R.L., Bourbon, W.T., Papanicolaou, A., 1994. Slow magnetic flux from human frontal cortex. *Electroencephalogr. Clin. Neurophysiol.* 90, 157– 165.

Bar, M., 2003. A cortical mechanism for triggering top-down facilitation in visual object recognition. *J. Cogn. Neurosci.* 15, 600-609.

Beauducel, A., Debener, S., Brocke, B., Kayser, J., 2000. On the reliability of augmenting/reducing: Peak amplitudes and principal component analysis of auditory evoked potentials. *J. Psychophysiol.* 14, 226-240.

Bennett, I.J., Golob, E.J., Starr, A. 2004. Age-related differences in auditory event-related potentials during a cued attention task. *Clin. Neurophysiol.* 115, 2602-2615.

Bishop, S., Duncan, J., Brett, M., Lawrence, A.D., 2004. Prefrontal cortical function and anxiety: Controlling attention to threat-related stimuli. *Nat. Neurosci.* 7, 184-188.

Bradley, B.P., Mogg, K., Falla, S.J., Hamilton, L.R., 1998. Attentional bias for threatening facial expressions in anxiety: Manipulation of stimulus duration. *Cogn. Emot.* 12, 737-753.

Brunia, C.H.M., van Boxtel, G.J.M., 2001. Wait and see. *Int. J. Psychophysiol.* 43, 59-75.

Carretié, L., Hinojosa, J.A., Mercado, F., 2003. Cerebral patterns of attentional habituation to emotional visual stimuli. *Psychophysiology.* 40, 381-388.

Carretié, L., Martín-Loeches, M., Hinojosa, J.A., Mercado, F., 2001. Emotion and attention interaction studied through event-related potentials. *J. Cogn. Neurosci.* 13, 1109-1128.

Carretié, L., Mercado, F., Hinojosa, J.A., Martín-Loeches, M., Sotillo, M., 2004a. Valence-related vigilante biases in anxiety studied through event-related potentials. *J. Affec. Dis.* 78, 119-130.

Carretié, L., Tapia, M., Mercado, F., Albert, J., López-Martín, S., de la Serna, J., 2004b. Voltage-based versus factor store-based source localization analyses of electrophysiological brain activity: A comparison. *Brain Topograph.* 17, 109-115.

Carretié, L., Iglesias, J., García, T., Ballesteros, M., 1997. N300, P300 and the emotional processing of visual stimuli. *Electroencephalogr. Clin. Neurophysiol.* 103, 298-303.

Chapman, R.M., McCrary, J.W., 1995. ERP component identification and measurement by Principal Components Analysis. *Brain Cogn.* 27, 288-310.

Cliff, N., 1987, *Analyzing multivariate data*, Harcourt Brace Jovanovich, New York.

Correa, A., Lupiáñez, J., Madrid, E., Tudela, P., 2006. Temporal attention enhances early visual processing: A review and new evidence from event-related potentials. *Brain Res.* 1076, 116-128.

Coull, J.T., Frith, C.D., Büchel, C., Nobre, A.C., 2000. Orienting attention in time: Behavioural and neuroanatomical distinction between exogenous and endogenous shifts. *Neuropsychologia* 38, 808-819.

Debener, S., Makeig, S., Delorme, A., Engel, A.K., 2005. What is novel in the novelty oddball paradigm? Functional significance of the novelty P3 event-related potential as revealed by independent component analysis. *Cog. Brain Res.* 22, 309-321.

Dien, J., 1998. Adressing misallocation of variance in principal component analysis of event-related potentials. *Brain Topograph.* 11, 43-55.

Dien, J., Spencer, K.M., Donchin, E., 2003. Localization of the event-related potential novelty response as defined by principal components analysis. *Cogn. Brain Res.* 17, 550-637.

Dien, J., Beal, D.J., Berg, P., 2005. Optimizing principal components analysis of event-related potentials: Matrix type, factor loading weighting, extraction, and rotations. *Clin. Neurophysiol.* 116, 1808-1825.

Donchin, E., Heffley, E.F., 1978. Multivariate analysis of event-related potential data: A tutorial review. In *Multidisciplinary perspectives in event-related brain potential research*, D. Otto, ed. US Government Printing Office, Washington, DC, pp. 555-572.

Duncan-Johnson, C.C., Donchin, E., 1977. On quantifying surprise: The variation of event-related potentials with subjective probability. *Psychophysiology* 14, 456-457.

Jasper, H., 1958. Report on the committee on methods of clinical examination in electroencephalography. *Electroencephalogr. Clin. Neurophysiol.* 10, 370-375.

Kaiser, J., Tenke, C.E., 2003. Optimizing PCA methodology for ERP component identification and measurement: Theoretical rationale and empirical evaluation. *Clin. Neurophysiol.* 114, 2307-2325.

Kartik, K.S., Amishi, P.J., 2007. Selective attention supports working memory maintenance by modulating perceptual processing of distracters. *J. Cogn. Neurosci.* 19, 32-41.

Kissler, J., Assadollahi, R., Herbert, C. 2006. Emotional and semantic networks in visual word processing: insights from ERP studies. *Prog. Brain. Res.* 156, 147-183.

Klein, C., Feige, B., 2005. An independent component analysis (ICA) approach to the study of developmental differences in the saccadic contingent negative variation. *Biol. Psychol.* 70, 105-114.

Kropp, P., Kiewitt, A., Göbel, H., Vetter, P., Gerber, W.D., 2000. Reliability and Stability of Contingent Negative Variation. *Appl. Psychophysiology Biofeed.* 25, 33-41.

Lang, P.J., Bradley, M.M., Fitzsimmons, J.R., Cuthbert, B.N., Scott, J.D., Moulder, B., Nangia, V., 1998. Emotional arousal and activation of the visual cortex: An fMRI analysis. *Psychophysiology* 35, 199-210.

Lang, P.J., Bradley, M.M., Cuthbert, B.N., 1997. Motivated attention: Affect, activation, and action. In *Attention and orienting: Sensory and motivational processes*, P. Lang, R. F. Simons. M. T. Balaban, eds. Erlbaum, Mahwah, NJ, pp. 97–135.

Lang, P.J., Bradley M.M., Cuthbert B.N., 2001. International affective picture system (IAPS): Instruction manual and affective ratings. *Technical report A-5. The Center for Research in Psychophysiology*, University of Florida, Gainesville, FL.

Lehmann, D., 1987. Principles of spatial analysis. In *Handbook of electroencefalography and clinical neurophysiology*, Vol 1, A.S. Gevins, A. Rémond, eds. Elsevier, Amsterdam, pp. 309-354.

Leynes, P.A., Allen, J.D., Marsh, R.L., 1998. Topographic differences in CNV amplitude reflect different preparatory processes. *Int. J. Psychophysiol.*, 31, 33-44.

Mangun, G.R., Hillyard, S.A., 1995. Mechanism and models of selective attention. In *Electrophysiology of mind*, M.D. Rugg, M.G.H. Coles, eds. Oxford University Press, Oxford, pp. 40-85.

McCallum, W.C., 1988. Potentials related to expectancy, preparation and motor activity. In *Handbook of electroencephalography and clinical neurophysiology*, Vol 3, T.W. Picton, ed. Elsevier, Amsterdam, pp. 427-535.

McCallum, W.C., Walter, W.G., 1968. The effects of attention and distraction on the contingent negative variation in normal and neurotic subjects. *Electroencephalogr. Clin. Neurophysiol.* 25, 319-329.

Miniussi, C., Wilding, E.L., Coull, J.T., Nobre, A.C., 1999. Orienting attention in time: Modulation of brain potentials. *Brain* 122, 1507-1518.

Mnatsakanian, E.V., Tarkka, I.M., 2002. Task-specific expectation is revealed in scalp-recorded slow potentials. *Brain Topograph.* 15, 87-94.

Mogg, K., Bradley, B.P., 1998. A cognitive-motivational analysis of anxiety. *Behav. Res. Ther.* 36, 809-848.

Montoya, P., Sitges, C., 2006. Affective modulation of somatosensory-evoked potentials elicited by tactile stimulation. *Brain Res.* 1068, 205-212.

Olton, D.S., Becker, J.T., Handelmann, G.E., 1979. Hippocampus, space and memory. *Behav. Brain Sci.* 2, 313-365.

Onoda, K., Okamoto, Y., Shishida, K., Hashizume, A., Kazutaka, U., Kinoshita, A., Yamashita, H., Yamawaki, S., 2006. Anticipation of affective image modulates visual evoked magnetic fields (VEF). *Exp. Brain Res.* 175, 536.543.

Pasqual-Marqui, R.D., Michel, C.M., Lehman, D., 1994. Low resolution electromagnetic tomography: A new method for localizing electrical activity in the brain. *Int. J. Psychophysiol.* 18, 49-65.

Picton, T.W., Bentin, S., Berg, P., Donchin, E., Hylliar, S. Johnson, Jr. R. et al., 2000. Guidelines for using human event-related potentials to study cognition: Recording standards and publication criteria. *Psychophysiology* 37, 127-152.

Picton, T.W., Lins, O.G., Scherg, M., 1995. The recording and analysis event-related potentials. In *Handbook Neuropsychology*, Vol 10, F. Boller, J. Grafman, eds. Elsevier, Amsterdam, pp. 3-73.

Ploghaus, A., Tracey, I., Gati, J.S., Clare, S., Menon, R.S., Matthews, P.M., Rawlins, J.N., 1999. Dissociating pain from its anticipation in the human brain. *Science,* 284, 1979-1981.

Posner, M.I., Petersen, S.E., 1990. The attention system of the human brain. *Annu. Rev. Neurosci.* 13, 13-25.

Proulx, G.B., Picton, T.W., 1984. The effects of anxiety and expectancy on the CNV. *Ann. N. Y. Acad. Sci.* 425, 612-617.

Regan, M., Howard, R., 1995. Fear conditioning, preparedness, and the contingent negative variation. *Psychophysiology*, 32, 208-214.

Richards, J.E., 2004. Recovering dipole sources from scalp-recorded event-related-potentials using component analysis: Principal component analysis and independent component analysis. *Int. J. Psychophysiol.* 54, 201-220.

Rohrbaugh, J., Gaillard, A., 1983. Sensory and motor aspects of the contingent negative variation. In *Advances in Psychology*, Vol 10, A. Gaillard, W. Ritter, eds. Elsevier, Amsterdam, pp. 269-310.

Rockstroh, B., Elbert, T., Canavan, A., Lutzenberger, W., Birbaumer, N., 1989. *Slow cortical potentials and behaviour* (2nd ed.). München: Urban and Schwarzenberg.

Rosahl, S.K., Knight, R.T., 1995. Role of prefrontal cortex in generation of the CNV. *Cereb. Cortex,* 2, 123-134.

Russell, J.A., 1979. Affective space is bipolar. *J. Pers. Soc. Psychol.* 37, 345-356.

Spencer, K.M., Dien, J., Donchin, E., 1999. A componential analysis of the ERP elicited by novel events using a dense electrode array. *Psychophysiology* 36, 409–414.

Spielberger, C.D., Gorusch, R.L., Lusthene, R.E., 1988. *Manual for the State-Trait Anxiety Inventory,* 3rd Edition Consulting Psychologists Press, Palo Alto, CA.

Talairach, J., Tournoux, P., 1988. Co-planar stereostaxic atlas of human brain. *Thieme*, Stuttgart.

Talsma, D., Slagter, H.A., Nieuwenhuis, S., Hage, J., Kok, A., 2005. The orienting of visuospatial attention: An event-related brain potential study. *Cogn. Brain Res*. 25, 117-129.

Van Boxtel, G.J.M., Brunia, C.H.M., 1994. Motor and non-motor components of the contingent negative variation. *Int. J. Psychophysiol*. 17, 269-279.

Vuilleumier, P., 2002. Facial expression and selective attention. *Curr. Op. Psych*. 15, 291-300.

Vuilleumier, P., 2005. How brains beware: Neural mechanism of emotional attention. *Trends Cogn. Sci*. 9, 585-594.

Vuilleumier, P., Schwartz, S., 2001. Beware and be aware: Capture of spatial attention by fear-related stimuli in neglect. *Neuroreport* 12, 1119-1122.

Walter, W.G., Cooper, R., Aldridge, V.J., McCallum, W.C., Winter, A.L., 1964. Contingent negative variation: An electric sign of sensoriomotor association and expectancy in the human brain. *Nature* 203, 380-384.

Weinberg, H., 1972. The contingent negative variation: Its relation to feedback and expectant attention. *Neuropsychologia* 10, 299-306.

Yee, C.M., Miller, G.A., 1987. Affective valence and information processing. *Electroencephalogr. Clin. Neurophysiol*. (Suppl. 40), 300-307.

In: Brain Mapping Research Developments
Editor: Lars N. Bakker, pp. 211-230
ISBN 978-1-60456-007-7

Chapter IX

Brain Electric Source Imaging by an Iterative Correlation Matrix Based Multiple Signal Classification Approach

Dezhong Yao [*]
Center of Neuroinformatics, School of Life Science and Technology,
University of Electronic Science and Technology of China,
Chengdu 610054, PR China

Abstract

How to localize the neural electric activities effectively and precisely from the scalp EEG recordings is a critical issue for clinical neurology and cognitive neuroscience. In the past 80s and 90s, suggested approaches included the dipole localization, cortical imaging, scalp Laplacian and 3D tomography. The 3D tomography may be realized by a direct linear inversion, or an indirect algorithm such as the subspace projection scanning method named MUltiple SIgnal Classification (MUSIC). However, the classical MUSIC algorithm is limited for its assumption of random noise. In this work, we propose to use a delay-correlation matrix instead of the previous zero-delay-correlation matrix in the signal-subspace estimate of the MUSIC algorithm to get a better performance over a spatial coherent but temporal random noisy disturbance. Then an Iterative application of the Delay-correlation MUSIC (IDM) is emphasized to derive a reasonable reconstruction of the multi-sources. The present simulation and empirical data experiment show that final promising results are obtained.

Keywords: Electroencephalography; inverse algorithm; delay correlation; multiple signal classification (MUSIC); subspace correlation; computer simulation; evoked potential; iteration.

[*] E-mail: dyao@uestc.edu.cn, www.neuro.uestc.edu.cn

Introduction

Noninvasive measurements of human brain functions have been attracting much interest. Such measurements often use various kinds of sensory stimuli, especially when measuring higher-order cognitive functions or identifying brain dysfunction. Among the different modalities that provide functional brain images, electroencephalogram (EEG) has a distinct characteristic that it can provide a temporal resolution less than 1 ms at a much less cost than the Positron Emission Topography (PET) or functional Magnetic Resonance Imaging (fMRI) and magnetoencephalography (MEG).

Recently, a considerable amount of effort has been made in the development of EEG–based source imaging and multi-sources localization techniques. Representative approaches in source-imaging include the low resolution electromagnetic topography (LORETA) [Pascual-Marqui et al., 1994; Yao et al., 1998; Yao et al, 2001b; Xu et al, 2007], scalp Laplacian [Yao, 2002a, 2002b] and the cortical imaging techniques [Sidman et al., 1992; Gevins et al., 1993; Srebro, 1993; Nunez et al., 1994; Yao et al., 1995, 1996, 2004a, 2004b].

Multi-sources localization from scalp-recorded EEGs provides quantitative three-dimensional information regarding electrical activities inside the brain, and it can be formulated in terms of finding a least-squares fit of a set of current dipoles with the observed data. A fundamental problem is that the least-squares cost function is highly non-convex with respect to the locations of the dipoles. Consequently, inverse methods such as gradient–based optimization or nonlinear simplex searches often become trapped in local minimums, yielding significant localization errors [Miltner et al., 1994; Supek et al., 1997a; Huang et al., 1998]. One of the attempt to overcome the difficulty of the least-squares fit is the application of the MUltiple SIgnal Classification (MUSIC) algorithm into EEG/MEG inverse problem [Schmidt, 1986; Mosher et al., 1992]. The canonical MUSIC-based EEG inverse algorithm localizes the multi-sources with a procedure in which a single dipole is scanned through a grid confined to a three-dimensional (3-D) head volume conductor. At each point on this grid, the forward model (transfer matrix) of a dipole at this grid point is projected against a signal subspace that has been estimated with the EEG/MEG data. The locations on this grid where the source model gives the best projections onto the signal subspace correspond to the dipole locations [Mosher et al., 1992]. The scanning manipulation instead of the non-linear multi-sources search makes it very attractive to the peers [Supek et al., 1997b]. However, the Canonical MUSIC (CM) algorithm suffers from two limitations (Yao et al., 1999): 1) the data are corrupted by additive spatial white noise; 2) the algorithm is based on the assumption that the data are generated by a set of asynchronous dipolar sources. To breakthrough these limitations, a few improvements have been made in recent years(Yao et al. 2000, 2001a). The nonwhite noise problem has been investigated under an assumption that the covariance of the background noise is known or it can be estimated [Soong et al., 1995; Sekihara et al., 1997, 1998], and a Recursive MUSIC (RM) was proposed to proceed synchronous activities [Mosher et al., 1998]. In the RM, the recorded EEGs are considered to be a sum of contributions from a fixed number of spatio-temporal independent topographies (IT), each IT being considered to be a source comprising one or more fixed dipoles which collectively have a single time-course.

In this paper, a Delay MUSIC (DM) based on a non-zero delay-correlation matrix instead of the CM on a zero-delay-correlation matrix is proposed as a novel algorithm for extracting the multi-sources from data corrupted by spatial coherent noise. And an Iterative/alternative idea is emphasized in the application of the DM (IDM) to get a promising result in practice.

IDM ALGORITHM

DM Algorithm

The EEGs may be formulated as the following mathematical model:

$$y(t) = A(L)x(t) + e(t), t = 1,\ldots, N \tag{1}$$

where, $y(t) \in R^{M\times 1}$ are the scalp recording potentials, M is the number of electrodes, $x(t) \in R^{L\times 1}$ are the multi-sources inside the brain, and L is the number of sources, $e(t) \in R^{M\times 1}$ are the noise which stem from environmental noise and random spontaneous electrical activities. A(L) is the transfer matrix accomplishing the transfer from the sources to the scalp electrodes, which is decided by the head model.

We may express the delay-correlation matrix of the scalp recordings as (Yao et al., 2000)

$$R(\beta) = < y(t)y^T(t+\beta) > = AP(\beta)A^T + W(\beta) \tag{2}$$

where $P(\beta) = < x(t)x^T(t+\beta) >, W(\beta) = < e(t)e^T(t+\beta) >$, T represents matrix transfer. β ranges from zero (CM) to other desired non-zero value (DM).

Suppose the following three notes hold for our problems:

Note 1: M>L , so rank(A)=L.

Note 2: Suppose the data is the evoked potential(EP) or evoked field(EF), and the main noise is the spontaneous EEG/MEG, then the delay correlation of the signal (EP/EF) will be much better than that of the noise. So β may be chosen approximately as the minimum delay corresponding to the zero-level delay correlation of the noise, hence equation (2) simplifies to

$$R = APA^T, W(\beta) = 0 \tag{3}$$

Note 3: The sources may be independent of each other, then we derive rank(P)=L, $rank(APA^T) = L$ [Mosher et al., 1992; Supek et al., 1997b; Yao et al., 1999]. If some of the multi-dipoles are synchronous, each synchronous set should be grouped as an “integrated source”, i.e., an “ independent topographies(IT)” model, then rank(P)=L_1<L,

$rank(APA^T) = L_1 < L$ [Mosher et al., 1998]. If some of the multi-dipoles are partly synchronous, we get rank(P)=L_2<=L, $rank(APA^T) = L_2 <= L$. Obviously, the first two are particular cases of the partly synchronous source model.

We may decompose the correlation matrix R as

$$R = U\Sigma V^T \tag{4}$$

where $\Sigma = diag[\lambda_1,...,\lambda_M]$, λ_i is the eigenvalues of the correlation matrix R, and $\lambda_i > 0, i = 1,..., L_s; \lambda_i \approx 0, i = L_s + 1,..., M$. The orthogonal matrix U and V are formed by the associated eigenvectors. Based on the eignevalues, the orthogonal matrix U or V may be decomposed into two parts, for example $U = [S \mid G] = [u_1,..,u_{L_s} \mid u_{L_s+1},...,u_M]$. The spans of the columns of matrix $S = [u_1,..,u_{L_s}]$ and matrix $G = [u_{Ls+1},...,u_M]$ are respectively called the signal subspace and the noise subspace. In theory, Ls should be one of the L, L_1 or L_2.

If the dipoles are independent of each other, we may calculate the Subspace Correlation(SC) between the subspaces spanned by the matrix S and transfer matrix A_i corresponding to a dipole at a grid point. The distribution of the SC or its function over a discrete grid of the solution space will show us the source locations [Mosher et al., 1992]. If the dipoles can be separated into a few independent synchronous set, i.e. a few IT models, the RM may be used, where the SC is between the subspaces spanned by the matrix S and transfer matrix A_{IT} [Mosher et al., 1998]. For the partly synchronous sources model, the following IDM may be used, where the SC is between the subspaces spanned by the matrix S and transfer matrix A_g, and the A_g is the transfer matrix of the partly synchronous sources configuration. In the IDM, not only the synchronous dipoles collectively with a single time-course but also the dipoles with a few partly synchronous time-courses are "grouped" as an " integrated source".

The subspace correlations(SC) are defined as

$$\{c_1, c_2,...\} = subcorr\{A_*, S\} \tag{5}$$

where the A_* may either be the A_i or A_{IT} or A_g. $\{c_1,...c_r\}$ are the ordered set of the SC, $1>=c_1>=...>=c_r>=0$, between the two subspaces spanned by the matrix A_* and matrix S.

The steps of computing the subspace correlations may be found in references [Golub et al., 1984; Mosher et al., 1998]. In practice, which to choose in the set $\{c_1,...c_r\}$ as the imaging metric still remains as a problem. Our opinion is stated in the following IDM algorithm (Yao et al., 2001a).

IDM Algorithm

IDM denotes an Iterative application of the Delay-correlation MUSIC algorithm. The steps are as follows:

(1) The delay-correlation matrix of the measured spatio-temporal data is calculated by $R = E\{yy^T(\beta)\}$, where β is decided by a prior judgement about the delay correlation of the signal and the noise or by a trial and error. If the noise is assumed to be white time-course noise, β =1.

(2) Singular Value Decomposition(SVD) of the matrix R performs as $R = U\Sigma V^T$, and the signal subspace is assumed being spanned by the eigenvectors correspond to the nonzero eigenvalues, and the number of the nonzero-level eigenvalues is called the Signal Subspace Dimensionality(SSD).

(3) Create a relatively dense grid of dipolar source locations in the solution space. In this work, a grid ranging from z=0.0 to z=0.80 with grid size 0.1 are created in the brain volume conductor (the solution space) whose surface radius is 1.0 and the total grid number is 1509.

(4) For index starts at 1.

(5) Let $G = [A_{*(1)}, A_{*(2)}, ..., A_{*(index-1)}]$ be the transfer matrix of the sources extracted out of the previous loops (It is a null matrix for the first loop).

(6) For index, concatenate the transfer matrix $A_{g(index)}$ (the A_i and A_{IT} are considered to be special cases of the A_g) to the present extracted model, $W = [G, A_{g(index)}]$. Calculate the subspace correlations(SC), $\{c_1, c_2, ...\} = subcorr\{W, S\}$.

(7) If c_{l-1} has been unit 1.0 (supposing l=1 and $c_{1-1}= c_0$=1.0 for the first loop), check the maximum of the c_l in the ordered set of the SC and the distribution map of the c_l or its function over the discrete grid of the solution space. If the maximum is closely enough to unit 1.0, and the map "clearly and simplely" shows local activities, they may be explained as effective activities. If the SC c_l has been used as the imging metric in the previous loops, i.e. the l is the same as that in these previous loops, the new identified activities is interpreted as (partly) synchronous activities with the sources which are extracted by the SC c_l in the previous loops; If the SC c_l has not been used in the previous loops, for example, the c_l in the first loop, the new identified local activities is interpreted as independent sources. If the c_l =1.0, let l=l+1. Finally let index=index+1, and back to step 5). If the map is blurred, there may be two reasons, one of which is that the source model of the A_g is simpler than the actual model, hence we should try a more complex model such as two dipolar sources instead of one dipolar source or three dipolar sources instead of two dipolar sources, etc. In such case, we should keep the index without change, and back to step 5) to start a new calculation with the new transfer matrix A_g. The other reason is that the next dipoles are asynchronous with the extracted sources. In such event, c_l to c_l mainly represent the SC of the previous extracted sources, then we should check the next SC c_{l+1}. If the maximum of the c_{l+1} is closely enough to unit 1.0, and the map of

the c_{l+1} or its function "clearly and simplely" shows local activities, the local activities is explained as new "independent sources", then let index=index+1, l=l+1, and back to step 5). If the actual "new independent sources" is an "integrated sources" with a more complex sources configuration, we should keep the index without change, and back to step 5) and increase the complexity of the transfer matrix A_g to start a new calculation. If both c_l and c_{l+1} can not give us any more reasonable source information through a trial and error, proceed to step 8). Apparently, l is a number without relation to the index and the source number. It is the number of the correlation coefficients of the SC that are equal to 1.0 or closely enough to 1.0.

(8) stop;

Obviously, the practice of the IDM is an interactive process between the man's assumption and the scanning results. In such sense, the "iterative" in the IDM is a more general concept than the "recursive" in the RM [Mosher et al., 1998]. The detail interactive process will be illustrated clearly in the following simulation and empirical data tests.

Besides, to get a reasonable reconstruction of the actual sources, there are a few problems to be considered in practice. First, the SSD should be carefully chosen. In theory, it is the number of independent sources, but, for a noisy data especially for a data corrupted by spatial coherent noise as shown in the following numeric tests, it had better to be chosen as a larger number than the actual independent signal number. In our practice, it is decided by the distribution of the singular values and assumed being the number of the non-zero level singular values, i.e. SSD=L_s, which is always equal to or larger than the L or L_1 or L_2.

The second is about the optimization of the sources assemblage with more than one dipolar source. The scanning of all the combinatories is a multidimensional search similar to the non-linear least-squares algorithm, and a random subset of the possible combinations is used in the RM[Mosher et al., 1998]. In this work, a similar subset search is utilized, however, the obtained scanning results are emphasized to be used as a prior information for choosing the next subset and searching region.

Finally, we'd like to point out the difference of the definitions of G in the IDM and RM. The whole transfer matrix of the sources extracted in the previous loops is concatenated to the current G in the IDM, it means that only the locations of the extracted sources are used as prior information in searching the next source(s) location. However, in the RD, both the dipole locations and orientations of the extracted sources are used as prior information in searching the next source(s), accordingly, where G is defined as $G=[a_{i(1)},a_{i(2)},...,a_{i(index-1)}]$, with $a_{i(k)}=A_{i(k)}\hat{u}_k$, $\hat{u}_k$ is the obtained unit dipole-orientation vector [Mosher et al.,1998]. In our numeric tests, we find that the reconstruction of location is more robust than that of orientation, and a wrong orientation of a extracted dipole may result in an ill reconstruction of the next source. So in our IDM algorithm, the orientations of the extracted dipoles are allowed of further adjustment with the new sources together. Another difference between the RM and IDM is that, in the RM, the extracted model is assumed to be fixed, and if the first one is wrong, the later will be influenced [Koles, 1998], while in the IDM, we may fix the later extracted sources and optimize the former sources again, therefore a more general "iterative" idea is involved in the IDM through the interaction between man's guess and the recursive application of the DM.

COMPUTER SIMULATION

Simulation Method

Volume Conductor Model and Electrode Configuration

The concentric three-spheres head model is used to represent the head volume conductor [Rush et al., 1969]. The radii of the brain, the skull, and the scalp spheres are taken as 0.87,0.92 and 1.0, respectively. The conductivity of the scalp and the brain is taken as 1.0, and that of the skull as 0.0125. The number of the scalp electrode is 120, and the configuration is derived from the Neuro SCAN electrode configuration projecting on the best-fit and normalized spherical surface of the group averaged head model over 10 subjects. About the Cartesian coordinate system of the Neuro SCAN electrode configuration, the midpoint between the left and right preauricular points is defined as the coordinate origin. The axis directed away from the origin toward the left preauricular point is defined as the +y axis, and that from the origin to the nasion is the +x axis. The +z axis is defined as the axis that is perpendicular to both these axes and directed from the origin to the vertex.

Signal Model

The time-course is supposed to be a Gaussian function modulated by a sine function, the waveform is controlled by adjusting the parameters [Yao et al., 1999]. The function is

$$f(t) = \exp(-(2\pi f_m (t - t_0)/\gamma)^2)\cos(2\pi f_m (t - t_0) + v) \tag{6}$$

Supposing dt=2ms,v=$\pi/2$, γ =3 and π=3.14159, the other parameters of source 1 used in the following simulation are f_m =5Hz, t_0=10*dt, and that of source 2 are f_m =15Hz, t_0=20*dt and that of source 3 are fm=10Hz, t_0=30*dt. The correlation coefficient between the source 1 and source 2 is –0.2925, and that between source 1 and source 3 is –0.0494. The total sample point is 150. In Figure 1 the three time-courses are shown.

Noise and Noise-Signal Ratio (NSR)

The time-course of the noise is white Gaussian. The spatial white (incoherent) noise denotes that the noise for each channel is generated independently, and the spatial color (coherent) noise means that the noise is same for all the 120 channels. The noise-signal ratio(NSR) is defined as the ratio of the squared Frobenius norm of the noise matrix to the squared Frobenius norm of the noiseless signal matrix.

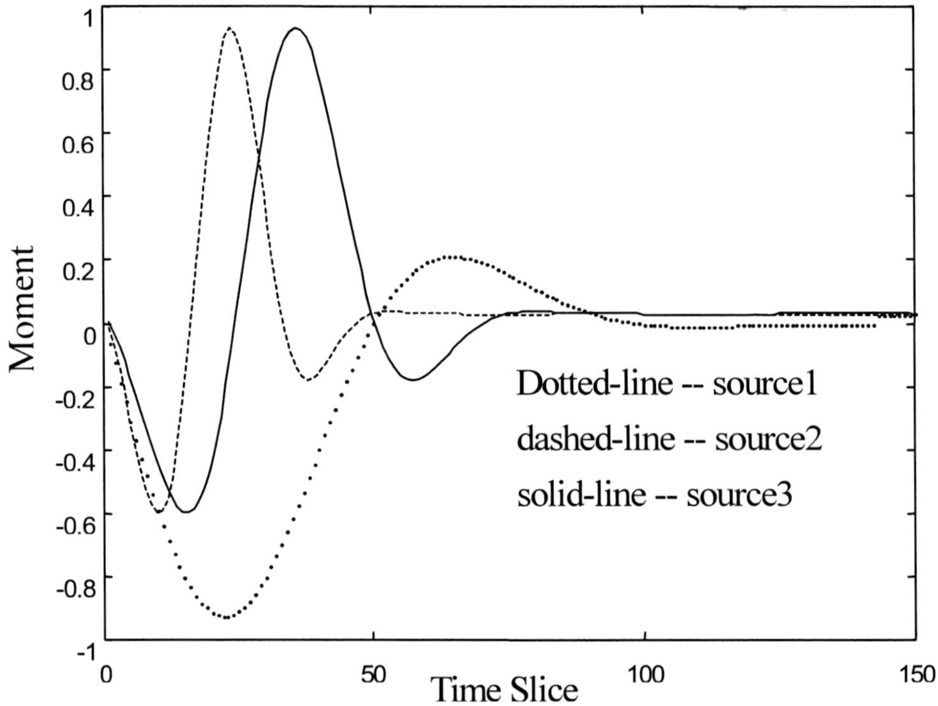

Figure 1. Time-courses of the simulated electrical generators.

Normalized Blurring Index (NBI)

A NBI of a function distribution is defined as to indicate the relative blurring level [Yao et al, 2001b; 1999), which is written as

$$NBI_i = \sqrt{\sum_k \|\vec{r}_k - \vec{r}_i\|^2 X^2(k) / \sum_k X^2(k)} \Big/ \sqrt{\sum_k \|\vec{r}_k - \vec{r}_i\|^2 / \sum_k 1} \quad (7)$$

where the order i denotes a grid point where the NBI is to be estimated and k denotes a grid point within a subregion of the point i, for example, within a subsphere originated at point i with radius equal to or smaller than 0.2. The $\vec{r}_i$ stands for the displacement of the grid point i. Apparently, if the distribution function X(k) is uniform in the subregion, the NBI will approach unit 1.0, and if the distribution is similar to a Dirc function $\delta(k-i)$, the NBI will approach to zero. Obviously, a smaller NBI is preferred in EEG inverse problem. Here the imaging metric X is defined as $X = 1./\sqrt{1.001 - c_l^{\,2}}$ in simulation study and $X = 1./(1.001 - c_l^{\,2})$ for empirical data test, where the 0.001 is introduced to remove the singular point when c_l=1.0. The c_l is the SC explained in the last section.

Simulation Results

The CM algorithm has been tested by a few authors [Supek et al., 1997; Yao et al., 2002]. Here the simulation will emphasize on the following items.

Effect of the SSD and the Delay

The signal-subspace estimate is the crux of the MUSIC-based algorithm. After the data acquisition, the remaining problems will be the selections of the delay parameter β and SSD. The signal subspace is spanned by eigenvectors associated with the non-noise level eigenvalues where the number of the non-noise level eigenvalues is believed to be the signal number [Schmidt, 1986]. However, due to the limited data length, low signal/noise ratio, the breakpoint between the noise level and non-noise level eignevalues is blurred, and because the (partly) synchronous sources and distributed source nature instead of the dipolar source model, it is difficult to determine the SSD in EEG inverse practice [Mosher et al.,1992; Greenblatt, 1993; Knosche, 1997]. In the following simulation, β=0(CM) and β=1(DM), SSD=2~6 are taken.

Supposing two radial asynchronous dipoles are located at (-0.3 -0.4 0.7) and (0.3 -0.4 0.7), whose time-courses are source 1 and source 2. The minimum delays are 1, 31 and 8 corresponding to the white time-course noise, source 1 and source 2, respectively, so β=1 is selected in the practice of the DM.

Table 1. Singular value distribution

	1	2	3	4	5	6
CM 0%	1.181794	0.546704	0	0	0	0
CM 10%nc	1.182127	0.545491	0.00477	0.000465	0.000438	0.000433
CM 10%c	1.183096	0.546621	0.012800	0	0	0
CM 80%nc	1.200860	0.551688	0.030564	0.029774	0.028000	0.027747
CM 80%c	1.550651	0.830970	0.411151	0	0	0
DM 0%	1.187160	0.539090	0	0	0	0
DM 10%nc	1.187320	0.537738	0.000313	0.000287	0.000280	0.000277
DM 10%c	1.186150	0.536900	0.000889	0	0	0
DM 80%nc	1.195314	0.533601	0.020022	0.018361	0.017963	0.017751
DM 80%c	1.172151	0.517173	0.059794	0	0	0

CM-Canonical MUSIC, DM –Delay MUSIC ; c- spatial coherent noise; nc – spatial non-coherent noise.

Table 1 shows the first six singular values of the delay-correlation matrix when different noise is added to the signal. Based on Table 1, actual rank 2 is revealed in results of the CM in cases of white spatial noises and in cases of spatial color noises with small NSR, and in results of the DM in all cases. Figure 2 shows the NBI of the reconstructed imaging maps, which is calculated around the known actual source locations, and the result is the average of the results on the two source locations. On the Figure, only the results of SSD=2 and 6 are shown, because the results from SSD=3 to 6 are similar to one another. Figure 3 shows the source imaging maps plotted according to the metric $X = 1./\sqrt{1.001 - c_1^2}$ when SSD=2, 3 and 6, where only the maps on slice with z=0.7 are shown for saving space.They are reconstructed by the CM and DM when different noise in type and content is added.

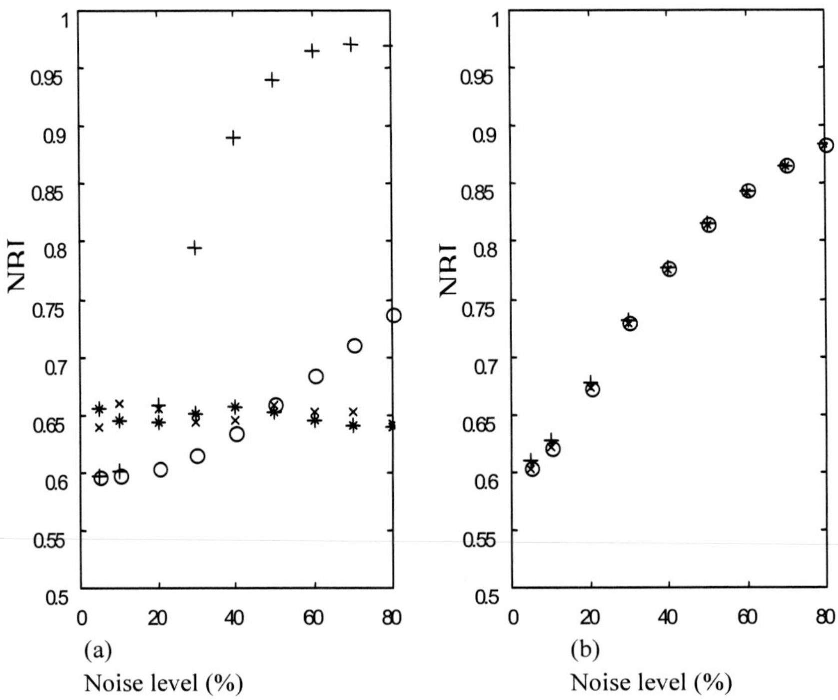

Figure 2. Normalized blurring index(NBI). The left figure corresponds to spatial coherent (color) noise, and the right figure corresponds to spatial incoherent (white) noise. O—DM, SSD=2; x—DM , SSD=6; + --NM, SSD=2; * --NM , SSD=6.

For spatial coherent noise, as shown by the point-curves (o,x) in Figure 2(a) and Figure 3(1,5,9,13,17), the DM conducts a very robust reconstruction no matter the rank is chosen equal to (2) or larger than (3,6) the true rank (2). The CM with the true rank 2 is sensitive to the NSR level as shown by the point-curve (+) in Figure 2(a) and Figure 3(3,7,11). When the NSR is equal to or larger than 50%, one source is missed (Figure 3(7,11)). However, if a larger rank (3,6) than the true rank (2) is chosen, the results of the CM are almost the same as that of the DM (the point-curve (*) in Figure 2(a) and Figure 3(15,19)).

For spatial incoherent noise, the performance of the CM and DM is similar to each other no matter the rank is equal to (2) or larger than (3,6) the true rank (2) (Figure 2(b), Figure 3(2,6,10,14,18) and Figure 3(4,8,12,16,20)). The differences among the Figure 3(2,6,10,14,18; 4,8,12,16,20) are due to the random spatial coherence of the white time-course noise. The random spatial coherence is almost equivalent to both the DM and CM, and this fact is shown by the wide singular value distribution of both the DM and CM (Table 1, *%nc). Besides, for the spatial incoherent noise, the imaging maps (Figure 3) shown again that nearly identical results are obtained with true or over-selected rank [Mosher et al., 1998; Supek et al., 1997b] and the larger the NSR is, the worse the map is [Yao et al., 2002].

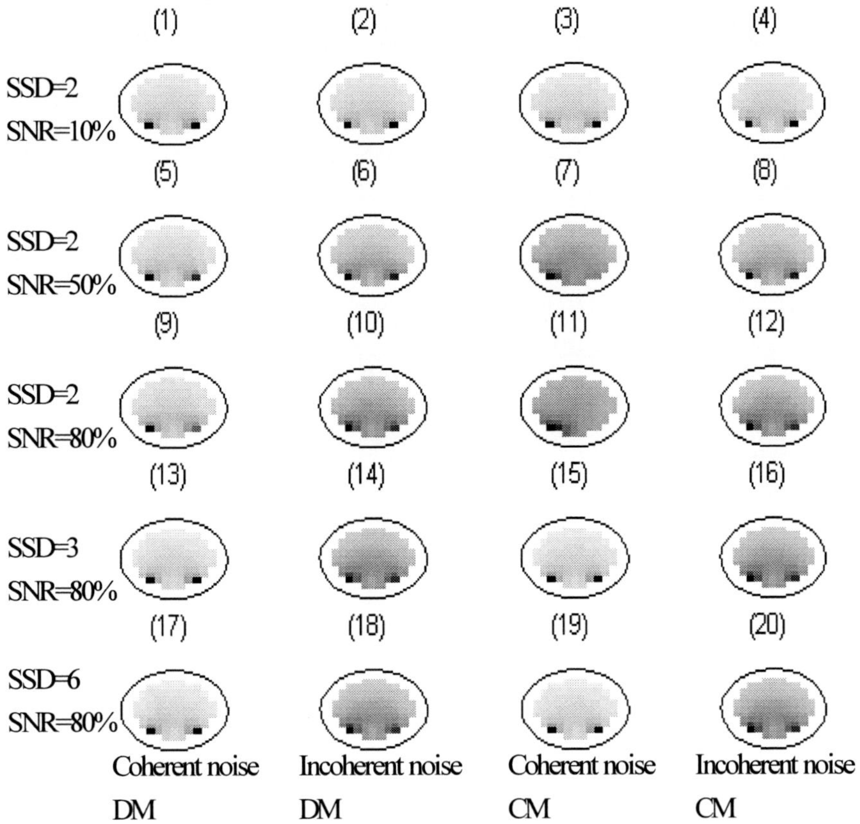

Figure 3. Maps of the metric $X = 1./(1.001 - c_1^{\ 2})$. The results are for slice with z=0.7 under different noise level, noise type (coherent/incoherent) and different SSD and method (CM/DM).

For the spatial coherent noise, due to its white time-course nature, it is depressed by the delay correlation no matter the content of the noise, and so the DM shows a very robust reconstruction when different NSR and SSD are involved. The bad performance, Figure 3(7,11), of the CM with true rank (2) is due to that the spatial coherent noise acts as a " signal" in the zero-delay-correlation matrix. In fact, rank 3 is implicated by the singular values (Table 1, CM 80%c). It means that the signal subspace should be spanned by its first three eigenvectors because these three eigenvectors can not be further divided into two groups with the first two pertaining to the "signal" and the third to the "coherent noise ". The similar performance between the CM with rank SSD=3 to 6 and DM may be due to that the extended signal subspace guarantees that the whole signal-subspace information is included. So on one hand, we can prove the subspace correlation between the actual source transfer matrix and the signal subspace. On the other hand, the noise subspace spanned by eigenvectors over-included by a larger SSD than the true rank does not correlate with an actual transfer matrix. It means that an over-selected eigenvectors do not change much of the correlation between the transfer matrix of a dipole at a grid point and the signal subspace.

Concretely, for the spatial coherent noise used here, though it acts like a "signal" in the zero-delay correlation as shown by the singular values of the " CM 80%c" in Table 1, it is not a dipole field, and it can not be extracted by the dipole scanning. Therefore, though a larger rank (3 to 6) is chosen, the resultant source number still is 2 (Figure 3). Finally, if the spatial coherent noise is not same in each channel, it can be considered as a combination of a spatial coherent noise and incoherent noise, and the results will be an intermediate state [Yao et al., 2002].

In summary, when the noise is spatially incoherent and the SSD is equal to or larger than the true rank, the performance of the CM and DM is similar to each other. If the noise is spatially coherent, the DM is very effective when a proper β is selected, the result of the CM pertaining to over-selected rank is better than that to true rank. So the DM and the CM with an over-selected SSD are more effective in repressing the spatial coherent noise than the CM with true rank. These results suggest that for data corrupted by unknown noise type, the DM is prefer to the CM, and an over-selected SSD is not a compromise [Mosher et al., 1998] but a necessary choice. Nevertheless, it can results in some false activities that the random subspace correlation (SC) between the transfer matrix of some grid-points and the "signal subspace" originated from an over selected SSD, so we do not commend that the larger the rank is, the better the result is. We choose the SSD based on the singular value distribution, and we believe that a trial and error is necessary in the choice of a proper SSD in some practices.

IDM Identifies Synchronous Activities

Supposing that there are three sources. One radial dipole locates at (0.0 0.0 0.6) with the source 1 time-course. The other two synchronous radial sources locate at (-0.3 –0.3 0.6) and (0.3 0.3 0.6) with the same source 3 time-course. The noise is the spatial coherent noise with NSR=80%. β=1 is used in the IDM because of the white time-course of the noise. The first six singular values are 1.153057, 0.066178, 0.010905, 0.0, 0.0, 0.0, they imply SSD=1~3. We choose SSD=3, and starting scanning with $W=A_i$, we get Figure 4(a). The maximum is $c_1=1.0$, which is located at the (0.0 0.0 0.6). Then after scanning the second dipole with $W=(A_{i(0.0,\ 0.0,\ 0.6)}$(extracted), A_i), we get figure 4(b), and its corresponding second maximum $c_2=0.974$ is at (0.1 0.2 0.0). Though the 0.974 is larger than the recommended criterion 0.95[Mosher et al., 1998], the map of the metric X is quite blurred which implicitly means the second dipole is not an independent dipole, so we start a two-dipoles scanning with $W=(A_{i(0.0,\ 0.0,\ 0.6)}$(extracted), A_i (fixed), A_i). We try to find some prior information from Figure 4(b). It is clear that there is a seriously deep blurred region and then is a "two sources" projection on slices z=0.6 and z=0.7. These facts implicitly tell us that the seriously blurred region should be an "equivalent source region" of two or more dipoles. And the actual dipoles may be within a sub-region around slices z=0.6 and z=0.7. We choose the maximum point on slices z=0.6 and 0.7 as the A_i(fixed), which is at (0.1 0.0 0.6) with $c_2=0.9536$, and we define a smaller scanning region which is composed by slices from z=0.5 to z=0.8. After a two-dipoles scanning with $W=(A_{i(0.0,\ 0.0,\ 0.6)}$(extracted), A_i (fixed), A_i), we choose the grid point where the maximum c_2 located at as the new A_i(fixed).

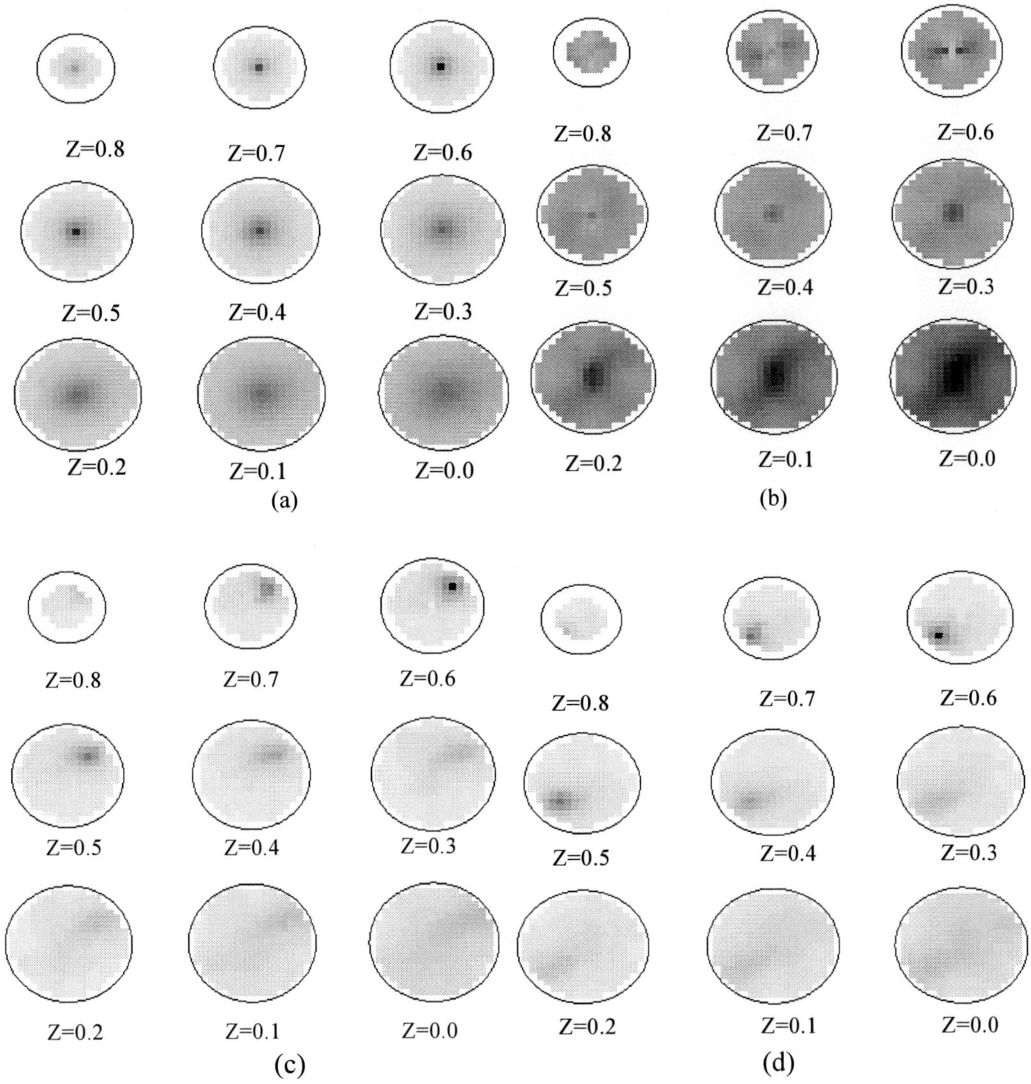

Figure 4. Maps of the metric X. Each map is a distribution of the imaging metric on a transverse plane, and the corresponding z-axis value is shown under the map. (a) Map of the $X = 1./\sqrt{1.001 - c_1^2}$ in an one-dipole scanning; (b) map of the $X = 1./\sqrt{1.001 - c_2^2}$ in a scanning after a dipole is assumed at (0.0 0.0 0.6); (c) map of the $X = 1./\sqrt{1.001 - c_2^2}$ in a two-dipoles scanning after a dipole is assumed at (0.0 0.0 0.6) and one of the two-dipoles is fixed at (-0.3 –0.3 0.6); (d) map of the $X = 1./\sqrt{1.001 - c_2^2}$ in a two-dipoles scanning after a dipole is assumed at (0.0 0.0 0.6) and one of the two-dipoles is fixed at (0.3 0.3 0.6).

Repeating this process, finally, we find that a two-dipoles scanning with W=($A_{i(0.0,\ 0.0,\ 0.6)}$(extracted), $A_{i(0.3\ 0.3\ 0.6)}$(fixed), A_i) results in maximum c_2=1.0 at (-0.3 –0.3 0.6) (Figure 4(d)); and a two-dipoles scanning with W=($A_{i(0.0,\ 0.0,\ 0.6)}$(extracted), $A_{i(-0.3\ -0.3\ 0.6)}$(fixed), A_i) results in maximum c_2=1.0 at (0.3 0.3 0.6) (Figure 4(c)). The maps, Figure 4(c) and Figure

4(d), are "simple and clear" and distinctly different from the Figure 4(b). And that the maximum points on Figure 4(a,c,d) are consistent with the actual source locations.

EMPIRICAL DATA TEST

Evoked by a check-board flashed to the right visual field on the horizontal line, the visual ERP data are collected. The check-board used as stimuli is shown in Figure 5. Volunteers sit in a sofa 60cm from the monitor, and fix his eyes on a cross at the center of the monitor. The visual angle is from 1.5° to 4.5°. The inter-stimulus intervals (ISIs) are from 250-550ms. The data used here is the grand average data over 10 healthy right-handed subjects with a mean age of 24. Subjects had normal or rectified-to-normal visual acuity. Due to an unreasonable singular waveform, the channel 86 is rejected.

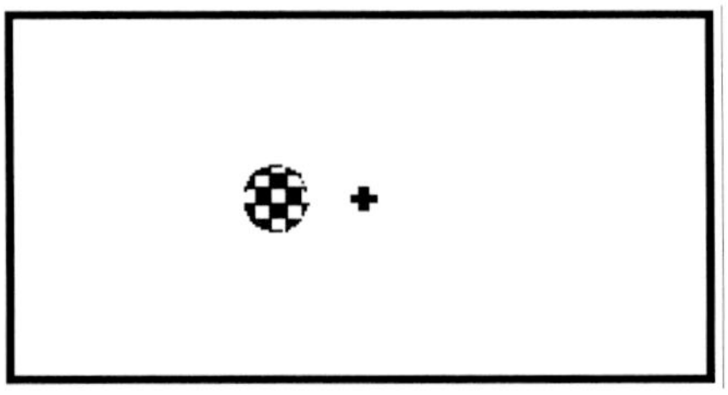

Figure 5. Visual stimulus pattern.

We are interested in source locations of the early visual electrical activities (t<160ms). Fig.6 shows scalp animations from post-stimuli 52ms to 140ms. It indicates three activities. They may be the C_1 before 80 ms on the visual cortex, and the P_1 after 60ms on left visual cortex and right visual cortex subsequently [Clark et al., 1995].

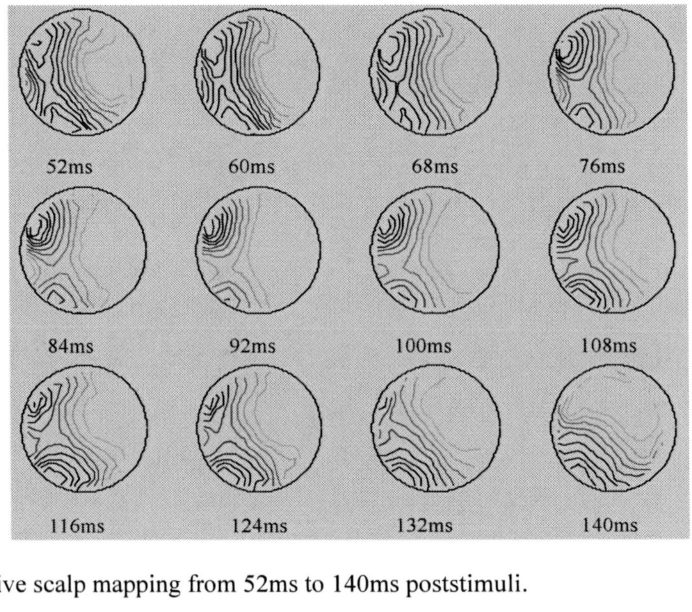

Figure 6. Successive scalp mapping from 52ms to 140ms poststimuli.

The first ten singular values of the delay-correlation matrix are 18.329, 10.3244, 0.40978, 0.2254, 0.18257, 0.09792, 0.05919, 0.03265, 0.02990, 0.02591. They hint two main signals and some small activities or distributed spontaneous activities in the data. Because there is not a clear breakpoint of the singular value distribution, we over-select SSD=5 and β=1.

We start scanning with W=A_i, and get the first maximum c_1=0.9903 located at the (-0.1 –0.1 0.6). However, the map, Figure 7(a), of the metric $X = 1./(1.001 - c_1^2)$ shows that there are two active regions. The other is centered on (-0.5 0.3 0.5) with c_1=0.9884. We note that these two active regions are the imaging result of the DM, and the active on the right visual cortex hinted by the animation, Figure 6, is lost. It means that the DM localizes fewer sources than the actual sources just as the CM does when synchronous sources existed [Supek et al., 1997; Mosher et al., 1998]. So an iterative search is necessary to improve the result of either the CM or the DM. Now, we choose the active on the left visual cortex centered on (-0.5 0.3 0.5) as the A_i(fixed), and do a scanning with W=($A_{i(-0.5,\ 0.3,\ 0.5)}$(fixed), A_i), we get the map of the metric $X = 1./(1.001 - c_1^2)$ (Figure 7(b)), which clearly shows an active on the right visual cortex centered on (-0.5 -0.5 0.5) with maximum c_1=0.9937, and we get a map of the metric $X = 1./(1.001 - c_2^2)$ (Figure 7(c)) with maximum c_2=0.9895 centered on (-0.1 0.0 0.6) — a point close the point (-0.1 –0.1 0.6). In order to affirm these three active regions, we choose the (-0.5 -0.5 0.5) as the A_i(fixed) , and get two activities centered on (-0.5 0.3 0.5) with c_1=0.9937 and on (-0.1 0.0 0.6) with c_1=0.9948 on the map of the metric $X = 1./(1.001 - c_1^2)$. And if the (-0.1 0.0 0.6) are chosen as the A_i(fixed), we get the maximum c_1=0.9949 at (-0.5 -0.5 0.5) and maximum c_2=0.9895 at (-0.5 0.3 0.5). These results repetitively affirm the three active regions centered on (-0.1 0.0 0.6), (-0.5 0.3 0.5) and (-0.5 -0.5 0.5). Their radii are 0.61, 0.77 and 0.87 in the unit sphere head model. These results are qualitatively consistent with the known early visual electrical generators, i.e. the early C_1, P_1 (left) and P_1 (right) [Clark et al., 1995]. However, the depth 1-0.61=0.39 of the C_1 is much deeper than the supposed region 17 and the depth 1-0.87=0.13 of the P_1 activity on the right visual cortex is shallower than the cortical surface. Such shortfalls may be due to the distributed nature of the actual sources, which is different from the dipole model used in the MUSIC scanning.

About the relations among the three activities, the activity centered on (-0.5 0.3 0.5) should be (partly) synchronous with the activity centered on (-0.5 -0.5 0.5), because when we choose one of them as the A_i(fixed), and do a scanning with W=(A_i(fixed), A_i), the other always appear on map of the c_1. It means that these two actives together respond to the SC c_1. The active centered on (-0.5 -0.5 0.5) should be (partly) synchronous with the active centered on (-0.1 0.0 0.6) due to the same reason. However, the actives centered on (-0.3 0.3 0.5) and (-0.1 0.0 0.6) should be asynchronous because both of them appear on the map of the metric X related to c_1 in the primary one dipole scanning (Figure 7(a)), and both them appear on the map of X related to c_1 when (-0.5 -0.5 0.5) is chosen as the A_i(fixed) . And because when one of them is chosen as the A_i(fixed), the other always appears on the map of the metric X related to c_2 . Based on these phenomena, the actives may be started in region centered on (-0.1 0.0 0.6). And then an (almost) independent active appears on the left visual cortex centered on (-0.5 0.3 0.5) (the stimuli is on the right visual field). At last, a secondary active appears on the right visual cortex centered on (-0.5 -0.5 0.5), and it may be a secondary evoked activity by the activities centered on (-0.5 0.3 0.5) and (-0.1 0.0 0.6).

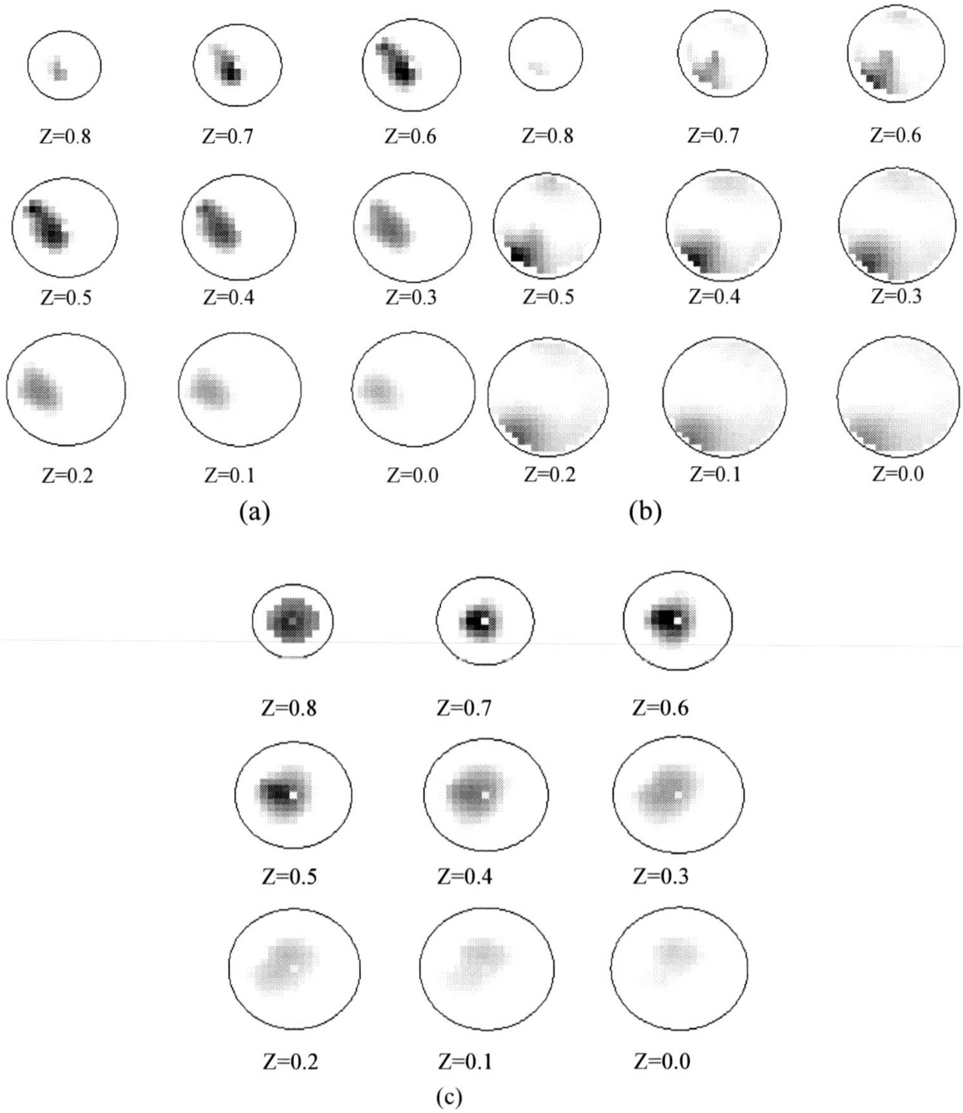

Figure 7. Maps of the metric X. Map of the $X = 1./(1.001 - c_1^2)$ in an one-dipole scanning; (b) map of the $X = 1./(1.001 - c_1^2)$ in a scanning after a dipole is assumed at (-0.5 0.3 0.5); (c) map of the $X = 1./(1.001 - c_2^2)$ in a scanning after a dipole is assumed at (-0.5 0.3 0.5).

Finally, the above result can be further improved if a finer grid and a realistic head model are involved. And due to the (partly) synchronous activities among the three source regions, a nonlinear multidimensional search is useful to further improve the location parameters of the three actives. However, since the nonlinear search algorithm is a problem under study, it is not included in this work.

Conclusion and Discussion

Based on the CM and the recently developed recursive framework, a new algorithm denoted as IDM is provided to localize the brain electrical activities. The non-zero delay correlation is introduced to replace the zero-delay correlation in the estimate of the signal subspace of the MUSIC-based algorithm. Numeric simulation shows a better performance of the new algorithm than that of the CM in repressing the spatial coherent noise. Numeric simulation also shows that a relative larger signal-subspace rank is preferred to the true rank, especially when the data are corrupted by spatial coherent or partly coherent noise. Besides, an iterative process is emphasized in the practice of the algorithm, and the iterative process is also an interactive process between man's guess and the practice of the DM. The results show that the IDM is a new choice in the EEG inverse problem.

The difference between the DM and the other pre-whitening methods is that the DM only requires the delay correlation is dramatically different between the signals and the noise [Yao et al., 2000], and the other methods require to estimate the noise covariance [Sekihara et al., 1997]. Reviewing the procedure to implement the IDM, the undesired subjective judgement is required in the selection of the SSD, and in the selection of a starting point of a muti-sources scanning, and some interactive guesses are required in the practice of the IDM. Meanwhile, for the coherent source imaging, there are some other methods are proposed in recent years, such as the frequency domain method [Gross et al., 2001], the fourth order cumulant matrix decomposition subspace method [Yao, 2000] and the multivariate correlation coefficient decomposition [Zhang et al, 2006], they are meaningful to evaluate these methods in the near future especially by empirical data.

Though an objective procedure has been the goal of the field for a long time, subjective participation still plays an important role in the current practice of EEG inverse problem like the BESA software [Scherg, 1990; Miltner et al. 1994]. Based on the state-of-the-art of the field, the non-unique of the EEG inverse problem has not been and may never be solved, we believe a positive barge is necessary for almost all the current dipole localization algorithms [Miltner et al., 1994; Supek et al., 1997a; Huang et al., 1998].

Acknowledgement

This work was supported by NSFC #30525030, #60571019 and #90208003, the 973 Project No. 2003CB716100. Te authors would like to thank the previous master students Min Zeng , Fansheng Meng, Xiao Hu, Yingchun Zhou for their contributions in programs and discussions, and Prof Lin Chen, Silu Fan and Dr Xinyu Ao for providing the ERP data.

REFERENCES

Cadzow JA (1998). A high-resolution direction –of- arrival algorithm for narrow-band coherent and incoherent sources. *IEEE Trans. ASSP* 36: 965-979.

Cadzow JA (1990). Multiple source location –the signal subspace approach. *IEEE Trans ASSP* 38:1110-1125.

Clark VP, Fan S, and Hillyard S (1995). Identification of early visual evoked potential generators by retinotopic and topographic analysis. *Human brain mapping* 2:170-187.

Gevins AS, Le J, Martin, NK, et al (1994). High resolution EEG: 124-channel recording, spatial de-blurring and MRI integration methods. *Electroenceph. Clin. Neurophysiol* , 90:337-358.

Golub GH and Van Loan CF (1984). *Matrix Computations*. 2nd ed. Baltimore, MD: Johns Hopkins Uni. Press.

Huang M, Aine CJ, Supek S, Best E, Ranken D, Flynn ER (1998). Multi-start downhill simplex method for spatio-temporal source localization in magnetoencephalography. *Electroenceph. Clin. Neurophysiol.* 108:32-44.

Greenblatt RE (1993). Probabilistic reconstruction of multiple sources in the bioelectromagnetic inverse problem. *Inverse Problem* 9:271-284.

Gross J,Kujala J, Hämäläinen M, Timmermann L, Schnitzler A, Salmelin R (2001). Dynamic imaging of coherent sources: study in gneural interactions in the human brain. *PNAS*, 98(2): 694-699.

Knosche T (1997). *Solutions of the neuroelectromagnetic inverse problem-- an evaluation study*. Ph.D thesis of Universiteit Twente.

Koles ZJ (1998). Trends in EEG source localization. *Electroenceph. Clin. Neueophysiol.* 106:127-137.

Miltner W, Braun C, Johnson R Jr, Simpson GV, Ruchkin DS (1994). A test of brain electrical source analysis (BESA): a simulation study. *Electroenceph. Clin. Neurophysiol.* 91: 295-310.

Mosher JC, Lewis PS, Leahy RM (1992). Multiple dipole modeling and localization from spatio-temporal MEG data. *IEEE Trans. BME* 39:541-557.

Mosher JC, Leahy RM (1998). Recursive MUSIC: A framework for EEG and MEG source localization. *IEEE Trans. BME* 45(11): 1342-1354.

Nunez PL, Silibertein RB, Cdush PJ, Wijesinghe RS, Westdrop AF et al (1994). A theoretical and experimental study of high resolution EEG based on surface Laplacian and cortical imaging. *Electroenceph. Clin. Neurophysiol.* 90:40-57.

Pascual-Marqui, RD, Michel, CM and Lehmann D (1994). Low resolution electromagnetic tomography: a new method for localizing electrical activity in the brain. *Int. J. Psychophysiol* 18:49-65.

Rush S, Driscoll DA (1969). EEG electrode sensitivity – An application of reciprocity. *IEEE Trans. BME* 16:15-22.

Scherg M (1990). Fundamentals of dipole source analysis. In: Grandori F, Hoke M, Roman GL (eds): *Auditory Evoked Magnetic Fields and Electrical Potentials.* Basel: Karper, 40-69.

Schmidt RO (1986). Multiple emitter location and signal parameter estimation. *IEEE Trans AP* 34:276-280.

Sekilhara K, Poeppel D, Marantz A et al (1997). Noise covariance incorporated MEG-MUSIC algorithm: A method for multiple-dipole estimation tolerant of the influence of background brain activity. *IEEE Trans. BME* 44(9):839-847.

Sekilhara K, Poeppel D, Marantz A, et al (1998). MEG covariance difference analysis: a method to extract target source activities by using task and control measurements. *IEEE Trans. BME* 45(1):87-97.

Sidman R, Vincent D, Smith D, et al (1992). Experimental tests of the cortical imaging techniques- applications to the response to median nerve stimulation and the localization of epileptiform discharges. *IEEE Trans. BME* 39:437-444.

Soong ACK and Koles AJ (1995). Principal-component localization of the sources of the background EEG. *IEEE Trans. BME* 42(1): 59-67.

Srebro R, Oguz RM, Hughlett K et al (1993). Estimating regional brain activity from evoked potential field on the scalp. *IEEE Trans. BME* 40:509-516.

Supek S, Aine CJ (1997). Spatio-temporal modeling of neuromagnetic data: I. Multi-source location versus time-course estimation accuracy. *Human Brain Mapping* 5: 139-153.

Supek S, Aine CJ (1997). Spatio-temporal modeling of neuromagnetic data: II. Multi-source resolvability of a MUSIC-based location estimator. *Human Brain Mapping* 5: 154-167.

Xu P, Tian Y, Chen HF, Yao D(2007). Lp norm iterative sparse solution for EEG source localization. *IEEE Trans Biomed Eng*, 54(3): 400-409.

Yao D (1995). Imaging of EEG by spherical harmonic analysis. *Journal of Electronics* (In Chinese) 17(5): 456-462.

Yao D (1996). The equivalent source technique and cortical imaging. *Electroenceph. and clin. Neurophysiol.* 98:478-483.

Yao D He B (1998). The Laplacian weighted minimum norm estimate of three dimensional equivalent charge distribution in the brain. *Proceedings of the 20th IEEE EMBS*, Hongkong.

Yao D, Fu S, Rao N, Zhou Y, Fan S, Chen L(1999). A computer simulation study of MUSIC algorithm for EEG inverse problem. *Chinese Journal of Biomedical Engineering* (In Chinese), 21(1): 53-58, 83.

Yao D (2000). Electroencephalography inverse problem by subspace decomposition of the fourth-order cumulant matrix. *Sheng Wu Yi Xue Gong Cheng Xue Za Zhi* (In Chinese), 17(2):174-8.

Yao D, Rao N, Fu S, Hu X(2000). A delay sub-space decomposition algorithm of electroencephalography sources localization. *Acta Electronica Sinica* (In Chinese), 28(4): 135-138.

Yao D, Zhou Y, Fan S, Chen L, Ao X(2001a). Multi-dimensional delay-correlation MUSIC: a new method to extract multi-sources of EEGs. *Acta Electronica Sinica* (In Chinese), 29(4): 522-525.

Yao D and He B(2001b). A Self-Coherence Enhancement Algorithm and its Application to Enhancing 3D Source Estimation from EEGs. *Annals of Biomedical Engineering*, 29(11):1019-1027.

Yao D (2002a). The theoretical relation of Scalp Laplacian and scalp current density. *Phys. Med.Biol.*, 47:2179-2185.

Yao D(2002b). High-resolution EEG mapping: a radial-basis function based approach to scalp Laplacian estimate. *Clin. Neurophysiol.*, 113(6): 956-967.

Yao D, Wang L, Nielsen KD, Arendt-Nielsen L,Chen CAN(2004a). Cortical Mapping of EEG Alpha Power Using a Charge Layer Model. *Brain Topogr*. 17(2):65-71.

Yao D, Yin Z, Tang X, Arendt-Nielsen L and Chen CAN(2004b). High-resolution Electroencephalogram mapping: scalp charge layer. *Phys. Med. Biol.*, 49: 5073-5086.

Zhang J, Yao D, Cui Y(2006). Multivariate Correlation Coefficient Decomposition and Its Application to Map the Coherent Sources in Human Brain. *Chinese Journal of Biomedical Engineering* (In Chinese), 25(1): 6-9.

INDEX

A

acclimatization, 46
accuracy, 14, 16, 134, 135, 141, 142, 145, 147, 229
acid, 53
activation, x, xi, xii, 1, 2, 5, 7, 8, 24, 32, 34, 38, 55, 58, 73, 74, 75, 76, 77, 82, 83, 84, 85, 86, 87, 88, 89, 90, 92, 93, 94, 95, 96, 99, 108, 112, 114, 115, 120, 122, 123, 124, 125, 126, 129, 130, 131, 132, 133, 135, 138, 141, 142, 145, 147, 148, 149, 150, 151, 153, 156, 157, 159, 170, 171, 172, 176, 207
activity level, 63
adaptation, 20, 21, 28, 30, 33, 34, 158, 186
ADC, 179, 180, 182, 183, 184, 190
adjustment, 216
administration, 133, 139
adults, 1, 2, 7
age, 2, 79, 116, 121, 143, 178, 224
aggregation, 136
aging, 114, 121, 125
algorithm, xii, xiii, 25, 34, 133, 135, 136, 152, 155, 158, 161, 163, 173, 181, 183, 186, 187, 188, 189, 190, 191, 192, 196, 203, 211, 212, 213, 214, 215, 216, 219, 227, 228, 229
alpha activity, 19
alternative, 20, 21, 23, 24, 33, 75, 93, 108, 205, 213
alternative hypothesis, 75
alternatives, 81
amnesia, 110, 111, 113, 114, 120, 121, 122, 123, 124, 126, 127
amplitude, ix, 13, 14, 16, 17, 18, 19, 20, 21, 22, 23, 24, 26, 27, 28, 29, 30, 31, 32, 33, 34, 38, 40, 133, 149, 160, 198, 200, 203, 204, 207
amygdala, 68, 69, 122, 124, 138, 151
anatomy, 70, 124
angiogenesis, 179, 186, 195
animals, 44, 45, 74, 109, 111
animations, 224
anisotropy, 193
annealing, 23
ANOVA, 20, 142, 145, 165, 171
anterior cingulate cortex, 204
anxiety, 206, 208
AP, 229
APC, 75, 82, 85, 87, 88
apoptosis, 180
appendix, 25
argument, 106
arousal, 199, 202, 207
aspartate, xii, 177
assessment, 38, 99, 106, 107, 111, 120, 194, 202
assignment, 184
assumptions, 20, 23, 25, 34, 110
asymmetry, xii, 123, 126, 155, 156, 157, 171, 172, 173, 176
atrophy, 113
attention, xiii, 26, 50, 76, 138, 174, 197, 198, 201, 203, 204, 205, 206, 207, 208, 209
audition, 36
auditory cortex, 16, 22, 26, 27, 28, 29, 31, 32, 33, 34, 36, 37, 38, 39, 40, 41
auditory evoked potentials, 39, 206
auditory stimuli, 25, 199
autobiographical memory, xi, 101, 102, 105, 106, 107, 108, 111, 112, 113, 114, 115, 116, 117, 119, 120, 121, 122, 124, 125
availability, 130, 180
averaging, 17, 18, 20, 21, 24, 35, 121, 167
awareness, 102, 104, 118, 198
axon terminals, 74

axons, 59

B

background noise, 160, 212
bandwidth, 27, 41, 141, 144
basic research, 147, 149
Bayesian, 174, 192
Bayesian estimation, 174
behavior, 54, 67, 151, 157, 186, 187
behavioral change, 67
Beijing, 162, 167
bias, 24, 174, 205, 206
biofeedback, 131, 137, 138, 147
blocks, 143, 146, 162, 166
blood, xii, 3, 5, 14, 80, 130, 133, 149, 156, 158, 176, 177, 179, 180, 183, 186, 194, 195, 196
blood flow, 3, 5, 156, 176, 194
Blood oxygenation level-dependent (BOLD), xii
blood supply, 179
blood vessels, 80, 149, 196
boredom, 18
brain activity, 14, 15, 18, 22, 32, 39, 138, 147, 149, 150, 198, 206, 229
brain asymmetry, 176
brain damage, 57, 107
brain functions, 106, 108, 137, 138, 149
brain imaging techniques, 2, 156
brain stem, ix, x, 26, 43, 44, 45, 58, 59, 60, 61, 62, 63, 64, 65
brain structure, 2, 107, 115
brain tumor, 180, 193, 194, 195
brainstem, 34, 61, 69
breathing, 133, 147, 179, 180, 194, 195
broadband, 30, 32
buffer, 53

C

C++, 151
cables, 16
calibration, 16
Canada, 14, 46, 153
cancer, xii, 177, 178, 180, 187, 193
capillary, 14
carrier, 31
case study, 121, 125, 194
cast, 198
categorization, 117
cats, x, 44, 46, 47, 49, 51, 52, 54, 55, 56, 57, 59, 60, 63, 64, 65, 66, 67, 68, 69, 74
cell, 63, 74, 180
central nervous system, 74, 95
cerebellum, 59
cerebral asymmetry, 40
cerebral blood flow, 1, 2, 58, 66, 149, 175
cerebral cortex, ix, x, 43, 44, 45, 46, 65, 67, 69, 70, 71, 96
cerebral function, xii, 2, 155, 172
cerebral ischemia, 196
cerebrospinal fluid, 191
cerebrum, 64, 68
certainty, 85
channels, 1, 4, 5, 6, 16, 19, 24, 29, 30, 190, 217
Chicago, 69, 145
childhood, 112
children, 2
China, 155, 173, 211
Chinese, 162, 167, 229, 230
chronic pain, 149, 153
classes, 19, 186, 189, 191, 192
classification, 178, 187, 188, 189, 191, 192, 193, 196, 211
classroom, 2
clinical examination, 207
clinical neurophysiology, 207
clinical trials, 196
cluster analysis, 196
clustering, 178, 187, 188, 196
clusters, 185, 187, 190
CNS, 65
CO2, 97, 179, 180
cochlea, 30
coding, 26, 29, 30, 34, 184, 186
cognition, 102, 111, 114, 119, 208
cognitive function, 109, 212
cognitive process, xiii, 106, 120, 197, 198, 200, 204
cognitive processing, xiii, 120, 197, 200
cognitive science, 122
cognitive set, 119
cognitive tasks, 22, 35
coherence, 26, 34, 102, 105, 220
commissure, xi, 23, 74, 76, 87, 90, 93, 94
communication, 65, 97, 99
communication systems, 65
complement, 204
complexity, xiii, 108, 123, 135, 177, 193, 199, 216
compliance, 131
complications, 137

components, 16, 20, 39, 40, 52, 97, 98, 109, 120, 127, 136, 137, 142, 143, 147, 151, 200, 201, 202, 203, 206, 209
computation, 134, 135, 136
computers, 132, 138
computing, 17, 19, 130, 135, 214
concentrates, 46
concentration, 1, 2, 4, 5, 6, 7, 8, 130, 138, 156
conception, 63
conditioning, 208
conduction, 141
conductivity, 217
conductor, 25, 212, 215, 217
configuration, 132, 166, 189, 200, 214, 216, 217
confounding variables, 116
confusion, 205
conjecture, 186
connectivity, x, 68, 73, 75, 95, 149, 186
conscious awareness, xi, 101, 105, 109, 118, 119, 120
consciousness, 35, 105, 118, 119, 121, 127
consensus, 108, 178
consolidation, 109, 110, 111, 113, 124, 125
constraints, 20, 23, 38, 189
construction, 53, 121
context memory, 109, 119
continuity, 33, 74, 93, 102
contralateral hemisphere, x, 17, 73, 75, 88, 90, 94, 184, 185
contrast agent, xii, 177
control, x, xi, 3, 6, 7, 16, 18, 19, 20, 25, 26, 30, 35, 43, 44, 45, 46, 52, 55, 56, 59, 62, 65, 66, 68, 69, 74, 77, 79, 80, 81, 82, 84, 85, 89, 90, 92, 108, 109, 116, 119, 137, 138, 139, 141, 143, 147, 148, 149, 151, 153, 229
control condition, 18, 25, 26, 30, 143
control group, 77, 79, 139
convergence, 130, 134, 187
cooling, 94
corpus callosum, x, 64, 73, 75, 76, 90, 92, 93, 94, 96, 97, 99, 113
correlation(s), xiii, 20, 27, 29, 34, 35, 36, 41, 136, 151, 173, 188, 194, 203, 211, 213, 214, 215, 216, 217, 219, 221, 222, 225, 227, 229
correlation analysis, 151
correlation coefficient, 136, 216, 217, 227
cortex, x, xi, 2, 7, 8, 9, 19, 22, 24, 26, 30, 34, 38, 42, 43, 44, 45, 46, 47, 55, 57, 59, 60, 61, 62, 63, 66, 67, 68, 69, 70, 71, 73, 74, 75, 80, 82, 84, 85, 88, 92, 93, 94, 95, 96, 97, 98, 99, 100, 113, 114, 115, 121, 123, 126, 133, 138, 156, 162, 163, 164, 165, 175, 207, 224, 225
cortical processing, x, 36, 44, 50, 52, 53, 56, 97
costs, 136
cotton, 1, 3, 80
covering, 113
craniotomy, 178
creatine, xii, 177
criticism, 94
CSF, 192
cues, 32, 39, 198, 200
cultural differences, 202
cultural norms, 118
cycles, 162, 166
cysts, 120
cytoarchitecture, 95
cytology, 127

D

danger, 93
data analysis, ix, 13, 131, 132, 133, 147
data processing, ix, 132, 138, 140, 147, 173
data set, 80, 81
data transfer, 140
database, 202
decay, 30, 158, 171, 172
decisions, 36
declarative memory, 103, 104, 109, 111, 123, 126
decomposition, 20, 227, 229
deficit, 55, 56, 57, 107, 120, 121, 124
definition, 196
deformation, 133
delivery, xiii, 16, 177
dementia, 114
density, 26, 180, 189, 203, 230
deoxyhemoglobin, 130, 156
desire, 17, 25
destruction, 121
desynchronization, 40
detection, 1, 9, 20, 26, 28, 31, 33, 36, 39, 40, 41, 118, 132, 133, 135, 152, 162, 167, 181, 182, 183, 186, 195, 203
developmental disabilities, 2
deviation, x, 44, 58, 61, 63, 167
differentiation, 107, 108, 114, 117, 119, 193, 199
diffusion, xii, 177, 179, 180, 183, 190, 193, 194, 195, 196
diffusion-weighted imaging, 195

dipole, ix, xiii, 13, 17, 20, 21, 22, 23, 24, 25, 26, 27, 29, 31, 33, 34, 35, 36, 40, 208, 211, 212, 214, 216, 221, 222, 223, 225, 226, 227, 228, 229
dipole moment, 21, 22, 26, 34
discharges, 50, 51, 229
discomfort, 14
discrimination, 7, 9, 35, 41, 53, 97, 158
discrimination learning, 97
discrimination tasks, 35
disorder, 9, 55, 123, 137, 204
displacement, 218
dissociation, 124, 200, 203
distracters, 207
distribution, 20, 23, 59, 60, 67, 95, 181, 188, 189, 214, 215, 216, 218, 219, 220, 222, 223, 225, 229
distribution function, 218
dominance, 7, 20, 31, 44, 58, 59, 61, 174
dorsolateral prefrontal cortex, 204
drowsiness, 18
drugs, 45
duration, 16, 17, 19, 21, 26, 27, 28, 31, 32, 33, 34, 38, 40, 41, 158, 171, 200, 206
dynamical systems, 174
dyskinesia, 55

E

early Contingent Negative Variation (eCNV), xiii
ears, 16, 17
earth, 14, 21
edema, xii, 177, 188, 192, 195
education, 1, 152
EEG, xiii, 4, 14, 18, 22, 23, 24, 26, 36, 41, 99, 138, 156, 176, 211, 212, 213, 218, 219, 227, 228, 229, 230
EEG patterns, 99
elaboration, 120
elderly, 8
electric current, 36
electrical power, 16
electrodes, 14, 16, 46, 138, 213
electroencephalogram, 138, 212
electroencephalography, 4, 14, 207, 229
electromagnetic, 38, 208, 212, 228
EMG, 50, 51, 53, 54, 56, 58
emission, 95, 126
emitters, 4
emotion, xiii, 102, 109, 113, 114, 123, 197, 198, 204
emotional reactions, 199, 201
emotional responses, 204
emotional stimuli, 201, 202, 204, 205
empathy, 109
encoding, xi, 38, 42, 101, 102, 104, 105, 106, 107, 108, 110, 112, 117, 118, 119, 120, 121, 122, 123, 125, 126, 198
energy, ix, 13, 19, 21, 26, 27, 28, 29, 30, 41, 138, 190
engagement, 110, 111, 114, 118, 124, 126
enlargement, 94
entorhinal cortex, 113, 123
environment, xii, 33, 114, 137, 177, 178, 179, 180, 181, 184, 185, 186, 190, 193
enzymes, 186
EOG, 200
epilepsy, xi, 74, 77, 86, 99
episodic memory, xi, 101, 102, 103, 104, 105, 106, 107, 108, 109, 110, 111, 112, 113, 114, 115, 116, 117, 118, 119, 120, 121, 122, 124, 125, 126
episodic memory tasks, 105, 106, 108, 109, 111, 112, 115, 117, 118, 119
EPR, 194
equipment, 147
ERD, 24, 35
ERPs, xiii, 197, 198, 201, 202, 203
estimating, 23, 163
Europe, 16
event-related brain potentials, 157, 175
event-related potential, xiii, 197, 198, 206, 207, 208
evidence, xi, xii, 27, 33, 34, 36, 38, 93, 95, 101, 102, 105, 107, 108, 111, 113, 114, 115, 117, 121, 125, 145, 149, 155, 157, 176, 206
evoked potential, x, 18, 73, 75, 97, 98, 157, 208, 211, 213, 228, 229
evolution, 93
examinations, xii, 129
executive function, 109, 121
executive functions, 109
exercise, 56
experimental condition, 112, 147
experimental design, 35, 116, 199, 200, 205
explicit memory, 103
exposure, 39
extraction, 182, 186, 206
eye movement, 200
eyes, 1, 3, 18, 224

F

facial expression, 138, 206
facial muscles, 52

failure, 187
fatigue, 17
fear, 123, 205, 209
feedback, xii, 45, 56, 129, 131, 132, 137, 138, 139, 142, 143, 144, 145, 146, 147, 148, 149, 152, 209
females, 2, 79
fibers, 59, 64
field theory, 35
filters, 19, 181
fish, 50, 54, 57, 58
fixation, 144, 162, 166, 167
flexibility, 35, 147
flexor, 61
fluctuations, 20, 21, 66
fluid, 14
food, 45, 47, 50, 51, 52, 55, 57
food intake, 57
forebrain, 98, 99
Fourier, 22, 133, 135, 150, 151
Fourier transformation, 133
fragmentation, 190
free recall, 104
freedom, 20
frontal cortex, x, 7, 8, 43, 44, 47, 95, 120, 205
frontal lobe, 7, 76, 123, 125, 126
fuel, 147
functional activation, 167
functional analysis, 140
functional imaging, 37, 99, 150
functional MRI, 142, 150, 151, 152, 156, 174, 175, 176
fusion, 99, 194

G

Gamma, xii
Gaussian, xii, 35, 155, 156, 158, 159, 161, 162, 163, 164, 165, 167, 172, 173, 174, 189, 217
gender, 108, 125
general knowledge, 115
generalization, 188
generation, 204, 208
genes, 186
Germany, 23, 101, 140
gingival, 48
glass, 82
glioblastoma, 193
glioma, 194, 195
glucose, 186
glycine, 65
glycolysis, 186
goals, 186
gold, 25
grants, 205
graph, 84, 86, 140, 143
gray matter, 133
Great Britain, 104
groups, 31, 82, 90, 135, 221
growth, 14, 44, 179, 186, 196
growth factor(s), 186, 196
gyrus, x

H

habituation, 39, 205, 206
handedness, 77, 91, 99
hands, 75, 76, 82, 91, 92, 93, 94
hardness, 50
harmonic frequencies, 28
health, 2
health care, 2
heart rate, 137, 147
heat, 95, 96
height, 20
helium, 14
hemisphere, 5, 6, 7, 17, 19, 23, 28, 32, 34, 50, 64, 74, 76, 84, 85, 86, 87, 89, 90, 91, 93, 157, 174, 176, 184, 185, 192
hemispheric asymmetry, 176
hemoglobin, 1, 2, 4, 5, 6, 7
heterogeneity, 173, 175, 178
high scores, 91
hippocampus, 102, 107, 109, 110, 111, 113, 114, 116, 119, 120, 122, 123, 124, 125, 126, 127, 208
histogram, 50, 112, 145, 146
histology, 187
host, xii, 177
human brain, 7, 8, 14, 36, 37, 39, 76, 95, 96, 98, 100, 104, 123, 147, 175, 208, 209, 212, 228
human cerebral cortex, 99
human condition, 97
human subjects, 107, 127, 149
hypoglossal nerve, x, 44, 58, 61, 63, 66, 67, 69
hypoglossal nuclei, x
hypothesis, x, xi, 25, 51, 52, 73, 74, 75, 77, 86, 121, 136
hypoxia, xii, 177, 179, 180, 182, 183, 184, 185, 186, 187, 188, 190, 192, 193, 195

I

identification, 67, 117, 206, 207
identity, 187
illusory contours, 171, 176
image analysis, 145
images, ix, xi, xii, 25, 35, 36, 79, 80, 81, 84, 86, 129, 134, 138, 147, 151, 152, 162, 167, 177, 178, 182, 183, 187, 188, 191, 192, 194, 195, 196, 202, 212
imaging, ix, xi, xii, xiii, 7, 8, 13, 26, 36, 37, 38, 41, 95, 125, 129, 130, 132, 137, 138, 140, 147, 149, 150, 151, 152, 156, 168, 169, 173, 177, 178, 180, 187, 188, 193, 194, 195, 196, 211, 212, 214, 218, 219, 220, 223, 225, 227, 228, 229
imaging techniques, xiii, 130, 177, 178, 180, 194, 212, 229
immunohistochemistry, 195
immunoreactivity, 96
impairments, 107, 110
implementation, 23, 132, 134, 137, 192, 199, 205
in vitro, 149
in vivo, xi, 76, 129, 130, 149, 162, 195
inattention, 174
inclusion, 28, 104, 190
independence, 29
indicators, 105
indices, 145
indirect measure, 14
indirect tasks, 201
individual differences, 24
induction, 69, 138
infants, 2
infinite, 23
information processing, xi, 67, 76, 101, 102, 103, 105, 108, 109, 115, 116, 118, 209
information retrieval, 119
informed consent, 2, 79, 141, 143, 178
infrared spectroscopy, 2, 8
infrastructure, 138
ingest, 47
ingestion, 50, 51, 52, 53, 54, 55, 56, 57, 58, 66
inhibition, 34, 39, 64, 65, 123
inhomogeneity, 130
initiation, 51
injections, 45, 66
injury, 126, 187
innovation, 99
insight, 195
instruction, 118, 143
integration, 17, 37, 40, 53, 76, 96, 117, 118, 126, 131, 132, 228
integrity, 92
intensity, 16, 26, 28, 30, 31, 33, 36, 40, 41, 42, 81, 82, 132, 133, 159, 160, 180, 181, 182, 184, 187, 188, 189, 191, 194, 205
interaction(s), 26, 27, 37, 41, 65, 114, 119, 145, 148, 153, 159, 176, 182, 188, 198, 204, 205, 206, 217, 228
interaction process, 159
interdependence, 36
interface, 150
interference, xii, 1, 4, 14, 16, 129, 142, 147
interneuron, x, 44, 64
interneurons, 64
interpretation, ix, xiii, 24, 174, 177, 186, 190, 202
interval, 18, 29, 33, 39, 141, 143, 156, 159, 200, 201
intervention, 25, 138, 178
interview, 150
intracortical microstimulation (ICMS), x
intracranial tumors, 194
intrinsic rhythm, 18
inversion, xiii, 211
ipsilateral, x, xi, 7, 17, 32, 56, 64, 68, 73, 74, 75, 76, 77, 82, 84, 85, 86, 87, 88, 89, 90, 91, 92, 93, 94, 96, 100
IQ scores, 77, 79
IR, 80
Italy, 73, 79
iteration, 134, 211

J

Japan, 1, 3, 4, 8, 43, 152
Java, 104, 122
joints, 63
judgment, 105
justice, 58

K

kinetic parameters, 193

L

labeling, 59, 186
labor, 180
lactic acid, 194
language, 26, 41, 94

laser, 75, 97
latency, ix, 13, 19, 20, 21, 26, 27, 28, 29, 31, 33, 36, 41, 42, 75, 93, 95, 98, 158, 174, 200
laterality, 20, 40, 48, 49, 52, 108
learning, 69, 76, 103, 104, 106, 111, 118, 119, 124, 126, 139, 176
learning task, 126
left hemisphere, 6, 20, 28, 108, 157
left visual field, 176
lesions, x, 43, 54, 55, 56, 59, 66, 67, 76, 97, 107, 110, 111, 120, 125, 127, 194
lexical decision, 157, 174
life experiences, 117
life span, 116
lifetime, 106, 126
likelihood, 23, 38, 184, 190
limitation, 205
linear function, 108, 159
linear model, 35, 36, 135, 152
links, 76
listening, 17, 18, 26, 32
literature, 18, 19, 22, 23, 76, 84, 96, 99, 148, 166
local area network (LAN), 132
localization, xiii, 9, 36, 38, 39, 52, 56, 59, 70, 82, 97, 105, 138, 203, 206, 211, 212, 227, 228, 229
location, 4, 14, 18, 20, 21, 22, 23, 24, 25, 26, 29, 30, 31, 32, 34, 36, 40, 45, 51, 55, 56, 97, 110, 156, 158, 192, 216, 226, 228, 229
locus, 174
long-term memory, 103, 125, 198
LTD, 3
lying, 82

M

magnet, 81, 139, 178
magnetic field, 9, 14, 15, 16, 21, 23, 24, 25, 36, 37, 38, 40, 41, 98, 130, 133, 138, 208
magnetic resonance, x, xi, xii, 2, 14, 15, 61, 73, 75, 95, 96, 98, 107, 122, 123, 125, 127, 129, 130, 138, 149, 150, 151, 155, 156, 157, 173, 174, 175, 194, 195
magnetic resonance spectroscopy, 194
magnetoencephalogram, 8
magnetoencephalography, ix, 13, 14, 38, 39, 42, 205, 212, 228
males, 2, 79
malignant cells, 186
mammal, 93
management, xii, 177, 178
manipulation, 52, 67, 119, 137, 147, 200, 212
MANOVA, 145
manufacturer, 14
mapping, iv, ix, xi, 13, 22, 26, 93, 95, 129, 130, 137, 175, 178, 190, 224, 228, 230
Marx, 39
masking, 20
masseter, 46, 50, 54, 56, 57, 58, 65
mastication, x, 43, 44, 45, 46, 47, 50, 51, 52, 53, 54, 56, 58, 59, 62, 63, 65, 66, 67, 68, 69, 70
mastication-related cortical areas, x
matching-to-sample, 38
matrix, xiii, 22, 24, 25, 26, 34, 141, 144, 162, 167, 180, 187, 203, 211, 212, 213, 214, 215, 216, 217, 219, 221, 222, 225, 227, 229
maxilla, 48
measurement, 1, 3, 4, 26, 35, 116, 141, 206, 207
measures, ix, xii, 14, 21, 29, 32, 33, 117, 133, 138, 142, 145, 177, 179
median, 23, 95, 96, 229
MEG, vii, ix, 13, 14, 15, 16, 17, 18, 19, 20, 21, 22, 23, 24, 26, 27, 28, 34, 35, 36, 37, 38, 41, 75, 156, 212, 213, 228, 229
memory, xi, 101, 102, 103, 104, 105, 106, 107, 108, 109, 110, 111, 112, 113, 114, 115, 116, 117, 118, 119, 120, 121, 122, 123, 124, 125, 126, 127, 136, 205, 208
memory processes, 109, 119, 205
memory retrieval, 108, 116, 117, 118, 123, 124, 125
mental image, 114
mental imagery, 114
meridian, 166
meta-analysis, 114, 127, 176
metabolism, 149, 180, 186
metacognition, 152
microscopy, 196
milk, 50, 54, 57, 58
Ministry of Education, 65
MIP, 82
misconceptions, ix, 13, 35
misunderstanding, 137
model system, 195
modeling, 106, 130, 135, 167, 228, 229
models, xii, 21, 23, 34, 133, 155, 158, 165, 167, 172, 173, 196, 204, 207, 214
monkeys, 46, 63, 67, 70, 74, 126
motion, xii, 32, 35, 81, 100, 129, 130, 131, 132, 133, 134, 135, 137, 139, 140, 141, 142, 143, 144, 145, 146, 147, 148, 150, 151, 152, 157, 167, 171, 173, 174, 175, 182

motion control, 142
motor activity, 94, 198, 207
motor behavior, 68
motor function, 69
motor neurons, 60, 63
motor skills, 69, 138
motor task, 93, 138, 150
motorneurons, 69
movement, ix, x, 15, 16, 17, 27, 43, 44, 45, 46, 48, 49, 50, 51, 52, 53, 54, 55, 59, 60, 61, 63, 64, 65, 69, 70, 81, 133, 138, 139, 175
MRI, x, xi, xii, 2, 14, 15, 61, 73, 75, 76, 83, 96, 98, 107, 129, 130, 131, 137, 150, 151, 153, 155, 156, 157, 162, 167, 173, 174, 177, 178, 193, 194, 195, 196, 228
mucosa, 48
multidimensional, 216, 226
multiple factors, 121
multiple sclerosis, 192, 196
MUltiple SIgnal Classification (MUSIC), xiii
multivariate, 135, 136, 203, 206, 227
muscles, ix, x, 16, 43, 44, 45, 47, 50, 51, 54, 57, 58, 59, 61, 64, 66
music, 16

N

naming, 157, 174
nasal cavity, 1, 2, 7
near-infrared spectroscopy, 1, 8, 9
necrosis, xii, 177, 180
negative mood, 138
negative valence, 112, 199
negativity, 19, 29, 33, 40
neglect, 174, 209
neocortex, 110, 112, 113
nerve(s), 30, 61, 67, 70, 95, 96, 98, 229
nervous system, 93, 99
Netherlands, 81
network, 27, 61, 102, 123, 132, 140, 142
neural mechanisms, 76, 118, 119, 125, 127
neural network(s), 122, 127, 191, 192, 193
neurofeedback, xii, 129, 130, 135, 138, 149, 150, 152
neuroimaging, ix, 7, 14, 16, 23, 24, 30, 38, 40, 102, 104, 107, 108, 109, 110, 111, 112, 114, 115, 117, 118, 121, 122, 123, 124, 130
neuroimaging techniques, 24
neurons, x, 18, 29, 31, 43, 44, 46, 48, 60, 61, 63, 64, 65, 66, 67, 68, 69, 71, 74, 94, 96, 100
neurophysiology, 41
neuropsychological tests, 77
neuroscience, ix, xi, xiii, 101, 129, 130, 147, 156, 157, 211
New York, 65, 68, 70, 95, 126, 206
NMR, 149, 151
nociception, 99
nociceptive, 94, 96
nodes, 136, 192
noise, xiii, 14, 16, 20, 24, 25, 27, 28, 29, 30, 32, 34, 37, 38, 39, 41, 42, 81, 165, 182, 188, 190, 191, 211, 212, 213, 214, 215, 216, 217, 219, 220, 221, 222, 227
non-human primates, x, 73, 75, 76, 88, 89, 103
nonlinear dynamics, 173, 175
normal distribution, 158
North America, 16
novelty, 206
nucleus(i), 44, 45, 50, 58, 59, 60, 61, 62, 63, 64, 70, 71, 75
null hypothesis, 25
nutrients, 179

O

object recognition, 205
observations, 39, 75
occipital lobe, 76, 157, 162, 163, 165, 172
occipital regions, xii, 155
oil, 1, 3, 15
olfaction, 205
olfactory nerve, 7
ontogenesis, 98
operator, 132, 137, 139, 182
optical fiber, 4
optimization, 151, 190, 196, 212, 216
optimization method, 196
oral cavity, 52, 57
organization(s), 36, 39, 40, 45, 46, 48, 50, 51, 52, 53, 58, 61, 63, 64, 67, 74, 76, 95, 97, 98, 126
orientation, 14, 22, 23, 24, 25, 26, 34, 40, 121, 216
outliers, 20
ownership, 105
oxygen, 130, 156, 179, 195

P

pain, xi, 74, 76, 77, 78, 79, 80, 83, 88, 92, 93, 94, 95, 97, 98, 99, 100, 153, 205, 208

panic disorder, 198, 205
parallel platform, 133, 150
parallel processing, 130, 133, 140
paralysis, 61
parameter, xiii, 23, 25, 34, 140, 158, 159, 161, 163, 165, 170, 171, 172, 177, 181, 182, 184, 185, 186, 187, 190, 203, 219, 229
parameter estimates, 23
parameter estimation, 163, 229
parietal cortex, 75, 84, 96, 97, 99
parietal lobe, 32
partition, 103
passive, 19, 32
pathology, 112, 114, 123, 126
pathways, x, xi, 48, 69, 73, 74, 75, 76, 88, 92, 94
PCA, 16, 203, 207
peers, 212
percentile, 184
perception(s), 2, 24, 28, 40, 55, 57, 100, 157, 171, 173, 176
perceptual processing, 174, 207
performance, xii, xiii, 18, 56, 68, 81, 91, 102, 107, 129, 130, 141, 142, 152, 157, 176, 211, 220, 221, 222, 227
performers, 176
perfusion, xii, 130, 155, 156, 158, 159, 160, 193, 194, 195, 196
periodicity, 31
permeability, 180, 186, 195
personal, xi, 18, 35, 101, 105, 109, 114, 115, 117, 118, 122, 130
personal computers, 130
phalanx, 81
phosphate, 53
physiological correlates, 205
physiology, xii, 65, 74, 150, 151, 177, 195
pigs, 45
pitch, ix, 13, 16, 17, 18, 20, 26, 28, 29, 30, 31, 37, 38, 39, 41
planning, xii, 63, 147, 177, 181, 192, 194
planum temporale, 27, 30
plasticity, 70, 95
PM, 63, 176
polarity, 26
polyethylene, 53
poor, 2, 14, 33, 59, 91, 176
ports, 142
positive correlation, 29
positron, x, 2, 24, 73, 75, 95, 107, 123, 125, 130
positron emission tomography (PET), x, 2, 7, 9, 24, 73, 75,95, 98, 100, 107, 121, 123, 125, 130, 152, 212
posttraumatic stress, 9
power, 14, 16, 18, 19, 22, 25, 27, 36, 130, 132, 137, 138, 176
prefrontal cortex, 9, 102, 107, 116, 122, 123, 124, 125, 127, 208
preparedness, 208
presylcian sulcus, x
primary visual cortex, 162, 163, 165, 167, 170, 172
primate(s), 63, 67, 68, 69, 70, 71, 95
priming, 103
principal component analysis, 203, 206
Principal Components Analysis, 206
probability, 29, 156, 158, 165, 167, 172, 189, 190, 192, 207
probe, xii, 4, 80, 177
procedural memory, 103
production, 70, 116
program, 120, 137, 140, 142, 143
promote, 65
protocol(s), xiii, 3, 79, 178, 180, 197, 198, 205
psychology, 106
pulse, 15, 141, 144, 156
pulses, 9, 47, 97
pyramidal cells, 46, 63

Q

quality assurance, xii, 129, 137, 139
quantitative technique, 186

R

radiation, xii, 177, 180, 181, 194
radiation therapy, xii, 177
radiotherapy, 178
radius, 215, 218
range, ix, 2, 13, 14, 18, 19, 22, 28, 31, 110, 178
ratings, 207
reaction time, xii, 33, 54, 141, 142, 145, 155, 157, 200
reading, 65, 127, 143
real time, xii, 129, 130, 131, 138, 139, 150, 151, 153
reality, 24
recall, xi, 101, 102, 106, 114, 115, 125
receptive field, 46, 57, 67, 74, 95
receptors, 1, 76, 80, 93, 99, 124

reciprocity, 228
recognition, xi, 55, 80, 101, 102, 104, 105, 114, 116, 122, 123, 125, 174
recollection, xi, 101, 102, 103, 104, 105, 106, 107, 108, 109, 111, 112, 114, 115, 116, 117, 118, 119, 120, 122, 125
reconstruction, xiii, 23, 34, 36, 117, 130, 131, 132, 135, 140, 211, 216, 220, 221, 228
recovery, 39, 57, 124, 147, 149
recurrence, 178, 179
reduction, xii, 25, 129, 137, 141, 142, 147, 171, 191, 203
reflection, 33
refractory, 86
regional, 58, 66, 124, 130, 150, 158, 179, 229
regression, 20, 136, 152, 174
regression analysis, 20
regulation, 138, 150, 152, 205
relationship(s), 31, 62, 67, 117, 125, 149, 156, 195
relaxation, 138
relevance, 118, 201
reliability, 137, 203, 206
repetitions, 18, 20, 33, 109
resection, xi, 74, 77, 78, 79, 86, 87, 89, 90, 92, 94, 178, 180
resolution, ix, xiii, 13, 14, 15, 17, 24, 25, 34, 40, 80, 82, 95, 130, 133, 136, 138, 144, 156, 165, 174, 176, 182, 195, 196, 197, 198, 205, 208, 212, 228, 230
resources, 132, 135, 201, 204
respiration, 1, 2, 4, 7, 9
respiratory, 2, 7, 136
response time, 33
retention, 76, 107, 118
retention interval, 107
retrograde amnesia., 121
returns, 28
RF, 46, 48, 49, 52, 53, 56, 74
rhythm(s), 16, 18, 22, 36, 45, 50, 51, 52, 65, 69
right hemisphere, 5, 6, 24, 28, 31, 32, 36, 81, 157
right visual field, 157, 173, 224, 226
rodents, 103, 104
ROI, 82, 84, 86, 137, 145, 148
root-mean-square, 19
rotations, 203, 206

S

SA, 95, 174
sadness, 138, 151
sample, 164, 178, 184, 191, 217
sampling, 14, 36, 159
saturation, 26, 162, 167
scaling, 188, 202
scheduling, 94
schema, 50, 52, 56, 59, 63, 64, 109
schizophrenia, 40
science, 68, 95, 165, 171, 173
scientific computing, 39, 151
scientific method, 204
scores, 82, 91, 92, 203
search(es), xi, 20, 35, 101, 102, 123, 157, 176, 212, 216, 225, 226
searching, 20, 216
segmentation, 182, 189, 190, 191, 192, 194, 195, 196
segregation, 26, 33, 102, 108, 109, 114, 115, 116, 118
selecting, 178, 184, 187, 203
selective attention, 18, 175, 198, 205, 207, 209
self-regulation, 137, 139, 150
semantic categorization, 118
semantic memory, 103, 104, 115, 124, 126
semantic networks, 207
sensitivity, 16, 25, 38, 76, 97, 133, 137, 174, 228
sensors, 14, 15, 16, 23, 24, 26, 34
sensory cortices, 76
sensory modality, 77
sensory systems, 22
separation, 56, 151, 173, 182, 203
series, xi, 6, 16, 26, 81, 104, 129, 133, 134, 141, 150, 152, 162, 167, 175, 188, 189
shape, 24, 29, 136, 160, 186, 203
shaping, 63
short term memory, 138
shoulders, 100
sign(s), 65, 209
signalling, 198
signals, 1, 14, 17, 23, 70, 94, 138, 149, 156, 163, 165, 225, 227
signal-to-noise ratio, 17, 138
significance level, 20, 162, 169, 170
SII, x, xi, 73, 74, 75, 76, 80, 82, 84, 86, 88, 90, 92, 93, 94, 97, 99
simulation, xiii, 149, 159, 160, 161, 176, 211, 216, 217, 218, 219, 227, 228, 229
sine wave, 157
sites, 4, 30, 37, 46, 47, 48, 52, 93, 110, 162, 167, 169
skin, 14, 47, 57, 80, 96, 100, 137
smoothing, 34, 136
smoothness, 25, 35

social cognition, 109
social perception, 122
society, 69
sodium, 46
software, 23, 25, 81, 130, 132, 135, 136, 138, 140, 143, 147, 150, 165, 167, 171, 174, 178, 182, 187, 191, 192, 193, 227
somatosensory, x, 43, 46, 47, 49, 50, 52, 55, 56, 57, 59, 64, 66, 67, 68, 70, 73, 74, 75, 76, 81, 86, 91, 92, 95, 96, 97, 98, 99, 100, 138, 149, 208
sounds, 16, 18, 32, 33, 37, 39
Spain, 197, 205
spatial frequency, 157, 162, 166
spatial learning, 124
spatial location, 16, 18, 166
spatial memory, 116
spatial processing, 26, 32, 42, 176
specialization, 97, 108, 127, 175
species, 44, 75
specificity, 40, 106, 133, 137, 149
spectroscopy, 194
spectrum, 16, 22, 39
speech, 16, 70, 138
speed, 21, 32, 132, 134, 136
spin, 86, 87, 90, 152
spinal cord, 60, 75, 100
splenium., xi
SPSS, 145, 165, 171
stability, 21
stabilization, 110
stages, 49, 77, 112, 113, 198
standard deviation, 163, 165, 167, 168, 170, 187
standard error, 192
standards, 208
stapes, 42
statistical analysis, 6, 20, 132, 133, 135, 138, 151, 202
statistical inference, 133
statistics, 36, 136
steel, 46, 53
stimulus, ix, xii, 1, 3, 4, 5, 13, 14, 16, 17, 18, 19, 20, 21, 22, 26, 27, 28, 29, 31, 32, 33, 34, 36, 38, 39, 40, 42, 50, 80, 81, 82, 85, 92, 93, 108, 114, 115, 117, 143, 150, 155, 156, 157, 158, 159, 160, 162, 165, 166, 167, 172, 198, 199, 200, 201, 203, 204, 206, 224
stimulus pairs, 38
stimulus perception, 198
storage, 109, 110, 132
strategic planning, 109
strategies, ix, xi, 13, 55, 101, 102, 109, 126, 134, 138, 149, 186, 193
stratification, 195
strength, 14, 22, 23, 24, 33, 35, 42, 133, 138, 167
striatum, 124
stroke, 3, 187
students, 227
subgroups, 85
subjectivity, 182, 186, 203
substitution, 42
substrates, 119
superior temporal gyrus, 145, 148
superiority, 157
suppression, xii, 31, 129, 131, 139, 142, 145, 147, 152
surgical resection, xi, 74, 77, 85
surprise, 207
survival, 186
susceptibility, 195
swallowing, 52, 62, 70, 133
Sweden, 175
switching, 29, 56
Sylvian sulcus,, x
symbols, 193
symmetry, 24, 74
symptom, 65
synchronization, 41, 69
synthesis, 126
systems, xiii, 14, 18, 69, 103, 104, 117, 123, 124, 125, 126, 173, 177

T

tactile stimuli, x, 73, 74, 75, 76, 77, 81, 88, 96
target stimuli, 199, 200, 201, 202
targets, 138, 198, 199, 201
task demands, 108
task performance, 147
TCP, 140
technology, 173
teeth, 47, 48, 66
teflon, 46, 53
temperature, 14, 137
temporal lobe, 2, 7, 19, 111, 113, 120, 122, 123, 124, 126
Tennessee, 177
tension, 51, 55, 179, 195
terminals, 58, 60
territory, 76
terrorism, 9

Tesla, 79
test scores, 82
test statistic, 162
tetanus, 47
thalamus, 59, 188
theory, 61, 109, 110, 111, 113, 122, 127, 134, 138, 176, 178, 214, 216
therapy, xii, 177, 193
threat, 123, 204, 206
three-dimensional space, 175
threshold(s), 16, 31, 40, 41, 42, 66, 80, 143, 144, 145, 182, 184, 185, 186
time resolution, 14
time series, xi, 129, 132, 133, 138, 152, 167
timing, 21, 56, 65, 143
tissue, xii, 113, 177, 178, 179, 180, 182, 186, 187, 188, 191, 192, 195, 196
tissue perfusion, xii, 177
Tokyo, 43, 69
tonic, 51
toxin, 65
tracking, 151, 152, 196
training, 16, 46, 139, 152, 153, 188, 191, 192
trajectory, 45, 53, 54, 132
transactions, 65
transcranial magnetic stimulation, 61, 69
transection, 122
transformation, 134
transition, 29, 52, 187
translation, 52, 135
transmission, xi, 74, 75, 92, 94
transport, 68
trauma, 9
trend, 4, 24, 136, 165, 171
trial, 4, 19, 27, 41, 138, 151, 192, 198, 200, 201, 215, 216, 222
trial and error, 215, 216, 222
tumor(s), xii, 97, 99, 177, 178, 179, 180, 181, 182, 184, 185, 186, 187, 190, 192, 193, 194, 195, 196

U

UK, 13, 39, 67, 81, 122, 124
ultrasound, 28
uniform, 218
updating, 140, 143, 190
users, 193

V

valence, 122, 199, 202, 205, 209
validation, 196
validity, 107
values, 6, 16, 20, 21, 23, 28, 58, 82, 92, 146, 162, 179, 180, 184, 186, 203, 216, 219, 221, 222, 225
variability, 20, 31, 173
variable(s), 16, 77, 92, 180, 200
variance, 206
variation, 20, 32, 33, 41, 108, 135, 187, 207, 208, 209
vascular endothelial growth factor (VEGF), 186
vasculature, 179, 186
vector, 24, 136, 151, 161, 187, 216
VEGF, 186
ventricle, 80, 120
vibration, 95, 97
virtual reality (VR), 117
vision, 143, 157
visual acuity, 166, 224
visual area, 116, 166
visual attention, 157
visual field, xii, 155, 156, 157, 171, 173, 174, 175, 176
visual field studies, 174
visual modality, 199
visual processing, 206
visual stimuli, 171, 199, 206
visual stimulus, xii, 155, 156, 165, 171, 172
visualization, ix, 80, 150, 174, 187, 195

W

wavelengths, 4
wavelet, 22
wavelet analysis, 22
wealth, 106
wheat, 58
wheat germ, 58
white matter, 133, 193
windows, 20, 203
wires, 46
Wisconsin, 70, 178
withdrawal, 196
word processing, 176, 207
workers, 61, 203
working memory, xii, 26, 108, 109, 119, 121, 123, 125, 127, 129, 142, 205, 207

workstation, 81

Y

yield, xii, xiii, 35, 94, 112, 177, 199